Springer

Paris
Berlin
Heidelberg
New York
Barcelona
Hong Kong
London
Milan
Santa Clara
Singapore
Tokyo

Gabriel N. Hortobagyi
MD Anderson Cencer Center
Cepartment of Breast Medical Oncology
University of Texas
1515 Holcombe Boulevard
Houston, Texas 77030
USA

David Khayat
Pitié-Salpétrière Hospital
SOMPS
47, bd de l'Hôpital
75651 Paris Cedex 13
France

ISBN-13: 978-2-287-59666-7   e-ISBN-13: 978-2-8178-0918-2
DOI: 10.1007/978-2-8178-0918-2

Spin: 107708595
CIP Requested

Gabriel N. Hortobagyi, David Khayat (Eds)

Progress in Anti-Cancer Chemotherapy

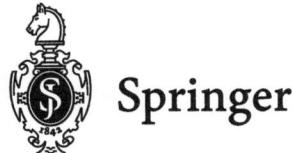 Springer

List of Contributors

Filiberto Belli
National Cancer Institute
Division of Surgical Oncology
Via Venezian 1, 20133 Milan – Italy

Diane R. Bielenberg
MD Anderson Cancer Center
Department of Cell Biology
1515 Holcombe Boulevard, Box 56
Houston, TX 77030 – USA

Christhian Brechot
Faculté de Médecine Necker – Enfants Malades
Laboratoire de Biologie Cellulaire – INSERM U370
156, rue de Vaugirard
75730 Paris Cedex 15 – France

Carleen A. Brunelli
MD Anderson Cancer Center
Departement of Breast Medical Oncology
1515 Holcombe Boulevard, Box 56
Houston, TX 77030 – USA

Paul A. Bunn Jr
University of Colorado
Cancer Center, Campus Box B 189
4200, East Ninth Avenue
Denver, CO 80262 – USA

Aman U. Buzdar
MD Anderson Cancer Center
Department of Breast Medical Oncology
1515 Holcombe Boulevard, Box 56
Houston, TX 77030 – USA

Natale Cascinelli
National Cancer Institute
Division of Surgical Oncology
Via Venezian 1
20133 Milan – Italy

Louis Denis
Oncologic Centre
Lange Gasthuisstraat 35-37
2000 Antwerpen – Belgium

Lawrence H. Einhorn
Indiana University Medical Center
Department of Medecine
Indianapolis, IN 46202-5289 – USA

Isaiah J. Fidler
MD Anderson Cancer Center
Departement of Cell Biology
1515 Holcombe Boulevard, Box 56
Houston, TX 77030 – USA

Bernard Fisher
Allegheny University of the Health Sciences
Four Allegheny Center, Suite 602,
Pittsburgh, PA 15212-5234 – USA

Emile Frei III
Dana Farber Cancer Institute
Binney Street, 44
Boston, MA 02115
USA

Anthony Greco
Sarah Cannon Cancer Center Columbia
250, 25th Avenue North, Suite 412
Nashville, TN 37203 – USA

Berverly Griffin
Imperial College School of Medecine
Division of Investigative Science
Hammersmith Hospital
Du Cane Road
London W 12 ONN – United Kingdom

John D. Hainsworth
Sarah Cannon Cancer Center Columbia
250, 25th Avenue North, Suite 412
Nashville, TN 37203 – USA

Jia-Qing Huang
Mc Master University Medical Centre
Division of Gastroenterology
1200 Main Street West, Room 4W8
Hamilton, Ontario, L8N 3Z5 – Canada

Richard H. Hunt
Mc Master University Medical Centre
Division of Gastroenterology
1200 Main Street West, Room 4W8
Hamilton, Ontario, L8N 3Z5 – Canada

Claudine Isaacs
Georgetown University Medical Center
Lombardi Cancer Center - Cancer Genetics
2233 Wisconsin Avenue NW, Suite 317
Washington, DC 20007-4104 – USA

Francesco M. Marincola
National Cancer Institute
Building 10, Room 2B42
Bethesda, MD 20892 – USA

Giovanni Motta
1st Department of General & Thoracic Surgery
Largo Rosanna Benzi, 8
16132 Genova – Italy

Raphael E. Pollock
MS Anderson Cancer Center
The University of Texas
1515 Holcombe Boulevard
Houston, Texas 77030 – USA

Beth N. Peshkin
Georgetown University Medical Center
Lombardi Cancer Center - Cancer Genetics
2233 Wisconsin Avenue NW, Suite 317
Washington, DC 20007-4104 – USA

Steven A. Rosenberg
National Cancer Institute
Building 10, Room 2B42
Bethesda, MD 20892 – USA

Ariel F. Soriano
University of Colorado
Cancer Center
Campus Box B 189
4200, Eats Ninth Avenue
Denver, CO 80262 – USA

Margaret Tempero
University of Nebraska Medical Center
Eppley Cancer Center
Omaha, NE – USA

Leonard A. Zwellig
MD Anderson Cancer Center
Department of Breast Medical Oncology
1515 Holcombe Boulevard, Box 56
Houston, TX 77030 – USA

Contents

Preface

This is the third volume of our series Progress in Anti-Cancer Chemo-therapy. Following the strategy of the first two volumes, it covers selected aspects of progress in this fast moving field of Oncology, with contributions from some of the world's best known leaders in both basic and clinical research.

This year we focused on seven areas:

Three prominent Clinical investigators reviewed conceptual advances in cancer research. Dr Buzdar presented a history and overview of the protection of human subjects who participate in clinical research, and the mechanisms developed to assure the ethical conduct of research on human beings. Frei reviewed an exciting and rapidly moving area of chemotherapy of solid tumors, including a cogent discussion of the issues related to dose-intensification. Fisher summarized conceptual advances in our therapeutic approach to breast cancer and the paradigm shifts that lead us to our current management strategies. From this summary he projected breast cancer research into the future, a daunting task under any circumstance.

Fundamental research in cancer biology has been responsible for our improved understanding of the development and progession of malignant disease. Such understanding will lead to improved diagnosis, therapy, and eventually, prevention. Isaacs reviews the area of hereditary breast cancer, a topic undergoing rapid transformation and with multiple implications in the daily practice of medicine. Fidler, an international expert in metastasis research reviews the potential utility of angiogenesis inhibitors in research and the therapeutic ramifications.

The next part covers progress in lung cancer. This clinically relevant part answers the "epidemic" of lung cancer in the western industrialized world and the approaching "epidemic" in the rest of the world. Despite important progress in biology and management, the loss of lives due to lung cancer continues to increase daily. This is the consequence of the extent of tobacco consumption around the world, and the lack of an effective, safe, and low-cost screening tool. Greco and Soriano independently review recent progress in the systemic and multidisciplinary management of lung cancer, while Motta provides a comprehensive overview of the surgical management of this disease. This latter issue is of interest and clinical utility, since for many years, whether to resect a tumor or not was based more on personal philosophy rather than factual information. The recent comprehensive revision of the staging system for lung cancer provided the impetus for a much more evidence-based surgical approach to the disease, and improved intergration of the various therapeutic tools (chemotherapy, radiotherapy and surgery) into a multidisciplinary approach.

In Part IV, Einhorn addresses the advances in the treatment of testicular cancer. This very visible accomplishment opened the era of modern medical oncology, and as such, it has become a model, or a paradigm of how concepts and therapeutic strategies must progress in a step-wise manner, based on hypothesis-bases clinical trials to treat, and eventually cure, malignant disease. The second chapter in this Part, prepared by Denis, evalutates the statuts of screening for prostate cancer, a critical review of this controversial and very important area for the most frequent cancer in western men.

The chapters by Cascinelli and Marincola (from S. Rosenberg's team) describe the latest advances in research and treatment of malignant melanoma. It is by now obvious that the emergence of immunotherapy has contributed to improving the efficacy of the treatments of advanced and early melanoma, event if the improvement has, to date, bee of a limited nature.

The role of interferon in the adjuvant treatment of cutaneous melanoma is of great interest and concern, not only because of its impact on the patient's quality of life, but also because of its significant cost. Therefore, it is of critical importance to determine the precise contribution of this intervention in the aduvant management of primary melanoma, and to identify those patient groups who are most likely to benefit from such intervention. Immunotherapy offers the hope of cure to a subset of patients with metastatic melanoma. However, much additional progress is needed to offer real chances of cure to most patients with this disease. The hope that some real progess will be made in the near future through the development of vaccines is critically addressed by Marincola and Ronsenberg.

It is becoming apparent that there is a strong epidemiological correlation between certain malignancies and specific infectious agents. Griffin summarizes the extensive information about the Ebstein-Barr virus and sereal neoplasias. The emerging date relating Helicobacter Pylori to gastrointestinal disease, including malignant tumors is reviewed by Huang and Hunt. Finally, Brechot presents a critical overview of potential etiological role of Hepatitis viruses in hepatocellular carcinoma. These chapters review the date pertaining to the causality of infection in the development of cancer, and the pathophysiological mechanisms elucidated during the past several years.

To complete the volume, the last two chapters review emerging progess in our understanding and management principles of pancreatic cancer (M. Tempero) and soft tissue sarcomas (R.E. Pollock), tumors that, because of their relative infrequency, are less publicized and discussed, even though serious and productive research is intensely pursued.

The editors hope that the chapters selected for this volume complement those offered in the previous two, and that the information presented is thought-provoking and useful to our readership.

Gabriel N. Hortobagyi
David Khayat

Part I
Conceptual Advances in Cancer Research

Protecting Human Subjects from Risk in the Performance of Clinical Research and the Informed Consent Process

A. U. Buzdar, C. A. Brunelli, L. A. Zwelling

Scientific research has produced substantial social benefits. It has also posed a number of ethical questions. Voluntary participation in clinical research and its potential for abuse of human subjects in biomedical experiments needs to be constantly reviewed. The modern history of protection of human subjects began with the Nuremberg code [1], which was developed as a universal standard by which to judge the ethical conduct of human experimentation. The code was a reaction to the abuses in human experimentation occurred in Nazi Germany and contained a number of principles for ethical conduct of clinical research. The first provision of the code stated that "the voluntary consent of human subjects is absolutely essential". This remains the cornerstone of all ethical experimentation involving human subjects. Other provisions required minimization of risk and harm, a favorable risk-benefit ratio, qualified investigators using appropriate research design, and freedom for the subjects to withdraw their consent from research at any time. Similar recommendations were made by the World Medical Association in its "Declaration of Helsinki Guidelines Involving Human Subjects".

In the United States, regulations protecting human subjects first became effective on May 30, 1974. These regulations established the Institutional Review Boards as one mechanism through which human subjects would be protected. In 1974, the passage of the National Research Act established the National Commission for Protection of Human Subjects from Biomedical and Behavioral Risk. This commission's report set forth the basic ethical principles that guide the conduct of biomedical research involving human subjects, and is entitled the "Belmont Report" [2]. These principles include respect for persons, beneficence, and justice, which are now accepted as the three essential tenets for the ethical conduct of research involving human subjects.

The distinction between research and medical practice at times is blurred. Practice is described as therapeutic interventions solely designed to enhance the well-being of an individual patient and that have a reasonable expectation of success. The purpose of medical or behavioral practice is to provide diagnosis, preventive treatment, or therapy for particular individuals. In contrast, research is an activity designed to test a hypothesis, permit conclusions to be drawn, and thereby develop or contribute to knowledge that can be generalized. Thus, the focus of practice is *always* on the individual patient, while research addresses the needs of individuals, groups, and society as a whole.

Institutional Review Boards

Institutional review boards are administrative bodies established to protect the rights and well-being of human subjects recruited into research activities conducted under the auspice of the institution with which it is affiliated. The IRB have the authority to approve, require modifications in, or disapprove all research activities that fall within their jurisdiction, as specified by both federal regulations and local institutional policies. A research reviewed and approved by an IRB may be subjected to review and disapproval by an official of the institution. However, those officials may not approve research, if it has been disapproved by the IRB. The IRB works independently and also in coordination with other committees. For example, an institution may have a research committee that reviews the scientific merit or financial impact of protocols to determine whether the institution should support the proposed research. The IRB, however, makes its independent determination whether to approve or disapprove a protocol, based upon whether or not human subjects are adequately protected.

In the United States each institution engaged in research involving human subjects and that is supported by a department or agency to which federal policy applies, and must establish an IRB to review and approve the research. Under the regulation, an institution can establish more than one IRB which may be necessary or appropriate, depending on the structure of the institution or the kind of human subjects research performed by that institution. Alternatively, an institution can designate another IRB to review its research for approval.

One of the IRB responsibilities is to review and approve the initiation of biomedical research involving human subjects in accordance with the FDA guidelines. The purpose of the review should be to assure that human research is performed using sound research design, avoiding unnecessary risks, evaluating the risk-benefit ratios, and selecting human subjects for the clinical study while minimizing risks to the subject. Informed consent should be sought from each prospective subject or legal representative and documented using an IRB-approved informed consent document signed by the patient, a witness and the investigator alike. Data should be prospectively collected to insure the safety of the subjects participating in the research and also protecting the confidentiality and privacy of the subjects. Another responsibility of the IRB is to monitor the welfare of particularly vulnerable groups such as children or prisoners.

The approval of clinical investigations with FDA-approved drugs is still under the IRB's purview, because it is research. IRB approval is required if investigators use a marketed drug for an indication for which there are no data about efficacy or safety in the literature. Community physicians who participate in clinical research also need to comply with these guidelines. They could submit their protocols to a hospital-based IRB or to an independent IRB; conversely, the sponsor of the research, who might have an established IRB, could provide IRB review and approval.

An IRB can have as many members as necessary to perform its duties effectively. Non-affiliated members (members who are neither hospital staff nor faculty) of the IRB should be drawn from the local community at-large; clergymen, teachers, attorneys, businesspersons, patients and homemakers are possible candidates. The persons selected should be knowledgeable about the local community and be willing to discuss research issues from that perspective.

One of the most important actions to be taken in establishing an IRB is selecting the individual who will act as the chairperson. The IRB chair should be an individual from within or outside the institution who is fully capable of managing the IRB and the matters brought before it with fairness and impartiality. An investigator can be a member of the IRB; however, there is a stipulation that must be adhered to without exception. An investigator as a member cannot participate in the review and approval process of any project in which he or she has a present or potential conflict of interest. An investigator member with a conflict of interest should be present only to provide information requested by the IRB, but should be absent from the meeting room during the discussion and voting phase of the review and approval process. IRB minutes should reflect that these requirements were met.

Informed Consent

Each approved protocol involving human subjects should have a written informed consent document (example of a model consent form from our institute is shown in appendix one), and the consent should be signed by each participant in triplicate. One form is for the medical record, one for the patient, and one must be kept by the investigator. The written consent document is an aid to provide appropriate and necessary information regarding the research. Ample opportunity should be provided to potential participants to consider all treatment options. Investigators should ensure that the subjects have comprehended and are voluntarily participating in the research. The consent form should identify the sponsor of the research, if exists. Subjects must be informed whether compensation for treatment and - related injuries is available, or the consent form should include a statement that the institution or IRB does not have to compensate a subject for injury for participation in research [3]. However, if funds are available from the sponsor for these types of injuries, that should be stated in the consent form. The consent form should also indicate whether the institution has the capability of providing care for potential complications related to research; it should include a statement confirming that confidentiality will be preserved. However, the FDA and the sponsor have the right to review the records to determine the accuracy of the data and, on rare occasions, may not be able to protect the privacy of subjects.

A copy of the consent form, completely filled in, signed and dated by the investigator, participant and witness, should be provided to each subject. Each informed consent document should have the following information:

- description of the research;
- purpose of the study;
- a detailed description of the risks, side effects, potential benefits, and alternative treatments;
- understanding that the patient, voluntarily participated, had the opportunity to ask questions, was able to withdraw consent, understood the limits of confidentiality, the recourse should injury occur, and any financial issues.

Consent forms should also include information on the person to contact for further information. This should be the Principal Investigator, and the chairman of the IRB who approved the study. All of this should be in language comprehensible to the average eighth grade reader.

Recent changes to federal regulations on informed consent

During past FDA audits of clinical trials, agency officials occasionally had difficulty verifying that informed consent was obtained prior to subjects being enrolled in studies because consent forms were not dated and the case histories contained insufficient documentation for verification. In December 1995, the FDA proposed to amend the regulations to require that informed consent documents be both signed and dated at the time consent is given and that adequate documentation of the consent process be entered in patient histories. The agency received positive comments on this proposal from patient advocacy groups, pharmaceutical and device manufacturers and private individuals. The new rule, effective December 1996, amended 21 CFR Parts 50, 312, and 812 and required that all informed consent documents be dated on the day of signing by the subject or his legal representative. The amended regulations also clarified the definition of case histories. The section of the federal code pertaining to investigator record keeping and record retention, 21 CFR § 312.62(b), was amended to include the following: "Case histories include the case report forms and supporting data comprising, for example, signed and dated consent forms and medical records including, for example, progress notes of the physician, the individual's hospital chart(s) and the nurses' notes. The case history for each individual shall document that informed consent was obtained prior to participation in the study".

Although this new rule was not in effect until December 1996, the open dialogue about the informed consent process throughout the year has had a positive influence on clinical investigators. Historically, inadequate consent forms were cited in 54 percent of clinical study site inspections. However, for fiscal year 1996, this proportion dropped to only 28 percent. The improved status of the informed consent was partially attributed to improved oversight by IRBs [4].

There have been instances in the last decade when the FDA has waived the informed consent rule. During Operation Desert Storm in 1990, in response to the U.S. Department of Defense, the FDA issued an interim rule stating that informed consent waivers could be authorized on a case by case basis; would apply only to investigational drugs; were to be used in military operations involving combat or the threat of combat; would expire after one year unless renewed at DoD's request. The arguments for the waiver were based on differences between military and civilian standards, the ethics of sending unprotected soldiers into battle, and the urgency of military action superseding normal rights. The waivers applied to the administration of tablets and vaccines to protect against biological and chemical weapons.

Retrospective analysis by both the Presidential Advisory Committee on Gulf War Veteran's Illnesses and the FDA found fault with DoD's application of the rule including inadequate record keeping and disclosure, failure to follow the protocol and failure to obtain review by an IRB external to DoD. A petition filed by citizen's and veteran's groups in response to these reports has been filed with the FDA to repeal the waiver. In response to the petition, the FDA sought public comment on issues including the scope, administration and ethical impact of the waiver. The FDA's final ruling has not yet been published.

In November 1996, the FDA implemented a final rule allowing investigators to treat patients with experimental therapies in emergency situations when they were unable to give their consent and their legal representatives were not available (21 CFR §50.24). This rule required the disclosure of risk and benefit information about the clinical trial information to the community from which the patients would be drawn. In addition, consultation with the communities was mandated to occur prior to the trials. The responsibility and burden of these activities was placed on the IRB and their institutions would have to support these activities. The rule has been described by many as a disincentive to the performance of research involving emergency treatment. The FDA plans to issue industry guidance on how to apply the rule. If the outcome of an investigation into the use and administration of the rule is not favorable, the FDA will reexamine the rule.

Current Issues of Informed Consent

The National Cancer Institute is currently involved in examining the issues surrounding informed consent for future research on banked tissue samples. This effort began in 1993 with the formation of the National Action Plan on Breast Cancer (NAPCB) and the recognition that availability of breast cancer specimens for future research was a high priority. It was recommended that consent be obtained at the time of tissue procurement to assure that specimens could be used for future research. An ethical subcommittee made up of ethicists, lawyers, pathologists, clinicians, laboratory researchers, patient advocates and office for Protection from Research Risks (OPRR) representatives were empanelled and guided by the need to protect patient confidentiality yet enabling medical research. A model informed consent document was prepared based on guidelines developed by the subcommittee addressing the issues of tissue collection, storage and distribution.

The document was presented by an outside agency to twenty six focus groups comprised of general consumers, cancer patients and their families, and members of the medical profession to obtain information regarding content and format of the document. The group's responses indicated that although the document was easy to understand, it left people confused and with many unanswered questions. NACPB was presented with the information from the focus groups as well as recommendations for improving the document and the informed consent process. An information sheet was prepared to be used as a tool during the informed consent process. The focus group comments, the IC document and the information sheet were well-received when presented to representatives of the IRB community in 1997.

To assess the feasibility of obtaining informed consent for future research use of tissue specimens from patients undergoing surgical procedures, the National Cancer Institute has embarked on a two phase project in which the University of Texas, M. D. Anderson Cancer Center (UTMDACC) is participating. The first phase of the project involved obtaining institutional approval for a new consent form for future use of tissues. This form has recently been approved by the UTMDACC IRB and Medical Records Committee (Appendix 2). Phase 2 will be an actual pilot project of collecting data from the care-givers who administer this consent to patients about the systems required to get consent, build a database to store the information, and retrieve the information prior to releasing tissue samples for research use. Data collection is slated to begin in September 1998.

There are other factors that further complicate the issue of obtaining consent for future research on banked tissues such as the potential for the development of commercial products from research done with these tissues. UTMDACC is currently examining all aspects of this issue, including what, if any, consent is required prior to sending material to business entities who may wish to develop products to be marketed at some time in the future.

Continuing Reviews of Clinical Research

Each research study approved by the IRB is only approved for a maximum of one year. At the end of the year the sponsor or the PI must submit a written report. This report should identify the risks (adverse events), if any, changes in the research design, if necessary, to ensure the safety of the subjects,and must be reviewed by the IRB. The IRB has the authority to suspend, terminate, or continue the research for another year.

Cooperative Group Research

Each institution is responsible for safeguarding the rights and the welfare of its human subjects. Thus, cooperative group protocols should be individually reviewed at each institution. During this review process some shortcomings of the study may be identified which may have been overlooked in the earlier reviews at other institutions.

Adverse Events

Investigators are responsible for prompt reporting of any unexpected adverse reactions occurring during the course of the research to the IRB. This allows the IRB to monitor the level of risk to the patients and to determine if there is significant toxicity on any individual study. The IRB has to reassess the situation on a continuing basis and determine whether to allow continuation of the protocol or require modification of the research based on these reports. The IRB is responsible for reviewing reports of adverse reactions involving subjects enrolled on protocols at their institution as well as reports involving subjects being treated with the same experimental therapies at other institutions. The internal adverse reaction reports are submitted to the IRB directly from the principal investigator within the institution. It is the responsibility of the sponsor of the research studies to forward adverse reactions reports to all principal investigators using the same therapy. These reports of external reactions are then submitted to the IRB to keep the committee apprised of the global view of the treatment's toxicity.

Clinical Investigations Regarding Medical Devices

Devices intended for use in diagnosis, treatment, or prevention of the disease, or other devices that may affect the function of part of the body, need to be evaluated in a fashion similar to that used to examine new drugs. Each device has to be reviewed on its own merit and its risk-versus-benefit ratio. IRB review is required for all devices. Devices that carry significant risk need to be approved by the IRB and the FDA prior to the initiation of the research. Non-significant risk devices do not require FDA approval but IRB approval is needed. The IRB acts as a surrogate for the FDA in these devices.

In conclusion, the Institutional Review Board's responsibilities are: to ensure that research is scientifically sound, risks are acceptable, alternative therapies are appropriately discussed in the consent process, and consent is voluntary from each subject.

References

1. Nuremberg Code, reprinted in trials of war criminals for Nuremberg Military Tribunal under control consular #10 (1949) Vol 2 pp 181-182 Washington, DC, US Government Printing Office
2. The Belmont Report (1978) Ethical principles and guidelines for protection of human subjects' research. Washington DC, US Government Printing Office, DHEW publication # (OS78-0012) reprinted in Federal Register 44 (April 18, 1979): 23192
3. Compensating for research injuries (1982) The ethical and legal implications for program to readdress injury subject. Washington, DC, US Government Printing Office, G.P.O. stack #040-000-00455-456
4. Guide to Good Clinical Practice (1997) Monthly Bulletin 4(6):6, Thompson Publ, Washington DC

The University of Texas
M.D. Anderson Cancer Center

Informed Consent for Treatment

Protocol Title:

1. _____   _____
    Participant's Name   ID Number

You have the right to know about the procedures that are to be used in your participation in clinical research so as to afford you an opportunity to make the decision whether or not to undergo the procedure after knowing the risks and hazards involved. This disclosure is not meant to frighten or alarm you; it is simply an effort to make you better informed so that you may give or withhold your consent to participate in clinical research. This informed consent does not supersede other consents you may have signed.

This clinical trial is so designed that no person shall on the grounds of race, color, gender, or national origin be excluded from participation in or be denied the benefits, or be otherwise subjected to discrimination through or under this study.

DESCRIPTION OF RESEARCH – (Items 2 thru 6 <u>must</u> be in 3rd person)

2. PURPOSE OF STUDY: @
3. DESCRIPTION OF RESEARCH: @
4. RISKS, SIDE EFFECTS AND DISCOMFORTS TO PARTICIPANTS: @
   This clinical research study may involve unforeseeable risks to the participant.
   4a. "This clinical research may involve unforeseeable risks to unborn children; therefore, the participants should practice adequate methods of birth control throughout the period of their involvement in the clinical study if they are sexually active. To help prevent injury to children, the female participants should refrain from breast feeding during participation in the clinical research study."
5. POTENTIAL BENEFITS: @
6. ALTERNATE PROCEDURES OR TREATMENTS: @

UNDERSTANDING OF PARTICIPANTS: (Choose appropriate options in items 7 and 9 and in the CONSENT section: choose 13 if 4a. is included).

7. I have been given an opportunity to ask any questions concerning the (survey/procedure/treatment/investigational drug regimen) involved and the investigator has been willing to reply to my inquiries. This (survey/procedure/treatment/investigational drug regimen) will be (executed/administered) under the above numbered, titled and described clinical research protocol at this institution. I hereby authorize Dr. _____, the attending physician/investigator and designated associates to (administer/perform) the (survey/procedure/treatment/investigational drug regimen).
8. I have been told and understand that my participation in this clinical research study is voluntary. I may decide not to participate, or withdraw my consent and discon-

tinue my participation at any time. Such action will be without prejudice and there shall be no penalty or loss of benefits to which I may otherwise be entitled, and I will continue to receive treatment by my physician at this institution.

Should I decide not to participate or withdraw my consent from participation in this clinical research, I have been advised that I should discuss the consequences or effects of my decision with my physicians.

In addition, I understand that the investigator may discontinue the clinical research study if, in the sole opinion and discretion of the investigator, the study or treatment offers me little or no future benefit, or the supply of medication ceases to be available or other causes prevent continuation of the clinical research study. The investigator will notify me should such circumstances arise and my physician will advise me about available treatments which may be of benefit at that time.

I will be informed of any new findings developed during the course of this clinical research study, which may relate to my willingness to continue participation in the study.

9. I have been assured that confidentiality will be preserved (except that, if applicable, qualified monitors from the Food and Drug Administration (FDA) or (Specify: National Cancer Institute or name(s) of sponsor(s) who finish(es) the drugs/ devices being utilized in this study)) may review my records where appropriate and necessary. Qualified monitors shall include assignees authorized by the Surveillance Committee of this institution provided that confidentiality is assured and preserved. My name will not be revealed in any reports or publications resulting from this study, without my expressed consent. In special circumstances, the FDA might be required to reveal the names of participants.

10. I have been informed that should I suffer any injury as a result of participation in this research activity, reasonable medical facilities are available for treatment at this institution. I understand, however, that I cannot expect to receive any credit or reimbursement for expenses from this institution or any financial compensation from this institution for such injury.

11. I have been informed that I should inquire of the attending physician whether or not there are any services, investigational agents or devices, and/or medications being offered by the sponsor of this clinical research project at a reduced cost or without cost. Should the investigational agent become commercially available during the course of the study, I understand that I may be required to cover the cost of subsequent doses.

Costs related to my medical care including expensive drugs, tests or procedures that may be specifically required by this clinical research study shall be my responsibility unless the sponsor or other agencies contribute toward said costs. I have been given the opportunity to discuss the expenses or costs associated with my participation in this research activity.

12. It is possible that this research project will result in the development of beneficial treatments, devices, new drugs, or possible patentable procedures, in which event I understand that I cannot expect to receive any compensation or benefits from the subsequent use of information acquired and developed through my participation in this research project.

13. Add if 4a is included:
    I understand that refraining from breast-feeding and practicing effective contracep-
    tion are medically necessary and a prerequisite for my participation in this clinical
    research study. Should contraception be interrupted or if there is any suspicion of
    pregnancy, my participation in this clinical research study will be terminated at the
    sole discretion of the investigator.
14. I may discuss questions or problems during or after this study with Dr. _____
    at 713-792-2817. In addition, I may discuss any problems I may have or any ques-
    tions regarding my rights during or after this study with the Chairman of the Sur-
    veillance Committee at (713) 792-2933 and may in the event any problem arises
    during this clinical research contact the parties named above.

CONSENT

Based upon the above, I consent to (participate in the research/undergo the described
procedure/participate in this survey) and have received a copy of the consent form.

_____   _____
Date   Signature of Participant

_____   _____
Witness other than Physician or   Signature of Person Responsible
Investigator   and Relationship

I have discussed this clinical research study with the participant and/or his or her authorized representative, using a language which is understandable and appropriate. I
believe that I have fully informed this participant of the nature of this study and its possible benefits and risks and I believe the participant understood this explanation.

                                            _____
                                            Physician/Investigator

Add if applicable:
"I was present during the explanation of the research to be executed under protocol @;
the child participant was also present. I feel that the child assented to the participation in
the research"

                                            _____
                                            Witness

I have translated the above informed consent into _____ for this patient.
                                            (name of language)

_____   _____
Name of Translator   Signature of Translator and Date

The University of Texas
M.D. Anderson Cancer Center

Disclosure and consent
Consent Form for Use of Tissue for Future Research

Tissue Collection For Research Purposes
With my consent, some of the tissues, blood or other body fluids that are left over after completing diagnosis will be kept and may be helpful for future research. Reports about research done with my tissues, blood or other body fluids will not be given to me or my physicians. Sometimes tissues, blood or other body fluids are used for genetic research (about diseases that are passed on in families). Even if these tissues, blood or body fluids are used for this type of research, results will not be put in my health records. No matter what I decide to do, it will not affect my care.

Benefits: The benefits of research using tissues. blood or body fluids include learning more about what causes cancer and other diseases, how to prevent them, how to treat them and how to cure them. Research with tissues, blood or body fluids by M. D. Anderson Cancer Center or others, including, but not limited to commercial entities, may result in the development of marketable treatments, devices, new drugs or patentable procedures, in which event I undestand that I cannot expect to receive any benefits or compensation.

Risks: These samples will have coded identifiers but will be kept in a secure and confidential tissue bank.

My tissue, blood, and other body fluids, *if not disposed of*, may be kept for use in research   YES   NO

Someone from this institution may contact me in the future to ask me to take part in more research   YES   NO

The research on my tissues, blood or other body fluids is not designed to produce information that would be medically useful to me as an individual. However, reasonable efforts will be made to contact me if such information should become available, unless I check 'no' here :   NO. I do not wish to be contacted

I (we) certify this form has been fully explained to me and that I (we) have read it or have had it read to me. I (we) understand its contents.

_____   _____
Date   Time

_____   _____
Patient/Other Legally Responsible Person   Witness Signature

_____   _____
Signature of Physician/PA or nurse   City   State

This form has been translated to the patient/other responsible person by:

                                              _____
                                              Signature of Translator

Progress and Perspectives in the Chemotherapy of Epithelial Solid Tumors

E. FREI III

Introduction

Major progress has been achieved in the curative treatment of the hematological malignancies, the childhood solid tumors, and in testis cancer [1-3]. These tumors comprise 10% of all cancers. The majority of tumors are epithelial solid tumors which occur in patients over 50 and include breast, bowel, lung cancer, head and neck, and selected genitourinary and gynecologic cancers. Cancer is the second cause of death in the US, after cardiovascular disease, and constitutes a major public health burden.

Selected advances and prospects in the therapy of epithelial solid tumors are the subject of this presentation.

Clinical Experimental Design Strategies

The evolution of clinical trial designs has been as follows:

The Chemotherapy of Overt Metastatic Solid Tumors

Treatment strategies that were successful in the leukemias-lymphomas such as combination chemotherapy and marrow transplantation have been less effective in the solid tumors [1-3]. Several reasons for this include the tumor burden [4] and the solid tumor microenvironment (see below) [5].

Adjuvant Chemotherapy

Perhaps the most compelling rationale for adjuvant chemotherapy is that, in essentially every preclinical tumor model, tumor size was inversely correlated with curability [4-6]. In addition to tumor burden, the rationale for adjuvant chemotherapy as compared to the chemotherapy of overt tumor relates to the microenvironment, angiogenesis, hypoxia, cytokinetics, drug resistance and other factors (see below).

Neoadjuvant or Induction Chemotherapy.

The principles and initial studies of neoadjuvant chemotherapy were formulated as a science and applied to head and neck cancer and osteosarcoma in the late 1970s and early 1980s [7, 8]. In the neoadjuvant design,
chemotherapy is administered initially with the intent of: 1) shrinking the
primary tumor and thus making it more amenable to local control; 2)
improving the quality of life by reducing the need for and extent of radical
surgery; 3) treating micrometastatic disease as early as possible, with the
intent of reducing the risk of mutation to resistance, and, finally, 4) to
serve as an *in vivo* (in the patient) assay of chemosensitivity [7-9a].

In stage III non-small cell lung cancer, a significant increase in cure
rate in definitive comparative studies has been achieved with a neoadjuvant approach [10]. In other tumors, there has been a questionable effect
on survival, though more recent studies are promising in that regard.

An important contribution of the neoadjuvant approach has been
improved quality of life as a result of reduced need for radical procedures
including, for example, amputation, laryngectomy, mastectomy, cystec-
tomy [11]. One dividend of neoadjuvant chemotherapy has been the
observation that solid tumors in general are much more chemosensitive
than previously appreciated on the basis of chemotherapy applied against
recurrent, overtly metastatic disease. Head and neck cancer is a notable
example wherein therapy involving combined fluorouracil, cisplatin and
leucovorin produces rapid and complete tumor regression in the majority
of patients many of whom will not, upon subsequent biopsy or resection
of the tumor area, have evidence of tumor on pathology examination [12].

Concomitant Radiotherapy and Chemotherapy

Another innovation in experimental design derives from the fact that
some chemotherapeutic agents are radiosensitizing. This approach may
expand with the advent of such potent radiosensitizers as gemcitabine
[13,13a,14]. How this compares to, for example, the neoadjuvant
approach is a subject of current quantitative studies. One might predict
that their concurrent use would be superior against the primary tumor, but
potentially inferior against systemic micrometastases because of potential compromises in the dosing of chemotherapy.

High-Dose - Stem Cell Rescue (HD-SCR)

Another clinical innovation is high-dose chemotherapy with autologous
myeloid stem cell rescue for selected epithelial solid tumors. Among all

of the variables that impact on experimental chemotherapy, dose is the most powerful, and dose increase in the form of high-dose - stem cell rescue (HD-SCR) has been curative for the leukemias and lymphomas [1, 2, 6]. There is controversy concerning its effectiveness in, for example, breast cancer where it has been extensively employed. That controversy was generated in part by the position that HD-SCR programs, because of their cost in morbidity, mortality and dollars, must have as their endpoint an increase in cure rate [14-16].

Advances in supportive care, particularly related to the use of peripheral blood stem cells, has reduced morbidity, time to marrow reconstitution, mortality, and the cost of this program. The most compelling parameter is mortality which has fallen from 10 to 15% in initial studies in the early 80's, to less than 4%, and indeed to less than 1% in major institutions [15]. While the jury is still out with respect to cure rate, the complete response rate in comparative and non-comparative studies is in the range of 50% with HD-SCR as compared to 5 to 15% for standard chemotherapy [17,18]. The acquisition of a high CR rate has historically been an important step in the direction of cure, for example, in the leukemias and lymphomas. Importantly, while essentially all systemic treatment modalities are more effective against microscopic as compared to macroscopic tumor, immunotherapy is particularly much more effective against a minimal tumor burden. Thus, the high complete remission rate afforded by high dose therapy of metastatic breast cancer provides the opportunity of introducing immunotherapy following complete remission with the intent of eradicating minimal residual tumor.

Why is Chemotherapy More Effective in the Leukemias-Lymphomas as Compared to the Solid Tumors?

In cancer chemotherapy research "the child is father to the man". Thus, many of the principles of systemic chemotherapy were first worked out in pediatric cancers. It is of interest to compare these two categories of cancer as a prelude to the possible understanding as to why the treatment of epithelial solid tumors has been less successful.

Chemosensitivity

A major difference is the intrinsic chemosensitivity of the leukemias-lymphomas as compared to the epithelial cancers. In the NCI, multiple

human tumor *in vitro* screens, the IC50 concentrations for the lymphoblastic tumors are fivefold lower than those for the epithelial solid tumors
[19a]. Thus, lymphoblastic leukemias are, indeed, intrinsically more sensitive than solid tumors. There is suggestive, but not statistically significant, evidence that the clinically more responsive epithelial solid tumors,
such as small cell lung cancer and breast cancer, are more sensitive *in
vitro* than are non-small cell lung cancer or melanoma, which are clinically resistant [19a].

The Solid Tumor Microenvironment

While the leukemias, certainly, and the lymphomas, to some extent, commonly begin clinically as disseminated disease (liquid tumors), the epithelial solid tumors, both the primary and metastasis, may grow locally
for some time before metastases develop. The multicellular construct of
epithelial solid tumors differs markedly from that of the leukemias. This,
along with tumor vascularity and matrix represents a newly appreciated
micropharmacologic challenge (see below).

Cytogenetics and Molecular Genetics

A second major difference between the leukemias-lymphomas, childhood solid tumors, and epithelial solid tumors relates to cytogenetics.
While cytogenetic abnormalities that are clonal have been found in essentially all of the leukemias-lymphomas, the genome compared to solid
tumors is relatively stable. In contrast, cytogenetics of many of the epithelial solid tumors, particularly when metastatic, is associated with multiple abnormalities. This is also found by molecular probing in the form
of LOH (loss of heterozygosity). Such instability of the genome would
be expected to markedly accelerate the clonal variation and selection of
more highly malignant and drug resistant cell lines [20]. For example,
small cell lung cancer responds initially with complete responses in the
majority of patients, but the development of drug-resistant relapse also
occurs rapidly in the majority. In contrast, a similar initial cytoreduction,
that is, a high complete remission rate, in the leukemias is more commonly durable. Hopefully, the advances in the molecular biology of
chemosensitivity and resistance will provide insight into the problem.

Resistance

Recent studies emphasize the downstream, multiple level, multi-drug and multi-factorial aspects of resistance [21-24]. Indeed, studies of apoptosis and antiapoptosis, genes and their products with respect to effect on chemosensitivity suggest that we may have pushed the envelop as far as possible with our classical approach to chemotherapy. Most of these studies indicate that cross resistance will be a substantially greater problem than was previously thought [22-26].

One way to overcome such resistance, which is almost always relative to dose, is to increase dose. This approach, that is, high dose therapy with stem cell rescue, has been clearly successful in a spectrum of tumors which is somewhat similar to the spectrum of response to classical combination chemotherapy.

Another major molecular difference between the solid tumors and the leukemias-lymphomas is the fact that the former more commonly result, at least in part, from tumor suppressor gene product dysfunction or deletion, whereas the leukemias-lymphomas more commonly derive from reciprocal translocations [20].

Holotherapy

We suggest this term for the predicted evolution of systemic therapy. While a magic bullet capable of destroying all of the tumor cells within a patient is possible and to be desired, tumor heterogeneity makes it unlikely that any target would be sufficiently represented on all the tumor cells.

While combination chemotherapy, based in part on heterogeneity and drug resistance, has been effective [28], we have a long way to go. The rationale for combination chemotherapy applies equally well to antisoil agents, such as antiangiogenesis, and anti-invasion compounds, such as metalloproteinase inhibitors. Some of these agents, particularly antiangiogenesis agents, are highly synergistic with chemotherapy and radiotherapy in experimental systems (see below). We use the seed and soil terms differently from Paget. He considered them in terms of the distribution of metastases. We define the seed as the tumor cells *per se* and the soil as the matrix/vasculature, the supporting structure of the tumor [27].

The evolution towards holotherapy is exemplified by acute lymphocytic leukemia in children, where there is a direct correlation between response and the number of chemotherapeutic agents employed. Thus, from 1 to 9 agents, there occurred a progressive increase in the complete remission up to 100%, followed by an increasing cure rate up to 80% [28-30, 36].

The following are examples of synergy between antiseed and antisoil agents. Teicher [34] has demonstrated that the antiangiogenic agents, TNP 470 and a collagenase inhibitor, used alone are inactive in a lung adenocarcinoma (Lewis lung) in the mouse. Cyclophosphamide has definite, albeit limited, activity. The two in combination produce cure in approximately 50% of the animals [31, 32]. Weichselbaum found that angiostatin and endostatin were synergistic with radiotherapy [13]. The basis for this synergism is incompletely understood. A three to five fold increase in distribution of cyclophosphamide into the tumor suggests that vascular damage by antiangiogenesis agents provides access to the tumor [34]. Similar, albeit somewhat less impressive, synergism has been demonstrated between the antisoil agents, that is, the metalloproteinases, and classical chemotherapeutic agents.

Modulators of the Tumor Microenvironment

Molecular oxygen is required for radiotherapeutic effect and for optimal effectiveness of many chemotherapeutic agents. Tumor hypoxia and areas of necrosis have been demonstrated to be a very common feature of epithelial solid tumors [34-36], and such hypoxia can be at least partially corrected by oxic agents such as perfluorocarbons and hemoglobin solutions [35]. Liquid tumors, such as the leukemias and lymphomas, do not have the microenvironment of solid tumors, and uncommonly exhibit hypoxia. Thus, hypoxia may be the obstacle that explains the generalization that solid tumors are less responsive than the leukemia-lymphomas to chemotherapy. Again, the ultimate rule for oxic/hypoxia correcting therapy may be in the holotherapy context (see below).

Holotherapy, with the multiple agents and approaches involved, provides a major challenge in the area of experimental design. Certainly, all variables cannot be subject independently to assessment of their effect. For example, surrogate endpoints, novel designs, the ongoing development of improved techniques for measuring minimal disease, these and other approaches must be integrated if holotherapy is to succeed.

Selected Areas of Basic Science and Cancer Therapy

The integration of basic science and clinical science in the construct of clinical trials, most particularly advances in molecular sciences, represent at once our greatest opportunity and challenge. I would re-emphasize the above comments on pluralism, that is, that basic science should be supported on a broad base since we can't predict which one or several will emerge as paramount in the curative treatment of solid tumors. The following represent areas of basic cancer science that are in process of impacting on therapy.

Angiogenesis and Antiangiogenesis

The critical role of tumor angiogenesis for the progressive growth of tumors beyond a few millimeters in diameter is established [36]. Such neovascularity is a target for chemotherapy in that the cytokinetic thrust, that is, the cell turnover of such tumor neovascularity, is markedly in excess of the normal vasculature [36]. In this sense, chemotherapy which targets prominently on the proliferative aspects of tumor biology has, unknowingly, represented antiangiogenic therapy. There are structural differences in the vessels of tumors which include uneven distribution of microvessels, fenestrations, blind ends, dynamic opening, and closing of vessels [35-37]. Importantly, there is evidence that the neovasculature of solid tumors can be targeted. Jain [38] has studied the pore size in tumor neovasculature. He has found an increased interstitial pressure which is maximal in the center of tumors and flows outward, thus inhibiting access of incoming therapeutic molecules. In addition to the proliferation target, some of the newer antiangiogenesis agents such as endostatin and angiostatin target on qualitatively unique targets in the neovasculature. There is experimental evidence that resistance does not develop to antiangiogenesis agents [39]. The synergism between such agents and chemotherapy and radiotherapy has been demonstrated in experimental models [31]. Clinical trials with these agents represent a unique and major opportunity and proper emphasis has been given to fast-tracking these agents to the clinic.

Another approach to targeting the vasculature of tumors is that involving the use of *in vivo* selection by phage displays libraries of peptides that hone specifically to tumor blood vessels. When coupled to the anticancer drug, doxorubicin, two of these peptides, one containing the integrin binding tripeptide motif, resulted in enhancement of doxorubicin antitumor specificity and decreasing toxicity. The results indicate that it may be possible to develop targeted chemotherapy strategies that are based on selective expression of receptors in tumor vasculature [38a].

The mesenchymal scaffolding is an intrinsic part of solid tumors and the extent and quality of the solid tumor mesenchyma may influence tumor invasiveness and growth. Thus, our therapeutic approach which, over the years, has been largely targeted on the tumor cells *per se*, that is, the seed, is being modified in a major way by the recognition of the importance tumor's soil and the therapeutic target it provides [39]. These include antiangiogenic agents metallo pro times inhibitors which prevent tumor invasion and agents which modify access to solid tumors [34].

Primarily because of the vasculature of solid tumors, hypoxia, often in major degree, is common. This is a therapeutic obstacle in that radiotherapy and many forms of chemotherapy require molecular oxygen for cytotoxicity. Red blood cell substitutes, such as perfluorocarbons and hemoglobin solutions, are much smaller and in the case of perfluorocarbon, much more deformable than stiff, large, red blood cells. This presumably is responsible for their better entry into hypovascular solid tumors where oxygen off-loading occurs. These oxic agents have been shown in experimental *in vivo* solid tumors to be capable of diminishing tumor hypoxia, and therefore increasing therapeutic effect of X-ray and chemotherapy. The areas of hypoxia and necrosis within solid tumors also contribute to genetic instability with increasing recombination and mutations, thus providing an environment for the acceleration of the neoplastic phenotype as well as variation that contributes to resistance [22].

The disregulation of apoptosis

Another discovery, largely in the last decade, is programmed cell death (apoptopsis) [33]. Prior to this decade, cell death was considered to be a passive process. A protein was discovered in the cells of patients with chronic lymphocytic leukemia and follicular lymphoma that was capable of inhibiting cell death, that is, apoptosis. This observation fit with other data to the effect that tumor enlargement in these diseases occurred as a result of lack of destruction rather than increased proliferation, that is, production of tumor cells [40]. Indeed, it is becoming increasingly evident that there are multiple regulatory proteins, stimulatory and inhibitory, involved in maintaining homeostasis of this system. It involves the balance between stem cell renewal, proliferation, differentiation, and apoptotic tumor cell death.

This field has altered our view of drug sensitivity and resistance. Essentially, all chemotherapeutic agents can induce apoptosis. The setpoint, that is, the sensitivity of the cell to apoptosis, can be influenced by the complex of gene products that regulate apoptosis/antiapoptosis.

Strategies for preventing or overcoming drug resistance will have to include the apoptosis setpoint. An example is bypassing the p53 pathway.

Molecular Cytokinetics

The science of the cell cycle clock has moved from cell biology to molecular biology with extraordinary thrust. Classical chemotherapeutic agents commonly affect proliferation mainly through inhibition of DNA synthesis. The cyclins and the cyclin-dependent kinases, determine the transit of cells through various stages of the cell cycle. The control of CDKs and relevant cyclins is, therefore, of central importance in the regulation of proliferation in normal and in neoplastic tissues. The molecular genetics and cytokinetics of cancer have come together in that the signal transduction pathways which controls the cell cycle at the level of cyclin-dependent kinases are paved with the products of oncogenes and tumor suppressor genes. Two factors of importance include the observation that normal cells may arrest at, for example, a G1/S interval to allow for repair of DNA damage induced by the environment or by chemotherapy. Tumor cells, on the other hand, may have lost that capacity to arrest, and as such, may have on one hand a proliferative advantage, and on the other, a more aggressive clonal evolution since the fixation of mutations by cells passing through DNA synthesis should increase tumor cell heterogeneity, progression of the neoplastic phenotype and drug resistance [41].

Telomerase

Normal stem cells have a limited stem cell renewal capacity, that is, human fetal tissue, for example, may be capable of approximately 50 divisions. This number is determined by the length of telomeres which, because of the special DNA polymerase, telomerase, are shortened with each successive division. Telomeres protect the ends of chromosomes from stickiness. When they become sufficiently shortened, senescence of the cells occurs in association with, and in part because of, the excess recombination and other DNA abnormalities which occur as a result of loss of telomere induced stickiness. The enzyme telomerase is present in tumor cells but not in normal cells (save for germ cells) which explains the maintenance of telomeres and immortality of tumor cells. Inhibitors of telomerase are under study [42, 43].

Immunotherapy

Immunotherapy has emerged as a highly sophisticated molecular science. Tumor specific antigens for a number of tumors, including melanoma, have been identified and molecularly cloned [44]. The specificity and complexity of arming the T cell with tumor cytotoxicity properties has been defined, and includes HLA restriction, antigen presentation, and co-stimulatory factors. Abnormalities of one or more of these mechanisms compromise immunologic restraint of the host against the tumor and may produce tolerance. Mechanisms of addressing such tolerance include genetic transfer and the fusion of dendritic cells with tumor cells. Consistent with holotherapy, we propose that immunotherapy will be integrated into a complex of agents and techniques. An example is the production of complete remission in breast cancer with high dose combination chemotherapy followed by immunotherapy in patients in complete remission [19].

Concluding Remarks

The field of oncology is full of promise and challenge. The opportunity relates to a growing number of agents with increasing specificity for the tumor, that is, increasing potency and decreasing toxicity. We would predict that given the success of combination chemotherapy and, most particularly, the obstacle represented by tumor cell heterogeneity and drug resistance, that the evolution of systemic cancer treatment strategy will be in the direction of holotherapy, that is, the integration of combined therapy across therapeutic sciences, such as combination chemotherapy, integrated immunotherapy, and antisoil agents, such as antiangiogenics, and antimatrix agents, such as metalloproteinase inhibitors. This will present a major, creative challenge to the clinical investigator, particularly in terms of experimental design.

References

1. Frei III, Antman KH (1997) Combination chemotherapy, dose and schedule. In: Holland J, Frei E III, Bast R, Kufe D, Morton D, Weichselbaum R (eds) Cancer Medicine. 4th Ed, Williams and Wilkins, Baltimore, 99.817-837
2. Thomas ED (1985) Current status of bone marrow transplantation. Transpl Proc 17428.
3. Armitage J, Antman K (eds.) In: High Dose Cancer Therapy. Second Ed, Williams and Wilkins, Baltimore,
4. Goldin A, Venditti J, Humphreys SB, Mantel N (1956) Influence of the concentration of leukemia inoculum on the effectiveness of treatment. Science 123:840
5. Jain RK (1998) Integrative pathophysiology of solid tumors: Role in detection and treatment. Cancer Journal Sci Am 4:S48-57
6. Frei E III, Canellos GP (1980) Dose a critical factor in cancer chemotherapy. Am J Med 69:585-594
7. Frei E III (1982) Clinical cancer research:an embattled species. Cancer 50:1979-1992
8. Frei E III (1988) What's in a name - neoadjuvant. J Natl Can Inst 80:1088-1090
9. Huvos A, Rosa G, Marcoue RC (1977) Primary osteosarcoma: Pathology aspects in 20 patients after chemotherapy, en bloc resection and prosthetic bone replacement. Arch Path Lab Med 101:14-18
9a. Goldie J (1987) Scientific basis for adjuvant and neoadjuvant chemotherapy. Semin Oncol 141
10. Dillman RO, Seagren SL, Propert KJ et al (1990) A randomized trial of induction chemotherapy plus high-dose radiation versus radiation alone in stage III non-small-cell lung cancer. N Engl J Med 323:940
11. Karp D, Vaughan C, Carter B, Willett B, Heeren T, Calarese P, Zeitels S, Strong MS, Hong W (1991) Voice preservation using induction chemotherapy (CT) plus radiation therapy (RT) as an alternative to laryngectomy in advanced head and neck cancer. Long term follow up. Am J Clin Oncol 14:273
12. Hong W, Choksi A et al (1990) Sequential induction chemotherapy and radiotherapy for advanced head and neck cancer: Impact of treatment on laryngeal cancer. Head and Neck Cancer 28:2-5
13. Weichselbaum R, Chen G, Hallahan D (1997) Biologic and physical basis of radiation oncology. In: Cancer Medicine, Fourth Edition. (eds.) JF Holland, E Frei III, RC Bast Jr, DW Kufe, DL Morton and R Weichselbaum. Williams and Wilkins, Baltimore, pp 697-727
13a. Clinical Investigational Brochure (1993) Gemcitabine HCl (LY188011 Hcl) Eli Lilly and Company
14. Bennett CL, Gulati SC, Smith TJ, Armitage JL (1995) A health policy perspective on high-dose cancer therapy: Cost, effectiveness, and cost-effectiveness. In: Armitage, JO Antman KH (eds) High-Dose Cancer Therapy. Second Ed, William and Wilkins, Baltimore pp 131-148
15. Kessinger A Reestablishing hematopoiesis after dose-intensive therapy with peripheral stem cells. In: Armitage, JO Antman KH (eds) High-Dose Cancer Therapy. Second Ed. William and Wilkins, Baltimore pp 196-210
16. Lee ME, Crawford J (1995) Delivery of high-dose chemotherapy with recombinant human granulocyte colony-stimulating factor support. In: Armitage JO, Antman KH (eds) High-Dose Cancer Therapy. Second Ed, William and Wilkins, Baltimore pp 342-371

17. Hendersen IC, Hayes DJ, and Gelman R (1988) Dose response in the treatment of breast cancer. J Clin Oncol 6:1501
18. Bezwoda WR, Seymour L, Dansey RD (1995) High-dose chemotherapy with hematopoietic rescue as primary treatment for metastatic breast cancer: a randomized trial. J Clin Oncol 13:2483
19. Gong J, Chen D, Kufe D (1997) Induction of antitumor activity by immunization with fusions of dendritic and carcinoma cells. Nature Medicine 3:558-561
19a. Weissman J Personal communication
20. Olufunmilayo I, Olopade O, and Rowley J (1997) Recurring chromosome rearrangements in human cancer. In: Cancer Medicine, Fourth Edition. (eds.) JF Holland, E Frei III, RC Bast Jr, DW Kufe, DL Morton and RR Weichselbaum. Williams and Wilkins, Baltimore pp 119-143
21. Ling V, Kartner N, Suda T, Siminovitch L, Riordan JR (1983) Multidrug resistance phenotype in Chinese hamster ovary cells. Cancer Treatment Reports 67:869
22. Fisher DE (1994) Apoptosis in cancer therapy: Crossing the threshold. Cell 778:539-542
23. Reed JC (1994) Bcl-1 and the regulation of programmed cell death. J Cell Biol 124:1-6
24. Morrow CA, Cowan K (1997) Drug resistance and its clinical circumvention. In: Cancer Medicine, Fourth Edition. (eds.) JF Holland, E Frei III, RC Bast Jr, DW Kufe, DL Morton and RR Weichselbaum. Williams and Wilkins, Baltimore pp 799-815
25. Kerr JFR, Winterford CM, Harmon BV (1994) Apoptosis - its significance to cancer and cancer therapy. Cancer 73:2013-2026
26. Harris CC, Holstein M (1993) Clinical implications of p53 tumor suppressor gene. New Engl J Med 329:13-18
27. Paget S (1989) The distribution of secondary growth in cancer. Lancet 1:571-573
28. Schnipper LE (1986) Clinical implications of tumor-cell heterogeneity. New Engl J Med 314:1423-1434
28a. Sallan S, Weinstein HJ (1987) Childhood acute leukemia. In: Nathan D, Oski F (eds) Hematology of Infancy and Childhood. Third Ed, WB Saunders Co, Philadelphia, pp 1028-1063
29. Reiter A, Schrappe M, Ludwig WD et al (1994) Chemotherapy in 998 unselected childhood acute lymphoblastic leukemia patients. Results and conclusions of the multicenter trial ALL-BFM 86. Blood 84:3122-3133
30. Frei E III, Elias A, Wheeler C, Richardson P, Hryniuk W (1998) The relationship between high dose treatment and combination chemotherapy: The concept of summation dose intensity. Clinical Cancer Research
31. Kakeji Y, Teicher B (1997) Preclinical studies of the combination of angiogenic inhibitors with cytotoxic agents. Invest New Drugs 15:39-48
32. Teicher BA, Sotomayor EA, Huang ZD (1992) Antiangiogenic agents potentiate cytotoxic cancer therapies against primary and metastatic disease. Cancer Res 52:6702-6704
33. Wythe AH, Kerr JFR, Currie A (1989) Cell death: The significance of apoptosis. Int J Cytol 68:251-306
33a. Mauceri HJ, Hanna NN, Beckett MA, Gorski DH, Staba MJ, Stellato KA, Bigelow K, Heinmann R, Gately S, Dhanabal M, Soff GA, Sukhatne VP, Kufe DW, Weichselbaum RR. Combined effects of angiostagin and ionizing radiation in antitumour therapy, Nature 1998; 394: 287-291.

34. Teicher BA, Herman TS, Frei E III (1992) Perfluorochemical emulsions: oxygen breathing in radiation sensitization and chemotherapy modulation. Important Adv Oncol 2:39-59
35. Teicher BA, Dupuis PN, Holden AS, Schwartz NG, Lester S, Frei E III (1994) Definition and manipulation of tumor oxygenation. Rad Onc Invest May(2):66-76
36. Folkman J, Shing V (1992) Angiogenesis. J Biol Chem 267:10931-10934
37. Fidler IJ, Ellis LM (1994) The implications of angiogenesis for the biology and therapy of cancer metastasis. Cell 79:185-188
38. Jain RK (1994) Transport phenomenon in tumors. Adv Chem Engineering 20:129-200
38a. Arap W, Pasqualini R, Ruoslahti E (1998) Cancer treatment by targeted drug delivery to tumor vasculature in a mouse model. Science 279:377-380
39. Kerbel RS (1991) Inhibition of tumor angiogenesis as a strategy to circumvent acquired resistance to anticancer therapeutic agents. BioEssays 13:31-36
40. Reed JC (1998) Dysregulation of apoptosis in cancer. Cancer Journal Sci Am 4:8-14
41. Morgan DO, Risher RP, Espinoza FH, Farrell A, Nourse J, Chamberlin H, Pin P (1998) Control of sukaryotic cell cycle progression by phosphorylation of cyclin-dependent kinases. Cancer Journal Sci Am 4:S77-83
42. deLange T (1998) Length control of human telomeres. Cancer Journal Sci Am 4:S22-25
43. Shay JW (1998) Telomerase in cancer: Diagnostic, prognostic, and therapeutic implications. Cancer Journal Sci Am 4:S26-34
44. Rosenberg SA (1998) New opportunities for the development of cancer immunotherapies. Cancer Journal Sci Am 4:S1-4

A Personal Perspective About the Future of Breast Cancer Research and Treatment

B. Fisher

It seems that, with the anticipation of a new millennium, there is keen interest in predicting what is likely to happen in almost every human endeavor once that boundary has been crossed, and the future of breast cancer research is no exception. At the request of the organizers of the February 1998 meeting of the International Congress on Anti-Cancer Therapy in Paris, I undertook the daunting, if not impossible, task of presenting a commentary on "the future of breast cancer research." This commentary is based primarily upon my presentation at the Paris meeting; it deals with the importance of understanding how current breast cancer management concepts were derived from past research and how the immediate future of brewit cancer research and treatment will be related to present findings. Because unknown events that occur in the immediate future are apt to shape the more distant future, long-range speculation is of limited value. In that regard, it needs to be emphasized that it is not in the best interest of either physicians or their patients to fécus exclusively on the future and disregard recent advances in the understanding and treatment of breast cancer.

Difficulty in Discussing the Future of Breast Cancer Research

Scientists who are immersed in one particular aspect of breast cancer research may be hesitalt about predicting the future direction of such research for several reasons. Not only may do g so inappropriately divert them from their own investigations, but they might also féel unqualified because they may be biased with regard to their own areas of research and less knowledgeable about the status of the investigations. of others. An event that occurred at a National Cancer Institute (NCI) Breast Cancer Progress Review Group Round Table Meeting in September 1997 is one case in point. Breast cancer researchers attended that meeting for the purpose of reviewing the NCI's research portfolio and for making recommendations about future investigations in the field. As objective as those scientists may have tried to be, it seemed to me that their recommendations were finked to their own areas of research and, particularly, to the conduct of investigations that would address questions that had arisen as a result of their individual accomplishments. Consequently, it seems that the ones to engage in such an ephemeral exercise as predicting the future should be those not personally involved in breast cancer research, but those who are superficially and broadly familiar with the "big picture."

My thoughts about the future of breast cancer research have been similarly conditioned by issues that have arisen as a result of my own research efforts. For me to attempt to divine th future would require that I be more intimately familiar with the work of others and be more prescient than I know myself to be. Consequently, it is my view that science is too complex and unpredictable for me to provide the reader with a list of predictions regarding future directions for breast cancer research that are unrelated to my own investigations. That is not to say, however, that I am unaware that the future of breast cancer research could well have ts origin in what is currently taldng place in a variety of settings. It is well recognized that there is no recipe for creativity or discovery in science. How a disease is treated relates to our comprehension of it and to the fact that understanding, for the most part, arises from both pet and current laboratory and clinical investigation. Just as to repair a watch one must understan,d the mechanisms responsible for its function, so, to treat breast cancer, one must understand how that biologie aberration is caused, or comes about. Consequently, any current or future investigation that can provide insight into some aspect of the complex mechanism associated with the initiation, progression, growth, and treatment of breast cancer should be vigorously pursued. With more precise identification of each new component of that mechanism, the greater the opportunity for devising new interventions that could damage one or more of the biologie systems responsible for maintaining the existence of tumor cells. This is an era when, at blinding speed, expanding technology, as well as advances in molecular, genetic, immunologie and viral research wül provide information about how that mechanism works. Many of the findings obtained could dramatically increase our understanding of breast cancer and have a major impact on the future treatment and prevention of the disease. As Napoleon is purported to have said, in affairs of magnitude, everything turns on a trifle. Other sources of discovery that may have a significant impact on the future often occur while investigators are looking for something else or when one scientist interprets an observation made by another to be more significant than was thought to be by the individual who made the original discovery.

In addition, many agents, such as anti-angiogenesis factors, Adriamy-cin-peptide conjugates, metalloproteinase inhibitors, HER-2 antibody, growth factor suppressors, and raloxifene, as well as studies related to the detection and nature of tumor metastatic cells in the bone marrow and to gene therapy and tumor vaccines are almost daily being touted in both the medical and lay press as being candidates for the future eradication of breast cancer. Certainly, when there is scientific justification for doing so, the design of such studies will be appropriate not only to determine if these agents are effective for treating breast cancer but also to obtain leads for future investigations.

Faced with an even greater array of laboratory and clinical investigations than the relatively few alluded to above, I cannot possibly provide, in this brief commentary, a meaningful list of candidates for further evaluation that are most apt to eliminate breast cancers in the next century. Whereas previously there was a relative paucity of new findings, and even fewer new testable hypotheses, there is now such a plethora of new data that it is becoming increasingly more difficult to prioritize and appropriately evaluate the information relative to its use in the clinical setting. How this is accomplished will, in no small part, determine the future direction of breast cancer research. Thus, the reason for my difficulty in discussing the topic assigned to me for my Paris talk should now be apparent.

On that note, it seems appropriate to share some of the thought processes that have guided my associates and me in obtaining and evaluating research findings that have altered the treatment of breast cancer over more than three decades. I believe that, because those guidelines are apt to have even greater relevance for the conduct of breast cancer research in the féresceable future, they should not be disregarded.

Pathways of Science and the Evolution of Treatment Paradigms: Their Role in the Future of Breast Cancer Research

On numerous occasions, 1 have indicated that future paradigms that will govern the treatment of breast cancer will arise from scientific achievement [1-3]. As the French physiologist, Claud4 Bernard, who focused on deductive scientific research, noted: "A hypothesis is ... the obligatory starting point of all experimental reasoning." Bernard himself insisted that a hypothesis is only of value if it can be tested. Only when reasonable hypotheses, formulated from the vast amount of laboratory and clinical observations currently available, are tested by appropriate laboratory experiments, or within randomized clinical trials, will it be possible to determine which of the findings are likely to play an important role in the future management of breast cancer. More attention must be given to the results obtained from testing a hypothesis than to the plethora of anecdotal reports of inductivist-generated information that continue to create so much confusion in the clinical setting. A few aphorisms wül emphasize the importance of testable hypotheses in the scientific process [4]. It has been noted that a belief that has not been logically tested and verified is, in a sense, irrational; thus, all hypotheses thet have not yet been tested may be considered to be so. In that regard, it has been stated that a hypothesis that has been constructed without an adequate program for its trial by experiment "is a burden to science and to the world," and that he who puts forth hypotheses that cannot be tested, "is a purveyor of rubbish." There should be no dogmas in science. There should also be no (or at least as few as possible) untestable assumptions.

As a consequence of appropriately conducted randomized clinical trials, information is obtainable that can lead to the rejection, modification, or support of a hypothesis. The greater the number of investigations that support a particular hypothesis, the more credible it becomes and the more likely it will be that a new paradigm for the treatment of a disease will result. It was Thomas Kuhn, a theoretical physicist, philosopher, and historian of science who described the developmental pathways of science as transitions from paradigm to paradigra that occur as the result of scientific revolutions [5]. Essentially, the terrn paradigm is used to encompass "all of the beliefs, values, and techniques shared by members of a [scientific or medical] community," e.g., the surgical paradigrn and/or the syst emic therapy paradigm that govem the treatment of breast cancer. Most important, a new paradigm is better than the one it replaces.

Since 1948, when Bradford Hill described findings from the first "modern" clinical trial conducted to evaluate the worth of streptomycin for the treatment of tuberculosis [6], the prospective randomized clinical trial has played an increasingly greater role in the scientific process as it relates to determining the future course of breast cancer therapy. Arguably, the development and use of that mechanism, which has become progressively more sophisticated in design and analysis during the past 25 years, has been one of the most important achievements of the twentieth century. As I have already pointed out, not only are clinical trials of value for hypothesis testing, but they have also been found to be of worth for obtaining natural history information, for determining the worth of therapies, and for conducting clinical research. Most important, new concepts and hypotheses not uncommonl arise from the findings that result from the conduct of clinical trials. I cannot too emphatically emphasize that clinical trials are a part of the discovery process in breast cancer research and are not solély for drug testing--a perception that has gained too much prominence in recent years.

Although critics of the clinical trials mechanism are numerous and their objections variable, e.g., that such trials take too long, are too cumbersome, too costly, and are in need of replacement by other mechanisms, until other alternatives become available, they continue to provide the most appropriate way of obtaining the Idnd of information necessary for verifying hypotheses and for evaluating therapies. It is unfortunate that many critics of clinical trials are those who do not participate in them, who do not understand the complexities and diligence necessary in their conduct to obtain credible data, and who would prefer to continue to believe in the worth of retrospective information for therapeutic decision making. On the other hand, there is little disagreement that there is a need for some clinical trials to be made simpler, that they be subject to less rigid rules and regulations, and that the media look upon them more favorably so as to eliminate the fear created by negative publicity, which inhibits women from participating in them.

As the physician and medical writer, Lewis Thomas, so aptly stated years ago [7], "From here on, as far as one can see, medicine must be building, as a central part of its scientific base, a solid underpinning of statistical knowledge. Hunches and intuitive impressions are essential for getting the work started, but it is only through the quality of numbers at the end that the truth can be told." That, indeed, sums up the purpose and value of appropriately conducted clinical trials.

The advances made by the National Surgical Adjuvant Breast end Bowel Project (NSABP) during the past four decades of this century were largely achieved by traversing the pathways of science briefly alluded to in this part of my commentary. Hypotheses were formulated from laboratory and clinical investigations, and clinical trials provided the mechanism for us to obtain information that could not have been gotten in any other way. Without them, the anecdotalism that had governed therapy for the first half of this century would have continued unabated, and the paradigm shifts that occurred based upon "the numbers" would have been unlikely.

The clinical trials process, which relates to the "scientific method," continues to be productive and must be permitted to continue as part of the research process as we proceed into the next millennium. It must not become trivialized or manipulated by nonscientific interests and must continue to be available for the conduct of investigator-initiated research rather than for only that resulting from impersonal programmatic planning. In order to justify my position, I will briefly review some of the highlights of our seminal findings that have been obtained by an adherence to these principles that, I believe, will continue to serve us well in the conduct of breast cancer research in the future.

Actual and Potential Paradigm Shifts in the Management of Breast Cancer Resulting from Hypothesis Testing in Randomized Clinical Trials

The purpose of this segment of my commentary is to briefly review some of the highâghts of the contributions to breast cancer research that my colleagues and I have made during the last four decades of the twentieth century--efforts that led to progress in understanding and managing the disease. I will note the ways in which our findings replaced the Halstedian paradigm for treatment of invasive breast cancer with another exemplar, gave rise to a paradigm that dictated the use of postoperative systemic adjuvant therapy, resulted in a unified paradigm for the management of stages I and II breast cancer, and led to a paradigm for the treatment of duct carcinoma in situ (DCIS). I will also describe findings recently obtained from clinical trials evaluating the worth of preoperative (primary or neo-adjuvant) systemic therapy and of tamoxifen in preventing breast cancer in women at high risk for the disease-findings that are likely to result in new paradigms that will dictate the future management of breast cancer.

Replacement of the Halstedian Paradigmfor Surgery: The observations of others in the mid-1950s that circulating tumor cells could be found in the venous blood of patients undergoing surgery, and speculation that arose regarding the significance of such cells, stimulated my studies in tumor metastases. During the decade from 1960 to 1970, my laboratory investigations relative to metastatic mechanisms led to my formulating a hypothesis contrary to that which gave rise to the Halstedian paradigm, the exemplar that had dictated the treatment of primary breast cancer for nearly three-quarters of this century. The Halstedian paradigm promulgated the concept that tumor cell spread was related to anatomic principles, and more expansive operations that could eradicate "one more tumor cell" would cure more patients. It was considered that "proper" cancer surgery removed a primary tumor with its regional lymphatics and lymph nodes by an en bloc dissection, the hallmark of the operation.

Cancer was considered to be a local-regional disease and, thus more "curable" if the surgeon broadly interpreted what constituted the "region." Local-regional recurrences were too often considered to be the result of inadequate application of surgical sldll rather than a manifestation of systemic disease. The use of postoperative regional radiation therapy was, similarly, based upon Halstedian principles. My alternative thesis formulated at that time contended that, because operable breast cancer was a systemic disease involving a complex spectrum of host-tumor interrelations, the ultimate outcome of the patient would unlikely be influenced solely by local-regional treatment. I was fortunate to have had the chance to, conduct two clinical trials, not only to obtain data regarding the credibility of my alternative hypothesis, but also to obtain the opportunity to either justify or reject Halstedian principles of cancer surgery.

The first trial, NSABP B-04, which was implemented in 1971, compared the outcome of clinically node-negative patients who were treated by a Halsted radical mastectomy with those who received a total (simple) mastectomy with local-regional irradiation but no axillary dissection, or total mastectomy with no irradiation and removal of axillary nodes only if these became clinically positive. Despite their therapeutie nonconformity and the finding that about 40% of patients in the latter two treatment groups had pathologically positive nodes left unremoved, no significant différence in overall treatment-failure, distant metastases, or survival has been noted among the three groups after almost 20 years of follow-up [8,9]. The B-04 findings continue to support our alternative hypothesis and corroborate our previous contention that tumor-bearing nodes are indicators of a tumor that has biologic properties for establishing metastatic disease. Moreover, they support our thesis that variations in the treatment of local-regional disease are unlikely to affect survival. That statement does not imply that I dismiss the idea that all efforts should be made to prevent local-regional metastatic tumor. I consider the B-04 trial to be the most important of my contributions because the findings from it caused physicians to doubt the merit of the Halstedian paradigm. Moreover, it promoted the realization that more patients would only be cured by the use of systemic treatment in conjunction with operation and it freed researchers, physicians, and the public from the shackles of scientific thought imposed by the Halstedian paradigm. The B-04 findings also éliminated most of the biologic considerations that might have contradicted evaluating breast-conserving operations by means of a randomized trial. Until the findings from B-04 became available, justification for breast preservation had been entirely based on arguments derived solely from anecdotal experience.

In October 1973, the NSABP began planning a study, B-06, to reevaluate the alternative hypothesis and, at the same time, to appraise the worth of lumpectomy and axillary dissection.

In that study, which began in 1976, nearly 2000 women were randomly distributed among three groups: total mastectomy, lumpectomy alone, or lumpectomy followed by breast irradiation. Women in all groups underwent an axillary dissection. Findings after more than 12 years of follow-up have indicated no significant différence in distant disease-free survival or survival among the three groups [10]. This was despite the fact that there was a 35 % cumulative incidence of ipsilateral breast tumor recurrence (IBTR) in women treated by lumpectomy without breast irradiation, a 10% incidence in women who underwent lumpectomy followed by breast irradiation, and zero incidence in women treated by total mastectomy. These findings provided further support for our alternative hypothesis and indicated that there is neither biologic nor clinical information to contradict our conclusion that almost all patients with stages I and II primary breast cancer should be treated by lumpectomy followed by breast irradiation. To continue to argue in favor of Halstedian principles of cancer treatment is to either ignore, deny, or be unaware of the validity of information obtained during the past two decades from laboratory investigations and from clinical trials that we and others who support our thesis have conducted. The Halstedian paradigm must now be permitted to assume its proper place in the annals of surgical history. Halstedian principles of cancer surgery are historic "milestones" against which progress in breast cancer treatment can be measured and nothing more. The total (modified radical or simple) mastectomy, which is considered the "radical" surgery of today, remains as a vestige of the Halstedian era. Surgeons who perform such operations should realize that the rationale for the procedure is no longer the same as it was at the time of its origin. Originally it was performed because it was believed that a curability rate similar to that achieved by the Halstedian radical mastectomy would result.

Today, it is performed to accomplish local-regional tumor control only when it is believed that lumpectomy cannot be as effectively used for that purpose. As has occurred with radical mastectomy, total mastectomy will ultimately be relegated to a position of historic significance. Similarly, axillary node dissection, which is no longer performed to enhance curability but rather to aid in determining the type of systemic therapy that should be used, will eventually become outmoded. Quadrantectomy might also be viewed, at least at the time of its origin, as a procedure that was aimed at fine-tuning the Halstedian paradigm. As originally described, it used an en bloc dissection and removal of the pectoralis minor muscle and fascia, whereas lumpectomy abandoned every principle of the Halstedian paradigm. In a lumpectomy, only enough normal breast tissue is removed to ensure that no gross tumor remains in the breast after operation.

Subsequent to the publication of the findings from both the B-04 and B-06 studies, an increasing number of physicians began to doubt the merit of the Halstedian paradigm and to alter their approach to treatment for breast cancer. They abandoned the principles of Halstedian surgery and have replaced them with those embodied in the paradigm for breast-conserving operations. One paradigm governing breast cancer management has been displacod by another, a sequence which represents an orderly scientific process.

Thus, in this section of my commentary, I have described how a radical shift in the treatment of primary breast cancer occurred in a relatively short time. Most significantly, the events described, which began in the laboratory and continued in the clinical setting via clinical trials, led to emancipation from "conventional" thinking regarding breast cancer and its treatment and set the stage for a multiplicity of new scenarios that were to occur in rapid fashion.

Paradigm Goveming the Use of Systemic Adjuvant Therapy: While progress against breast cancer was occurring on the surgical front as a result of hypothesis testing by means of randomized clinical trials, a new, independent, paradigm was maturing: the era of systemic adjuvant therapy was evolving. As awareness increased that only through systernic therapy could breast cancer be cured, interest in that therapeutic approach achieved prominence. Observations in the mid-1950s indicating that cancer cells could be found in the circulating blood during surgical removal of tumors and that chemotherapeutic agents had a cytotoxic effect on disseminated tumor cells in experimental animals led to the hypothesis that adjuvant chemotherapy would lower tumor recurrence and improve the survival of breast cancer patients. That hypothesis was first tested in a clinical trial by the NSABP in 1958. Although study results demonstrated both a decrease in tumor recurrence and an improvement in survival. of premenopausal, node-positive patients after 10 years of follow-up, disappointment with the overall findings because all patients were not cured caused practitioners to be slow to adapt to systemic adjuvant therapy [11]. Consequently, no paradigm arose to govem its use. Nevertheless, the observations observed provided the first evidence that the natural history of breast cancer could be perturbed by adjuvant chemotherapy and that différences in the respo se of patient cohorts occurred--a prediction of future findings.

After a hiatus of almost a decade, we launched a new trial to evaluate adjuvant therapy. A new set of concepts, based mainly on Idnetic princi-ples of tumor growth elucidated from animal experiments conducted in the 1960s and early 1970s, provided a rational basis for formulating another hypotheses that could be tested by clinical trials. The first trial to evaluate adjuvant chemotherapy and to test the hypothesis that supported the use of such therapy was begun by the NSABP in 1971. In that study (B-05), L-phenylalanine mustard was administered to patients with posi-tive axillary nodes. The results, first reported in 1975, indicated that such therapy could alter the natural history of patients with primary breast can-cer [12]. That conclusion was confirmed, by findings from the Milan study carried out by Bonadonna and associates using cyclophosphamide, methotrexate, and 5-fluorouracil [13]. As a consequence of our findings and of those by Bonadonna and, subsequently, by a multiplicity of other investigators, a new paradigm regarding the management of breast cancer arose. Treating patients. who were free of identifiable metastatic disease with systemic adjuvant therapy because some of thera might develop dis-tant disease in the future was a revolutionary departure from prior treat-ment strategy and became a new exemplar.

Further support for the validity of the systemic therapy paradigm was provided by a demonstration of the efficacy of the anti-estrogen, tamo-xifen. Extensive study of that drug in experimental systems and its dem-onstrated benefit in patients with metastatic breast cancer provided the justification for conducting randomized clinical trials to evaluate the worth of the drug for the treatment of stages I and Il breast cancer. NSABP trials provided evidence to justify the use of tamoxifen for the treatment of axillary node-positive and node-negative patients with estro-gen receptor (ER)-positive tumors [14-17]. We also found that the addi-tion of chemotherapy to tamoxifen was more effective than tamoxifen alone in node-positive and node-negative patients with ER-positive tumors. As a result of those findings, I concluded around 1980 that the treatment of breast cancer was governed by two independent paradigms. One was concerned with eradicating local manifestations of the disease without compromising prospects for cure, while maintaining the best possible cosmesis. The other served as the exemplar for the eradication of systemic disease.

Origin of a Unified Paradigm: The two-paradigm concept changed when it was observed that the rate of ipsilateral breast tumor recurrence following lumpectomy was significantly decreased when systemic adjuvant therapy, i.e., chemotherapy or tamoxifen, was administered. Use of such therapy enhanced the acceptance of lumpectomy for the treatment of primary breast cancer, even for the treatment of women with large tumors and positive nodes. There was reason to conclude that the two independent paradigms for breast cancer management had converged into a single, unified paradigm. Thus, it was no longer possible to consider the surgical management of breast cancer without considering how other therapeutic, modalities would influence that treatment and vice versa. Within the short space of less that two decades, patients with primary breast cancer were given both the opportunity of preserving their breasts *and* the potential of experiencing an improved disease-free survival and survival.

A Paradigmfor Governing the Management of DCIS: Despite the evolution of new paradigms for the treatment of invasive breast cancer, the management of DCIS remained uncertain. (It was mainly dictated by anecdotal information collected at a few major cancer centers.) Whereas, for example, breast conservation was being used with increasing frequency for treating the former, breast removal remained the choice for managing noninvasive cancers. In 1985, the NSABP initiated a clinical trial (B-17) to test the hypothesis that excision of DCIS with tumor-free specimen margins (referred to as *lumpectomy,* although most women did not have a palpable mass) followed by radiation therapy of the breast was more effective than lumpectomy alone in preventing the occurrence of a second tumor in the ipsilateral breast (IBT). In 1993 we reported findings through 5 years of follow-up and in 1998 we updated the findings through 8 years [18, 19]. In both reports, the event-free survival. was significantly better for women who received radiation therapy after lumpectomy than for those treated by lumpectomy alone. Although the incidence of noninvasive IBT was reduced, of particular importance was the marked reduction in the occurrence of an invasive IBT as a result of the use of postoperative breast irradiation. When the outcome of patients was examined relative to an array of pathologic and mammographic characteristics, we failed to identify a discriminant that selected DCIS patients who did not require postoperative radiation therapy.

Thus, once again through hypothesis testing in a randomized clinical trial (the first to provide data relative to DCIS), we provided the basis for rational consideration of what should be considered appropriate treatment for that disease. Until a prognostic marker is available to select patients who do not need postlumpectomy irradiation for the treatment of localized mammographically detected DCIS, we recommend its use. For a variety of reasons, we believe that there is no reasonable justification for treating such lesions with mastectomy.

Recent unpublished findings from a second NSABP randomized trial (B-24) have demonstrated that the risk of a woman's developing a subsequent invasive breast cancer in the ipsilateral breast was further decreased when tarnoxifen was given in conjunction with surgery and breast irradiation. Those findings further diminish the justification for performing mastectomy to treat DCIS.

Establishing the Role of Preoperative Chemotherapy in Breast Cancer Management: Hypotheses formulated from biologic and clinical information obtained during the 1980s led the NSABP to initiate a clinical trial (B-18) to evaluate the worth and role of preoperative chemotherapy (PROP) for the treatment of primary operable breast cancer. The primary objective of that study was to determine if such therapy could more effectively prolong disease-free survival and survival than did the same therapy administered postoperatively. A second objective was to determine whether the response of a primary tumor to PROP could be correlated with disease-free survival, recurrence-free survival, and overall survival rates. If a correlation could be demonstrated, then breast tumor response might serve as an indicator of the response of micrometastases to the therapy. Moreover, it was considered that it might be possible to use local tumor response to determine whether or not more of the same therapy--or other systemic therapy--should be administered. A third aim was to, determine if the use of PROP would permit more patients to become candidates for lumpectomy when they were initially considered to, require mastectomy. Finally, an additional objective was to ascertain whether PROP downstaged axillary lymph node status, i.e., increased the frequency of patients with negative nodes.

The use of PROP failed to improve the overall benefit from chemotherapy beyond that of patients who were randomized to receive the same therapy (Adriamycin, cyclophosphamide) postoperatively [20,21]. On the other hand, findings indicated that PROP could be used without fear of decreasing the disease-free survival or survival of patients who received such therapy.

The most compelling findings were those indicating that the response of a primary breast tumor to PROP related to subsequent patient outcome. Those whose tumors displayed a pathological complete response to

PROP had a more favorable outcome than did those whose tumors displayed either a clinical complete response or a clinical partial response. Thus, the findings indicated that the response of a breast tumor to PROP could serve as a surrogate or intermediate end point for determining the response of micrometastases to systemic therapy. Because breast tumor response can be determined within weeks after giving PROP, it, thus, becomes possible to predict a patient's outcome and then to provide her with information so that she and her physician can consider other treatment strategies without having to wait for years to determine if a treatment failure occurs and then to treat her.

As a result of these findings with PROP, it is now justifiable to evaluate, in that setting, new chemotherapeutic regimens alone, in combination, or in sequence with those that have already been proven to be effective [22]. Conclusions regarding their worth can be drawn on the basis of their effect on the intermediate end point, i.e., breast tumor response. In addition, it now seems appropriate to evaluate the worth of promising new therapies such as growth-inhibitors, antihormonal agents, and anti-angiogenesis factors in the preoperative setting rather than in patients with advanced disease. Finally, findings indicated that the downstaging of large tumors after the use of PROP permits more patients to be treated with lumpectomies. As a consequence, I have proposed that women with tumors judged by surgeons to be too large for lumpectomies, or whose surgeons are ambivalent about performing that procedure, should initially have the option of receiving PROP followed by lumpectomy and irradiation rather than mastectomy in an attempt to enhance their quality of life. There will, of course, always be patients whose lack of tumor response to such therapy will preclude breast-conserving surgery.

These findings represent the first obtained from a randomized clinical trial conducted to test hypothesis that PROP is advantageous for treating women with breast cancer. Additional studies are underway evaluating other systemic therapy regimens and accumulating additional information in the PROP setting. Whether or not PROP plays a sufficiendy important role for practitioners to embrace it so that it becomes a paradigm which will replace the use of postoperative systemic therapy remains to be ascertained. At least at this time, there is ample justification to suggest its use in certain circumstances.

Establishing the Role of Tamoxifen in the Prevention of Breast Cancer: During the late 1970 s and 1980s, tamoxifen was shown to be of value when used to treat advanced breast cancer, and when administered as postoperative adjuvant therapy in stages I and II disease. It also significantly reduced the incidence of contralateral breast cancer, was found to interfere with the initiation and promotion of tumors in experimental. systems, and inhibited the growth of malignant cells by a variety of mechanisms. Most patients used tamoxifen safely and with good compliance and minimal side effects. Consequently, a testable hypothesis was formulated by us to justify considering tamoxifen as a chemopreventive agent. On June 1, 1992, the NSABP implemented the P-1 prevention trial, the primary aim of which was to determine whether tamoxifen administered for 5 years prevented invasive cancer in women at increased risk for the disease. Additional objectives were to assess the benefits and risks from the drug, as well as to obtain information with regard to breast cancer genetics. At the time of the Paris meeting in February 1998, the results of the P-1 study were as yet unknown. Consequently, at that time, I presented a general overview of the trial indicating that it was another endeavor conducted by the NSABP which demonstrated how a clinical trial could be used to test hypotheses formulated from laboratory and clinical data. Two months later the results became known. Once again, they indicated the importance of that scientific course for making progress. The following briefly comments on some of the findings, even though they were not presented at the meeting. A more complete presentation is in the recently published paper [23].

The results of the P-1 study clearly indicated that tamoxifen reduced the risk of developing breast cancer in a substantial number of women at high risk for the disease. Through 69 months of follow-up, the risk of invasive breast cancer was reduced by 49%. The decreased risk was observed in women of all ages and in those with a history of LCIS or atypical hyperplasia. The risk of microinvasive breast cancer was also reduced by 50%.

Although an increased rate of endometrial cancer, predominantly in women ≥50 years of age, was observed in the tamoxifen group, all were stage I (localized), and there were no deaths attributed to endometrial cancer. No liver cancers or increase in colon, rectal, ovarian, or other tumors occurred in the tamoxifen group. Somewhat higher rates of stroke, pulmonary embolism, and deep-vein thrombosis were observed in women ≥50 years of age who received tamoxifen.

Although the results of the P-1 study clearly indicate that tamoxifen reduces the risk of developing breast cancer in a substantial number of women at high risk for the disease, whether the findings are sufficient for the creation of a new paradigm will relate to their acceptance by physicians who counsel women at high risk for developing breast cancer, as well as by the women themselves. At this time, it is my view that the primary hypothesis which led to the conduct of the P-1 trial has been supported, thus permitting the conduct of future investigations relative to breast cancer prevention.

Summation and Comment: This portion of my commentary has provided a cursory overview of six areas of accomplishment by the NSABP during the past four decades that have altered our understanding and management of breast cancer. It has described how each was attained by using prospective randomized clinical trials to test the efficacy of hypotheses that were created from information obtained by scientific and clinical investigations. Again I emphasize that this formula remains worthy of use in the conduct of future breast cancer research, provided it remains a scientific effort and does not become an entrepreneurial exercise.

Subsequent to each of the achievements that I have noted, an identical paradoxical situation occurred that has relevance for the conduct of future breast cancer research. Because awareness of the unknown is most often enhanced in direct proportion to the degree of knowledge that is attained, it was not surprising that, subsequent to each demonstration of a therapeutic advance in breast cancer management, additional issues arose that could not immediately be resolved. That consequence of accomplishment has, all too often, resulted in confusion and pessimism regarding the meaning and worth of the results obtained, and, thus, uncertainty arises with regard to the clinical application of the findings. As a result, it has become evident that a new era of medicine has occurred in which success may create more havoc than does failure. This circumstance is, indeed, unfortunate because those putative uncertainties do not detract from either the credibility or the importance of the findings that gave rise to them. It is, indeed, rare, if not impossible, for a single study to provide enough information to eliminate all uncertainties associated with positive achievement. In essence, every answer generates a whole set of new questions.

Only when the findings obta'ined from an investigation support a hypothesis being evaluated and, thus, provide justification for adopting a new paradigm for breast cancer management do those questions and issues generated become relevant. Then, those questions, issues, and controversies that have arisen provide the agenda and road map for carrying out future studies that aim to strengthen and expand the worth of existing paradigms. Unfortunately, however, there may be less inclination for those in charge of research programs to support research that arises from both current and prior accomplishments, often because their relevance to progress may seera trivial. They may be more apt to express the opinion that, "Unquestionably, progress has come through earlier diagnoses, healthier lifestyles, and better cancer care. But, where are the real medical breakthroughs?" [24] While efforts to achieve "big breakthroughs" obviously must be supported, so must the research that builds upon small, incremental gains. That approach cannot be discarded while a new idea that will completely and simply eradicate or prevent all breast cancer is awaited. The following section of this commentary outlines some areas of research that should be investigated to seek a resolution to some of the questions that have arisen as a result of 'the contributions made by me and the NSABP.

Future research arising from recent accomplishment

Subsequent to the reporting of each NSABP investigation that has resulted in a therapeutic benefit, uncertainty and confusion has occurred. With demonstration of the worth of a) systemic adjuvant therapy for the treatment of invasive breast cancer; b) postoperative breast irradiation after lumpectomy for the treatment of DCIS; and c) tarnoxifen for reducing the incidence of invasive and noninvasive breast cancer in women at high risk for the disease, the same questions have arisen. They relate to who will benefit from treatment and who will not, who will not need the therapy because they will never demonstrate a treatment failure, how much of a benefit is worthwhile, and whether or not the toxicity and mortality encountered justify its administration. Despite these uncertainties, the use of adjuvant therapy was considered to be a major advance in the treatment of early stage breast cancer, as is exemplified by the outcome of patients with negative axillary nodes and estrogen-receptor positive tumors (Fig. 1). Similarly, the use of breast irradiation following lumpectomy for the treatment of DCIS has been a major advance in treating that disease despite the questions that have arisen. The use of a chemopreventive agent (tamoxifen) denotes a similar advance in th at it is being employad at an even earlier stage of disease, i.e., during the origin and development of a phenotypically expressed cancer before its diagnosis. Nevertheless, research directed toward identifying cohorts of patients who, either do or do not benefit frorn those therapies that demonstrate an overall advantage must be vigorously pursued because such information will permit identifying patients according to their need for and response to therapy.

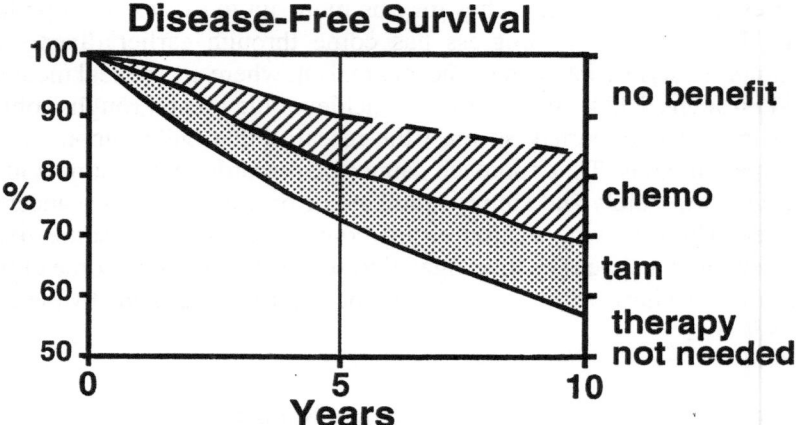

Fig. 1. Magnitude of the Disease-Free Survival Benefit Achieved from Chemotherapy in Axillary Node-Negative Patients With ER-Negative Tumors

Another series of investigations that need to be carried out as soon as possible are those that serve as a sequel to the NSABP prevention trial. The primary aim of those studies would be to obtain genetic information from. women enrolled in the trial to answer such questions as: 1) What proportion of participants carry inherited BRCA1 and BRCA2 mutations? 2) What is the risk of developing breast cancer among women with those mutations compared with that of non-gene carriers in the stud y population? 3) Does the effect of tamoxifen differ in women with or without inherited mutations? What is the change in the 5-year breast cancer incidence rate due to tamoxifen in women with these mutations? The answers to these and similar questions are necessary for expanding our knowledge regarding the use of tamoxifen and à ther SERMs (selective estrogen receptor modulators) in the prevention setting.

Breast Cancer Management in the Near Future

Although I have hesitated to predict future direction of breast cancer research, the following are a few general thoughts regarding how breast cancer is apt to be managed during the next decade or so. It is highly likely that surgery for the disease will continue to diminish in and importance, as improved methods of detection and tumor cell eradication are more common. However, it is unfortunate, but likely true, that surgery, as we have known it, will continue in those environments where recent improvements in breast cancer management have not been implemented.

I also believe that there will be a redefinition of the use of radiation therapy for the treatment of the disease. Its effect on biologically altered breast cells before the phenotypic expression of a tumor may be looked upon as another preventive agent. Also, refining the ability of radiation to eradicate tumor cells may necessitate alterations in its current use.

In addition, it seems likely that primary systemic therapy (PROP) will play a substantial role in further elucidating our understanding how a primary breast cancer responds to therapy. It will also be used to evaluate the worth of new therapeutic agents. Thus, its use for treating the disease is likely to become more expansive than is currently the case.

More effective systemic therapies and biological agents, used alone or in combination, will be used. That therapeutic approach will attain prominence, however, only if toxicity can be minimized.

It seems possible that there could be a change in our perception of the biology of breast cancer which would alter current paradigms used for its management. However, the probability of i that occurring within the next decade seems highly unlikely. Moreover, it seems unlikely that such modalities as gene therapy, immunotherapy, or the use of biological modulators of tumor growth will become paradigms for breast cancer management during that time.

Prevention of breast cancer will play an increasingly greater role in breast cancer management. Since breast cancer is a public health problem, this approach will not only employ the use of chemopreventive agents but will also attempt to identify and eliminate etiologic agents (primary prevention) and to detect and eliminate phenotypically expressed breast tumor cells and their predecessor cells as early as possible (secondary prevention). Success in those endeavors would radically alter the use of all other efforts that have been considered.

Summary

In this commentary I have indicated why I consider it difficult to predict what the future course--beyond the short term--of breast cancer research might be and why I do not believe that being involved in such predictions is a very useful exercise. On the other hand, I have briefly indicated how the combination of scientifically based hypotheses and the use of welldesigned clinical trials for testing the credibility of those theses has resulted in a dramatic alteration of our understanding and mana-gement of the disease over the last three decades. I believe that the continued use of this scientific process is imperative for making future progress. I have presented herein a few examples of how each accomplishment that we have made has resulted in numerous questions and issues which set the stage for important new lines of investigation. Finally, I have made a few generic predictions, not of research directions but of the status of breast cancer management strategies that I think are likely to occur in the not-too- distant future.

References

2. Fisher B: Laboratory and clinical research in breast cancer - A personal adventure: The David A. Karnofsky Memorial Lecture. *Cancer Research 40:3863-3874, 1980*
3. Fisher B: The evolution of paradigms for the management of breast cancer: A personal perspective. *Cancer Research 52:2371-2383, 1992*
4. Fisher B: Personal contributions to progress in breast cancer research and treatment. *Seminars in Oncology 23:414-427, 1996*
5. Root-Bernstein RS: Discovering. Harvard University Press, Cambridge, MA, 1989, p. 501
6. Kuhn TS: The Structure of Scientific Revolutions, ed. *2*. Chicago, University of Chicago Press, 1970
7. Silverman WA: Where's the Evidence? Controversies in Modem Medicine. Oxford University Press, Oxford, *1998,* Chapter 24, p. 98, pps. 259
8. Thomas L: Quoted in: Redmond C and Fisher B: Design of the controlled clinical trial. In: Yosef H. Pilch, Tapas Das Gupta, eds. Surgical oncology. New York, New York. McGraw Mill Book Company, 1994
9. Fisher B, Redmond C, Fisher ER, et al: Ten-year results of a randomized clinical trial comparing radical mastectomy and total mastectomy with or without radiation. *NEngl.r Med* 312:674-681, 1985
10. National Surgical Adjuvant Breast and Bowel Project: NSABP Progress Report. 1997, pp. 17-23
11. Fisher B, Anderson S, Redmond C, et al: Reanalysis and results after 12 years of follow-up in a randomized clinical trial comparing total mastectomy with lumpectomy with or without irradiation in the treatment of breast cancer. *N Engl J Med* 333:14561461, 1995
12. Fisher B, Ravdin RG, Ausman RK, et al: Surgical adjuvant chernotherapy in cancer o the breast: Results of a decade of cooperative investigation. *Ann Surg* 168:337-356, 1968
13. Fisher B, Carbone P, Economou SG, et al: L-phenylalanine mustard (L-PAM) in the management of primary breast cancer: A report of early findings. *N Engl J Med* 292:117-122, 1975
14. Bonadonna G, Brusamolino, E, Valagussa P, et al: Combination chemotherapy as an adjuvant treatment in operable breast cancer. *N Engl J Med* 294:405-410, 1976
15. Fisher B, Redmond C, Brown A, et al: Treatment of primary breast cancer with chemotherapy and tamoxifen . *N Engl J Med* 305:1-6, 1981

16. Fisher B, Redmond C, Brown A, et al: Adjuvant chemotherapy with and without tamoxifen in the treatment of primary breast cancer: 5-year results from the National Surgical Adjuvant Breast and Bowel Project trial. *J Clin Oncol* 4:459-471, 1986

17. Fisher B, Costantino J, Redmond C, et al: A randomized clinical trial evaluating tamoxifen in the treatment of patients with node-negative breast cancer who have estrogen-receptor-positive tumors. *N Engl J Med* 320:479-484, 1989

18. Fisher B, Dignam J, Wolmark N, et al: Tamoxifen and chemotherapy for lymph node negative, estrogen receptor-positive, breast cancer. *J Natl Cancer Inst* 89:1673-1682, 1997

19. Fisher B, Costantino J, Redmond C, et al: Lumpectomy compared with lumpectomy and radiation therapy for the treatment of intraductal breast cancer. *N Engl J Med* 328:1581- 1586, 1993

20. Fisher B, Dignam J, Wolmark N, et al: Lumpectomy and radiation therapy for the treatment of intraductal breast cancer: Findings from National Surgical Adjuvant Breast and Bowel Project B-17. *J Clin Oncol* 16:441-452, 1998

21. Fisher B, Brown A, Mamounas E, et al: Effect of preoperative chemotherapy on localregional disease in women with operable breast cancer: Findings from National Surg Adjuvant Breast and Bowel Project B-18. *J Clin Oncol* 15:2483-2493, 1997

22. Fisher B, Bryant J, Wolmark N, et al: Effect of preoperative chemotherapy on the outcome of women with operable breast cancer. *J Clin Oncol* 16:2672-2685, 1998

23. Fisher B, Mamounas EP: Preoperative chemotherapy: A model for studying the biology and therapy of primary breast cancer. *J Clin Oncol* 13:537-540, 1995

24. Fisher B, Costantino JP, Wickerham DL, et al: Tamoxifen for prevention of breast cancer: Report of the National Surgical Adjuvant Breast and Bowel Project P-1 study. *J Natl Cancer Inst* 90:1371-1388, 1998

25. Bulletin: American Association of Retired People. AARP, 1998, p. 10

Part II
Ethic and Fundamental Research in Cancer

Hereditary Breast Cancer: an Overview

C. J. D. Isaacs, B. N. Peshkin

Introduction

It is estimated that hereditary breast cancer accounts for up to 10% of all cases of breast cancer [1]. Thus, of the 180,000 cases of breast cancer diagnosed yearly, up to 18,000 may be due to an inherited predisposition to this disease. To date, several genes have been identified that account for different hereditary breast cancer syndromes. BRCA1 and BRCA2 mutations are thought to account for the majority of inherited breast cancer. Although less frequent, hereditary breast cancer may be a feature of Li-Fraumeni and Cowden syndrome and may also occur in Ataxia Telangiectasia heterozygotes. In addition, it is likely that other rare, as yet unidentified, genes exist.

This chapter will provide an overview of the major genes responsible for hereditary breast cancer and will focus on the following aspects of the BRCA1 and BRCA2 genes: 1) clinical features of individuals and families with a mutation in one of these genes; 2) the process of genetic testing including a review of the benefits, limitations and risks of such testing; 3) interpretation of genetic test results; and 4) management options for individuals who are found to have a mutation.

BRCA1 AND BRCA2

BRCA1 was localized to chromosome 17q21 in 1990 and identified in 1994 [2]. It extends over approximately 100,000 base pairs of DNA, encodes a very large protein of 1,863 amino acids, and is believed to function as a tumor suppressor gene. Mutations are inherited in an autosomal dominant fashion. BRCA2 was identified more recently, in December 1995 [3]. Like BRCA1, mutations are inherited in an autosomal dominant fashion, and it too is believed to be a tumor suppressor gene. It has 11,385 nucleotides and encodes a protein of 3,418 amino acids. However, the exact mechanisms of action of BRCA1 and BRCA2 remain unclear. The normal BRCA1 gene has been shown to suppress the growth of ovarian and breast cancer cell lines [4]. Recent studies have suggested that BRCA1 and BRCA2 may play a role in transcription and DNA repair [5, 6].

It is not surprising, given the large size of both BRCA1 and BRCA2, that multiple disease-conferring mutations have been identified, many of them unique to individual families. To date, over 400 BRCA1 and BRCA2 mutations that are scattered throughout the gene have been documented [7]. Some of these mutations have been found to occur more frequently, particularly in certain ethnic groups. For example, two BRCA1 mutations, 185delAG and 5382insC, and one BRCA2 mutation, 6174delT, have been noted with increased frequency in individuals of Ashkenazi Jewish descent [8]. In addition, numerous BRCA1 and BRCA2 benign polymorphisms and variants of unknown significance have been identified [7].

Clinical Features of Hereditary Breast Cancer

The majority of identified cases of hereditary breast cancer appears to be associated with mutations in BRCA1 and BRCA2. Cancer risks conferred by BRCA1 and BRCA2 mutations are derived largely from highly selected families in which multiple women have developed early onset breast and ovarian cancer [9, 10]. Data from individuals with less striking family histories are beginning to emerge and suggest that on average, cancer risks are lower than those observed in the highest risk families [8]. Thus, while no single number can quantify precise cancer risks for an individual who tests positive, the risks should be interpreted within the context of a specific medical and family history. Information about risks associated with particular BRCA1 or BRCA2 mutations is not yet available, but ranges of cumulative risk estimates are summarized below (see Table 1).

BRCA1 and BRCA2

Cancer Risks

Women who inherit a BRCA1 mutation have a significantly elevated risk of developing both early onset breast and ovarian cancer. The lifetime risk of breast cancer in mutation carriers is estimated to range between 55-85%, with over 50% of these women being diagnosed by age 50 [8-10]. In addition, by age 70, 15-60% of BRCA1 carriers will have devel-

Table 1. Estimated cancer risks associated with BRCA1 and BRCA2 mutations*

Type of Cancer	Estimated Lifetime Risk in BRCA1 Mutation Carriers [8-12]	Estimated Lifetime Risk in BRCA2 Mutation Carriers [3, 8, 13-17, 41]	Lifetime Risk in General Population
Breast cancer (female)	55% - 85%	55% - 85%	13%
2nd Breast cancer (contralateral)	Up to 65%	Probably similar to BRCA1 risks	Up to 1% a year (leveling off at up to 25%)
Ovarian cancer	15% - 60%	15% - 27%	1.4%
Ovarian cancer after breast cancer	Up to 30%-55%	Comparable to BRCA1 risks	2-3% (approximately twice the average risk)
Colon cancer	Possible relative risk of 4	Possible increased risk	Approximately 6%
Prostate cancer	Increased risk, possibly up to a relative risk of 3	Probable increased risk	At least 10% but risk is difficult to quantify due in part to the presence of clinically undetectable cancers
Breast cancer (male)	A few reported cases	Approximately 6%	Extremely rare
Pancreatic cancer	Not increased	Associations noted	Rare

Note: These risks are cumulative and are not mutation-specific. In general, early ages of onset have been associated primarily with female breast cancer and ovarian cancer. However, there are some reports of early onset pancreatic cancer associated with BRCA2 alterations. Relative risks, such as those associated with prostate and colon cancer in BRCA1 carriers, are not directly translatable to absolute risks. It is also important to note that general population risks include some patients with hereditary cancer. All risks must be evaluated in the context of the patient's medical and family history.

*Modified from [42]

oped ovarian cancer [8, 9]. In the general population, the risk of ovarian cancer is between 1–2%. In addition, mutation carriers with a prior history of breast or ovarian cancer appear to have an increased risk of developing a second malignancy. For example, the risk of contralateral breast cancer for mutation carriers who have already had a diagnosis of breast cancer has been estimated to be up to 65% by age 70 [10]. In comparison, for patients with sporadic breast cancer, the risk of contralateral breast cancer is thought to be 0.5–1% annually [18]. Little information exists on the risk of ipsilateral breast cancer recurrence in BRCA1 carriers who undergo breast conserving surgery. However, given the high rate of contralateral breast cancer in this population, the rate of in-breast recurrence in mutation carriers appears to be elevated also [17]. In addition, the risk of ovarian cancer after a diagnosis of breast cancer is elevated up to 44% by age 70 [10]. For women in the general breast cancer population, this risk is about 3%. In male mutation carriers, prostate cancer has been noted with increased frequency [8,10], although the absolute risk compared to the general population is not clear. There is some controversy about whether colon cancer is associated with BRCA1 mutations [8,10], and it is expected further studies will clarify this issue. When observed in mutation carriers, both prostate and colorectal cancer appear to have the same age distribution as is seen in the general population [10].

BRCA2 mutations are associated with a markedly elevated risk of breast cancer in women and in men. Whereas the risk of breast cancer in women has been estimated to vary between 55% and 85% [8,16], the risk of male breast cancer in BRCA2 mutation carriers is estimated to be about 6% [13]. However, in the general population, male breast cancer is extremely rare, with only 1600 cases of this disease diagnosed yearly in the United States [19]. Although BRCA2 is not as strongly associated with ovarian cancer as is BRCA1, the risk in mutation carriers is still elevated above that seen in the general population and the lifetime risk is estimated to be between 15–27% [8, 16]. Little information exists on BRCA2 carriers' risk of developing a second malignancy (e.g. contralateral breast cancer or ovarian cancer after a diagnosis of breast cancer), though these risks appear to be elevated also [17, 41]. Prostate cancer, though not diagnosed at an early age, also seems to be associated with BRCA2 alterations [8]. In addition, some studies have reported an increased frequency of pancreatic cancer [15, 20].

Cancer Prognosis

Recent studies have indicated that the breast tumors seen in BRCA1 and BRCA2 carriers appear histopathologically more "aggressive" than those observed in the general breast cancer patient population. These tumors have a higher histologic grade, are more frequently aneuploid, and have a higher S-phase fraction than tumors seen in women with sporadic breast cancer [21]. Despite this finding, some studies in BRCA1 carriers have shown the same or better prognosis than what is noted in the general breast cancer patient population when matched for age at diagnosis [22] and stratified for stage of disease [21]. A more recent study however, suggested that the breast and ovarian cancer prognosis in BRCA1 carriers was the same or worse than that for an age- and stage-matched control group [23]. The BRCA2 breast cancer phenotype appears to be more heterogeneous than what is noted for BRCA1, and for BRCA2 carriers the breast cancer prognosis may be worse [21].

It is important to stress that the information on the prognosis of tumors in BRCA1 and BRCA2 carriers is derived from small studies and is therefore limited. In addition, it is possible that ascertainment and screening biases may have influenced the results obtained in these studies. Therefore, before integrating this information into clinical practice, it will be necessary to conduct larger studies to validate the findings of these reports.

Cancer Risk Modifiers

Investigators have begun to examine the impact of environmental factors and gene-gene interactions on the cancer risks of mutation carriers. In a study of 333 BRCA1 carriers from 28 different hereditary breast-ovarian families, Narod et al. [24] found that the risk of breast cancer was increased in carriers who underwent early menarche (relative risk 1.57 for menarche <12) and those who had had fewer than three live births (relative risk 2.04) when compared with carriers with an otherwise similar history. It was also observed that the risk of ovarian cancer was higher with increasing parity, but the risk was lower the older a woman was at last live birth [24]. With respect to oral contraceptives (OCPs), a recent study of 50 young Ashkenazi Jewish breast cancer patients suggested that long term OCP use (i.e. > 48 months), particularly before a first full-term pregnancy, was associated with higher breast cancer risks in BRCA1/2 mutation carriers versus non-carriers [25]. That study did not determine whether OCP use decreases the risk of ovarian cancer in mutation carriers; however, a recent case-control study revealed that six or more years of OCP use was associated with a 60% decrease in ovarian cancer risk in BRCA1/2 mutation carriers [26]. It is also possible that modifier genes may affect gene penetrance. For example, one group found that the risk of ovarian cancer in BRCA1 carriers with one or two rare *HRAS1* alleles was about two times greater than noncarriers with common alleles [27].

The studies described in this section are based on relatively small sample sizes; therefore, these results will need to be validated in larger series. If the findings are substantiated, then it may be possible to determine more specifically an individual carrier's cancer risks and to devise strategies to minimize these risks.

Li-Fraumeni Syndrome

Although less frequent, breast cancer may be a feature of other hereditary diseases or syndromes which together probably account for fewer than 1% of all breast cancers. Among the most recognized of these is the Li-Fraumeni cancer syndrome—an autosomal dominantly inherited condition characterized by sarcomas, brain tumors, early onset breast cancers (often diagnosed < 30), leukemias, and adrenocortical cancer [28]. For individuals at risk, it is estimated that up to 50% will develop some form of cancer by age 30, and over 90% will develop cancer by age 70. Mutations in the p53 gene have been associated with Li-Fraumeni syndrome, and predictive testing may be available if a p53 mutation is identified in the family.

Ataxia Telangiectasia

Ataxia telangiectasia (AT) is an autosomal recessive syndrome characterized by cerebellar degeneration, immunodeficiency, telangiectasias, and predisposition to both solid tumors and hematologic malignancies. AT may occur in as many as 1/40,000 live births, and has an estimated carrier frequency of 1% [29]. DNA testing is now available for the gene implicated, known as ATM, which is located on chromosome 11q [30]. Although it has been suggested that over 8% of breast cancer patients in the United States may be carriers of the ATM gene and have an estimated relative risk of 4 compared to noncarriers for the development of breast cancer [31], others have refuted the idea that such carriers face an increased risk for early onset breast cancer [29]. Some concern has also been raised that breast cancer susceptibility in female heterozygotes may be increased by exposure to ionizing radiation. It is hoped that large scale population studies will address this issue further.

Cowden Disease

Cowden disease is a rare autosomal dominant familial cancer syndrome that predisposes women to a high risk of breast cancer and an elevated risk of thyroid cancer. Hamartomas of the oral mucosa, such as multiple oral papillomas, are pathognomonic. Some estimates suggest that breast cancer may affect 20–30% of females with Cowden disease, often at an early age, and that there may be a higher than average incidence of bilateral cancer [32]. The gene for Cowden disease has been localized to chromosome 10q and clinical DNA-based testing may soon be possible [33].

Identification of High Risk Families

The clinical features suggestive of hereditary breast and ovarian cancer due to BRCA1 or BRCA2 mutations include the occurrence of breast and/or ovarian cancer, especially when noted in two or more first-degree relatives or in at least two generations; early onset breast and ovarian cancer; the presence of associated malignancies in other family members (particularly ovarian cancer but also male breast cancer, pancreatic, prostate, or bilateral breast cancer); multiple primaries in the same individual; and ethnic ancestry associated with a founder mutation (see Table 2). It is important to note that despite the fact that BRCA1/2 mutations are inherited in an autosomal dominant fashion, cancers can skip generations due to the fact that about 15-45% of female carriers never develop cancer, and that male carriers have a low risk of developing cancer. Such a situation may obscure the detection of an autosomal dominant pattern of inheritance; nonetheless, these carriers can still pass on the mutation to their offspring.

Ethnic ancestry has been noted to be predictive for detecting a BRCA1/2 mutation within a family. While so-called "founder" mutations have

Table 2. Characteristics of high-risk BRCA1/2 families

- Early onset breast and/or ovarian cancer
- Multiple primary breast and/or ovarian cancers in the same individual
- Associated cancers (e.g. male breast, pancreatic)
- Autosomal dominant pattern of inheritance
- Ethnic ancestry associated with founder mutations

been observed in specific populations (e.g. Icelandic, Swedish), the strongest founder effects have been noted in Ashkenazi Jews (descended from Eastern or Central Europe) [34]. Two BRCA1 mutations, 185delAG and 5382insC, and one BRCA2 mutation, 6174delT, have been observed with increased frequency in Ashkenazi Jews both with and without a strong family history of cancer. A recent study has shown a high gene frequency for all three of these mutations in a Jewish population unselected for a family history of cancer – about 0.8% for 185delAG, 0.4% for 5382insC and 1.2% for 6174delT [8]. This finding translates to a carrier frequency for these three mutations of about 1 in 45 in Jewish women and men. In comparison, the combined frequency of all BRCA1 mutations in non-Jewish populations is estimated to be between 1 in 500 to 1 in 833 [35]. Because BRCA2 mutations appear to account for a lower proportion of hereditary breast cancer than BRCA1, it is likely that carrier frequency of BRCA2 in the general population is even lower.

Studies in Jewish cancer patients have also demonstrated a high carrier frequency rate for the common mutations – 21% of Jewish breast cancer patients unselected for family history diagnosed at age 40 or less [36], and 38% of Jewish ovarian cancer patients diagnosed prior to age 50 carried the 185delAG mutation [37]. Another study carried out in Israel examined the frequency of the three common founder mutations in 199 Ashkenazi Jewish women with breast and/or ovarian cancer [38]. Of these women, 99 had no family history of breast or ovarian cancer. It was observed that 30% of the breast cancer patients under the age of 40 and 62% of the ovarian cancer patients tested positive for one of the three mutations. Of note, 10% of the patients without any family history of cancer had one of these mutations. Thus, for individuals of Jewish descent, simply having one family member with early onset breast or ovarian cancer appears to be associated with a reasonable likelihood of finding a BRCA1 or BRCA2 mutation. In addition, in such families, the likelihood of finding one of the three common mutations increases dramatically when there is a very strong family history of breast and particularly ovarian cancer in a pattern consistent with dominant inheritance. However, it is important to note that novel BRCA mutations have been reported in individuals of Jewish descent and that an increasing number of high-risk Jewish families do not harbor any detectable mutations in BRCA1 or BRCA2 [39]. Earlier studies had predicted that up to 90% of Jewish families with a strong history of breast and ovarian cancer would have one of the three founder mutations [20].

Studies that have systematically assessed the probability of detecting a BRCA1 or BRCA2 mutation have been published [40, 41]. For example, a large multi-institutional study used logistic regression to determine that women with breast cancer before age 50 who also have at least one relative with breast cancer diagnosed less than age 50 or ovarian cancer at any age have at least a 25% chance of carrying a BRCA1 or BRCA2 mutation (the odds increase with the number of affected relatives) [41]. The observed probabilities also showed, as predicted, that Jewish ancestry in high-risk women was associated with a significant likelihood of harboring a BRCA1 or BRCA2 mutation, usually one of the three founder mutations (43% in this series) [41]. Although not formally addressed in the cited studies, the observation of rare cancers such as male breast cancer and pancreatic cancer should alert the clinician to the possibility of detecting a BRCA2 mutation.

Although mathematical models have been developed to assist the clinician in predicting BRCA1/2 carrier probabilities, an important, albeit subtle point that patients must understand is that there is a difference between the chance that the cancers in their family are hereditary and the chance that a detectable mutation will be found in their family, thereby maximizing the likelihood of an informative test result [42]. In fact, the study of 238 high-risk women by Frank et al. [41] revealed that only 39% carried deleterious BRCA1 or BRCA2 mutations, suggesting that other susceptibility genes are likely to account for a proportion of the remaining cases [41]. As testing progresses, further data should emerge to guide clinicians in ascertaining a particular individual's risk of carrying a deleterious mutation in either BRCA1 or BRCA2. Given the expense of testing and the limitations of test result interpretation in low-risk women, probabilistic information is helpful in determining which individuals have the most potential to gain risk information as a result of genetic testing.

Implications of Genetic Testing

It is crucial for patients to understand fully the complexities of genetic testing prior to providing a blood sample for testing. Thus, as part of the informed consent process, a review of the potential benefits, limitations and risks of testing is essential. In addition, unlike most medical procedures, the implications of genetic testing extend not only to the individual being tested, but also to his or her family members.

Benefits of Testing

It is important to note that the benefits of genetic testing for hereditary cancer are as yet unproven. However, potential benefits include:

Increased Knowledge about Cancer Risks

The information gained from genetic testing may help tailor an appropriate cancer screening regimen, as well as allow more informed decision-making about cancer prevention options, including prophylactic surgery and chemoprevention. For individuals who test positive, more intensive screening and consideration of prevention options is recommended. Standard screening guidelines are recommended for those with true negative test results. In addition, some individuals may wish to use genetic testing results to help guide decisions about childbearing and other lifestyle issues.

Information for Family Members

The information obtained from testing may enable close relatives to learn more about their cancer risks. This is particularly true for the relatives of individuals with an alteration in BRCA1 or BRCA2, given that these family members may now be offered the opportunity to be tested. In addition, children of individuals who are found to have true negative test results (i.e. individuals from families with known mutations who are found to test negative for that mutation) can usually be reassured that their cancer risks are now those seen in the general population.

Psychological Relief

The reduction in uncertainty derived from obtaining a test result is a potential benefit of testing.

Insurability

Members of high-risk families who test negative for a known mutation in their family may be less likely to compromise their insurability. Because these individuals would now face the general population risks for cancer instead of the elevated risks noted in mutation carriers, it is possible that insurance companies would be less likely to consider these individuals poor candidates for coverage.

Risks and Limitations of Testing

There are risks and limitations for testing not only for those who test positive but also for those who test negative. These risks and limitations include:

Insurance and Employment Discrimination

The possibility of health insurance discrimination is one of the major issues facing individuals considering testing in the United States. At the present time, fewer than half of the states have laws restricting the extent to which genetic information may be used by health insurers. Almost all states allow life and disability insurers to ask questions about genetic predisposition to cancer and use the answers in their underwriting decisions. However, recently enacted federal legislation may help to protect those individuals who decide to undergo genetic testing. The Health Insurance Portability and Accountability Act of 1996 recognizes "genetic information" as protected medical information, and forbids those who provide health care coverage from using such information to deny access to individuals who must change health plans when they change jobs.

The Act also states that, based on genetic information, a group medical plan cannot require an individual to pay a premium or contribution that is greater than that for a similarly situated individual enrolled in that plan. A limitation of the Act is that the premiums charged for individual health insurance are not restricted by the Act, and need only comply with state law. These insurance reform provisions of the Act went into effect on July 1, 1997. Other federal legislation, such as the Genetic Information Nondiscrimination in Health Insurance Act of 1997, is expected to expand on these protections.

Emotional Implications

It has been observed clinically that individuals who test positive often experience some feelings of mild depression, anger, or anxiety. One study documented that mutation carriers with no history of cancer or cancer-related prophylactic surgery had higher levels of psychological distress compared to noncarriers [43]. However, in another study of high-risk kindreds who received genetic counseling in a research setting, individuals who tested positive had no significant increase in either depression or functional impairment within one month of receiving their test result [44]. While non-carriers with true negative results may be relieved about their results and actually show statistically significant reductions in depressive symptoms [44], some adverse effects are possible such as the manifestation of "survivor guilt." In addition, these individuals may experience a false sense of security about their remaining cancer risk. Therefore, counseling should reinforce the need for them to adhere to the standard cancer screening recommendations.

Impact on Family Dynamics

Unlike most medical procedures, results of genetic testing affect not only the individual being tested, but also his or her relatives. This impacts the approach both to initiating testing within a family and to communicating test results. If a mutation is identified, careful pedigree analysis may reveal that, in addition to siblings and children, a significant number of more distant relatives may be at risk for inheriting the identified mutation. While it is important to convey this knowledge to the patient, it is also important to recognize that communicating such information may place a large burden on the patient, who may not want to contact these relatives or compromise the privacy of information relevant to her test result or cancer history. Family communication patterns are highly variable, and although some individuals may want to share test results openly, others may not. Clinicians must balance the need to respect the patient's wishes regarding this issue while also ensuring that patients are informed about the implications to their family members. Genetic counseling often allows the patient to explore ways in which family communication and overall coping can be facilitated.

Possibility of a False or Inconclusive Result

In addition to a small chance of laboratory error, the possibility of obtaining either a false negative, false positive, or inconclusive test result exists. The interpretation of these findings will be discussed in greater detail in the section on testing outcomes. It is important to note that there are possible psychological ramifications and medical implications that arise in these situations. For instance, individuals from very high-risk families who test negative for mutations in both BRCA1 and BRCA2 may experience some distress due to lingering uncertainty about the etiology of the cancer in their family as well as the cancer risks for themselves and their relatives.

Lack of Proven Methods of Screening and Prevention

The suggested guidelines for medical management for BRCA1 and BRCA2 mutation carriers are outlined below. At present, none of the suggested interventions has been proven to be effective in these individuals. In addition, these procedures may not be covered by insurance carriers.

Logistics of Testing

The cost of commercial testing can be prohibitively high—ranging from about $300 to $2400. Not only is it unclear to what extent insurance companies will reimburse this expense, but many individuals are reluctant to seek reimbursement for fear of divulging information about testing to their insurers. The turnaround time for obtaining test results has decreased significantly in the last couple of years, although in some instances, the waiting time may still be considerable. For those patients hoping to use this information to guide medical decision-making, this wait may still prove to be too long.

Process of Genetic Testing

Once a high-risk family is identified, genetic counseling and testing should be offered first to a family member with a diagnosis of early onset breast or ovarian cancer. Such an approach maximizes the likelihood of obtaining an informative test result. For example, if a family member with breast or ovarian cancer diagnosed at a young age tests negative after complete BRCA1 and BRCA2 gene analysis, then it is less likely that a BRCA1/2 mutation explains the cancers observed in the family. If, on the other hand, an unaffected family member undergoes testing first and tests negative, it would not be possible to determine if this result was obtained because there is no BRCA1/2 mutation present in the family or simply because he or she is a non-carrier. Thus, such a finding would not exclude the possibility that a mutation was present in another family member.

The actual testing consists of a blood test. The testing process differs from laboratory to laboratory—some do complete BRCA1 and BRCA2 testing, whereas others test first for the most commonly identified BRCA1/2 mutations. If a disease-conferring mutation is found, then testing may be extended to other at risk relatives. This includes first-degree relatives, and in many cases, more distant relatives such as aunts, uncles, and cousins. The standard approach is to test these family members only for the presence or absence of the specific mutation identified in their kindred.

In high-risk families of Ashkenazi Jewish descent, if it is not possible to initiate testing in an affected individual, it is reasonable to test an unaffected relative for the three mutations commonly identified in Jewish individuals (185delAG, 5382insC, and 6174delT). A negative test result in this situation, however, does not rule out the possibility of an inherited cancer susceptibility. In addition, in Jewish families in which a BRCA1/2 mutation has been identified, it is recommended that at-risk relatives receive testing for all three common mutations, not just the mutation already found in the family [20].

As part of the process of offering genetic testing, it is essential that genetic counseling be made available to all individuals seeking testing. This should be provided both before testing is undertaken and at the time of the disclosure of the test result.

BRCA1 and BRCA2 Testing Outcomes

There are several possible outcomes from genetic testing. These include a true positive, a true negative and an inconclusive result. A true positive result occurs when a disease-conferring mutation is identified, which is clearly associated with increased risks for breast, ovarian, and possibly other cancers. When a disease-conferring mutation has been identified in the family (usually in a close relative such as a parent or sibling), and is not found to be present in the individual being tested, the result is classified as a true negative, as illustrated in Fig. 1. However, as demonstrated in Fig. 2, the absence of BRCA1 or BRCA2 mutation in the affected proband may be interpreted as an inconclusive finding. This is true whether the patient received only partial testing (e.g. for alterations in only one gene or for common mutations in one or both genes) or complete BRCA1/2 analysis. Possible explanations for this include: 1) the occurrence of a sporadic, non-hereditary cancer; 2) if only partial testing is performed, it is possible that a mutation is present in an untested portion of BRCA1/2; or 3) if complete testing is performed, a mutation could be present in either a regulatory region of the gene or in another gene predisposing to hereditary breast cancer. A second type of inconclusive result occurs when a BRCA1 or BRCA2 alteration is identified, but is of unknown clinical significance. This alteration may be a benign polymorphism or may be a deleterious mutation.

Ashkenazi Jewish

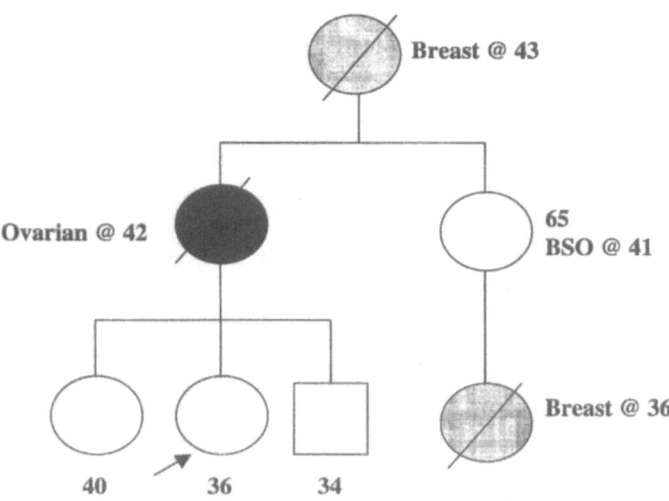

Fig. 1. This pedigree illustrates several different issues. In many families there are no living affected individuals available for testing. Because this family is Jewish, testing for the 3 common mutations was first offered to the proband (↗). She tested negative for these mutations. This result was therefore considered inconclusive. Her older sister was then tested and found to be positive for the 185delAG mutation. Given this finding, the proband's result can now be interpreted as a true negative and she can be reassured about her cancer risk. In addition, their maternal aunt, who is alive without cancer at age 65, is now presumed to be an obligate carrier. The fact that she had a bilateral oophorectomy (BSO) in her 40s may, in part, explains why she is a non-penetrant carrier

Medical Management for Mutation Carriers

Screening and prevention options

At present, there are no proven methods of cancer screening or prevention in individuals with an inherited susceptibility to cancer. The guidelines outlined below were modified from those set forth by Cancer Genetics Studies Consortium, a group of experts convened by the National Institutes of Health [45].

Irish

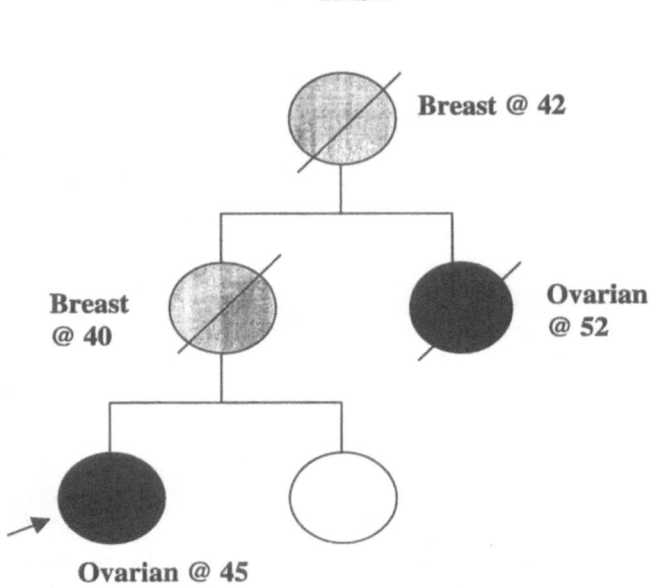

Fig. 2. Complete BRCA1 and BRCA2 testing was performed on the proband (↗) and no mutation was identified. Given the strong family history of early onset breast and ovarian cancer, this finding does not rule out the possibility of an inherited predisposition to breast and ovarian cancer. The potential reasons for this finding are outlined in the text

Breast Cancer

Screening Guidelines

Monthly breast self-examination, clinician exams every 3 to 6 months, and annual mammography. It is recommended that annual mammography begins between the ages of 25 and 35. The efficacy of breast self-exam, clinician exam, and mammography in BRCA1/2 carriers has not yet been demonstrated.

Prevention Options

It is recommended that prophylactic bilateral total mastectomy be discussed with mutation carriers. At present, little data exist to evaluate the efficacy of this surgery. However, it is clear that such an approach does not completely eliminate the risk of developing breast cancer. Two groups have reported their experience with prophylactic mastectomy. A study from the Mayo Clinic of 950 women who underwent prophylactic bilateral mastectomy used the Gail model to predict the expected numbers of cases of breast cancer. This study included 287 women who had a family history strongly consistent with hereditary breast cancer. With a median follow-up of 17 years, a highly significant 90% reduction in risk of breast cancer was noted in all groups of patients including those with a very strong family history [46]. A second study demonstrated that in a group of 510 high risk women, of which 210 had a positive family history, 1.18% went on to develop invasive breast cancer after either prophylactic total or subcutaneous mastectomy [47]. It is important to note that there are significant limitations in applying the results of these reviews to the anticipated outcome in BRCA1/2 carriers. First, it is now widely agreed that subcutaneous mastectomy is not an acceptable option for prophylaxis, given that a significant amount of residual breast tissue remains. Second, the definition of family history used in these studies was quite broad. Thus, it is likely that many women who chose to undergo this procedure were not members of true hereditary breast cancer families. In addition, given that these studies took place before genetic testing was available, even for those members of high risk families, one would anticipate that at most one half inherited an alteration in a breast cancer susceptibility gene. Studies focusing on known mutation carriers who have undergone prophylactic mastectomy are planned and should provide clearer answers on the efficacy of this approach. Another possible prevention option for high-risk women is participation in chemoprevention trials. Early results from a large randomized trial of tamoxifen, carried out by the NSABP, demonstrated that tamoxifen reduced the risk of breast cancer by 49% in high-risk healthy women [48]. A subset analysis will evaluate the impact of tamoxifen in BRCA1/2 carriers. In addition, other chemoprevention trials will become available in the future.

Ovarian cancer

Screening Guidelines

The current recommendations for ovarian cancer screening include pelvic exam, CA-125 blood tests, and transvaginal ultrasound with color Doppler every 6–12 months beginning at age 25-35. In the general population, these measures have not proven to be very sensitive in detecting early stage ovarian cancer. It is unclear how efficacious these procedures are in a high-risk population.

Prevention Options

It is recommended that prophylactic oophorectomy be considered in women with a BRCA1 alteration or BRCA2. An NIH consensus conference convened in 1994 recommended prophylactic oophorectomy at age 35 or when childbearing is complete for women from hereditary ovarian cancer families [49]. A more recent review by the Cancer Genetics Studies Consortium recommended that such an approach be considered, but did not endorse it given the lack of evidence regarding its efficacy [45]. Observational studies have documented a residual risk of primary peritoneal carcinomatosis in members of high-risk families who have undergone prophylactic oophorectomy. A report from the Gilda Radner Familial Cancer Registry demonstrated a 2% (6 cases among 324 women) failure rate [50]. An NIH study of 12 breast/ovarian families showed 2 cases of peritoneal carcinomatosis in 460 person-years in a group of oophorectomized women as compared with 8 cases of ovarian cancer in 1665 person-years in family members who had not undergone oophorectomy. This translated to a 24-fold excess risk of ovarian cancer in non-oophorectomized family members, versus a 13-fold excess of "ovarian" cancer in those who underwent oophorectomy [51]. This difference, however, was not statistically significant. Thus, the extent to which prophylactic surgery reduces the risk of ovarian cancer is unclear. Further research, including a large international study, is planned to address this issue.

Other possible prevention options include the use of chemoprevention agents. It has been demonstrated that women in the general population who have taken the oral contraceptive pill for at least five years reduce their risk of ovarian cancer by about 40% [52, 53]. In addition, a recent study suggested that the oral contraceptive pill reduces the risk of ovarian cancer in BRCA1/2 carriers [26].

Colon Cancer

Screening Guidelines

Fecal occult blood testing coupled with flexible sigmoidoscopy or colonoscopy is recommended beginning at age 50. The endoscopic exams should be repeated every 3-5 years if normal, and the fecal occult blood testing should be performed annually. These recommendations are no different from the screening guidelines for the general population; however, they may be modified in the setting of a family history of colon cancer.

Prostate cancer

Screening Guidelines

Rectal exam and PSA annually beginning at age 50 is recommended. This guideline is no different from the screening recommendation for the general population.

Hormone Use

Oral Contraceptives (OCPs)

The long term use of oral contraceptives in younger women appears to be associated with an increased risk of developing breast cancer before age 40 [54, 55]. Overall, however, OCPs are not associated with a significantly elevated risk of breast cancer [55]. It is unclear if the risk of breast cancer is further increased in OCP users who have a close relative with breast cancer [54, 56]. As discussed previously, a recent study has suggested that among young breast cancer patients, long-term use of OCPs increases the risk of breast cancer significantly more in mutation carriers than in non-carriers [25]. However, studies have demonstrated consistently a protective effect of OCPs on ovarian cancer risk in the general population, which appears to increase with duration of use of OCPs [52, 53]. These findings seem to apply also to mutation carriers [26]. Thus, in the setting of limited knowledge, one must balance the potential benefits of the pill in terms of reduction in risk of ovarian cancer against the possible increase in breast cancer risk in BRCA1/2 carriers. Studies are underway to determine whether risks for breast or ovarian cancer in BRCA1 and BRCA2 carriers are modified by other known reproductive history risk factors.

Hormone Replacement Therapy

Studies have demonstrated that, in women in the general population, long-term use of hormone replacement therapy (HRT) with estrogen alone or estrogen and progesterone, increases the risk of breast cancer (relative risk of 1.2-1.5) [57, 58]. Again, it is important to note that little information exists on the effect of HRT in women who are BRCA1/2 carriers. These women are often considering having prophylactic oophorectomy at an early age and therefore the question about HRT for protection against heart and bone disease as well as relief from menopausal symptoms frequently arises. Some clinicians do not believe that HRT is necessarily contraindicated for BRCA1/2 carriers who have prophylactic mastectomy and oophorectomy performed at a young age. However, at present there is little information available to guide patients and their physicians who are considering this option.

Individualizing a Screening/Prevention Program

It is important for individuals undergoing genetic testing to understand that there are no proven means of cancer prevention or screening in mutation carriers. Thus, each carrier should be encouraged to take the time to fully weigh the implications of different management approaches prior to deciding on a particular plan. It is also not infrequent for an individual's approach to change over time. For example, a young woman may choose surveillance for ovarian cancer if she has not yet completed childbearing. Once her family is complete, she may then wish to consider prophylactic surgery.

Conclusion

While it took many years to clone BRCA1 and BRCA2 after the initial identification of high-risk families, much information has been elucidated about these genes in the short time since then. The molecular structure of BRCA1/2 has been characterized and research is underway to learn more about the BRCA1/2 protein products, how they function as tumor suppressors, and how these proteins may interact with biologic and environmental modifiers of gene expression. It is also likely that more precise genotype-phenotype correlations will emerge. With the identification of hundreds of mutations in these genes, new technologies are being developed to improve the sensitivity and specificity of testing. All of this information will be critical in providing more accurate risk assessments, particularly for those individuals with less striking family histories.

Increasing knowledge about the clinical manifestations of BRCA1/2 alterations will help practitioners determine who is an appropriate candidate for testing based in part on the likelihood of finding a mutation in the family. Patients, particularly those with a strong family history of cancer, appear to accept the ambiguity in what is known with respect to cancer risks. However, long-term data regarding the effectiveness of the available screening and preventive strategies for mutation carriers are eagerly awaited. In addition, it will be important to initiate or continue prospective studies regarding the impact of potential risk modifiers in mutation carriers (e.g. hormone replacement therapy, oral contraceptives, tamoxifen, etc.).

In the meantime, individuals considering genetic testing must do so in the context of the uncertainties that exist in the present time. Aside from limited knowledge about cancer risks and management options, the psychological effects of risk notification are relatively unknown, especially in the long term. Because of the magnitude of information that patients must assimilate and the potential psychological sequelae of testing, it is critical that patients have access to genetic counseling before and after testing. This process enables patients to provide properly obtained informed consent, and to make their own choices about getting tested and about management options based on currently available information. To guide the clinician, several organizations, including the American Society of Clinical Oncology and the National Society of Genetic Counselors, have published position statements regarding the indications for testing and the components of genetic counseling [59, 60]. The general principles set forth in those statements, as well as in this and other documents, will no doubt be considered as we prepare for the inevitable isolation of additional breast and ovarian cancer susceptibility genes and the subsequent patient interest in testing.

References

1. Claus EB, Schildkraut JM, Thompson WD, Risch NJ (1996) The genetic attributable risk of breast and ovarian cancer. Cancer 77: 2318-2324
2. Miki Y, Swensen J, Shattuck-Eidens D et al (1994) A strong candidate for the breast and ovarian cancer susceptibility gene BRCA1. Science 266:66-71
3. Wooster R, Bignell G, Lancaster J et al (1995) Identification of the breast cancer susceptibility gene BRCA2. Nature 378:789-792
4. Holt JT, Thompson ME, Szabo C et al (1996) Growth retardation and tumor inhibition by BRCA1. Nature Genet 12:298-302
5. Sharan SK, Morimatsu M, Albrecht U et al (1997) Embryonic lethality and radiation hypersensitivity mediated by rad51 in mice lacking BRCA2. Nature 386:804-810
6. Scully R, Chen J, Plug A et al (1997) Association of BRCA1 with rad51 in mitotic and meiotic cells. Cell 88:265-275
7. Breast Cancer Information Core (1998) http://www.nhgri.nih.gov/intramural_research/Lab_transfer/Bic
8. Struewing JP, Hartge P, Wacholder S et al (1997) The risk of cancer associated with specific mutations of BRCA1 and BRCA2 among Ashkenazi Jews. N Eng J Med 336:1401-1408
9. Easton DF, Ford D, Bishop T and the Breast Cancer Linkage Consortium (1995) Breast and ovarian cancer incidence in BRCA1-mutation carriers. Am J Hum Genet 56:265-271

10. Ford D, Easton DF, Bishop DT, Narod SA, Goldgar DE and the Breast Cancer Linkage Consortium (1994) Risks of cancer in BRCA1-mutation carriers. Lancet 343: 692-695
11. Serova OM, Mazoyer S, Puget N et al (1997) Mutations in BRCA1 and BRCA2 in breast cancer families: are there more breast-cancer susceptibility genes? Am J Hum Genet 60:486-495
12. Struewing JP, Brody LC, Erdos MR et al (1995) Detection of eight BRCA1 mutations in 10 breast/ovarian cancer families, including 1 family with male breast cancer. Am J Hum Genet 57:1-7
13. Easton DF, Steele L, Fields P et al (1997) Cancer risks in two large breast cancer families linked to BRCA2 on chromosome 13q12-13. Am J Hum Genet 61:120-128
14. Friedman LS, Gayther SA, Kurosaki T et al (1997) Mutation analysis of BRCA1 and BRCA2 in a male breast cancer population. Am J Hum Genet 60:313-319
15. Phelan CM, Lancaster JM, Tonin P et al (1997) Mutation analysis of the BRCA2 gene in 49 site-specific breast cancer families. Nature Genet 13:120-122
16. Ford D, Easton DF, Stratton M et al (1998) Genetic heterogeneity and penetrance analysis of the BRCA1 and BRCA2 genes in breast cancer families. Am J Hum Genet 62:676-689
17. Seynaeve C, v.d. Bosch LMC, Brekelmans LC, et al. Local recurrence following lumpectomy and irradiation in familial and hereditary vs sporadic breast cancer patients. Proc Am Soc Clin Oncol 1998; 17: 457 (abstract)
18. Hayes DF, Kaplan W (1996) Evaluation of the patient after primary therapy In: Harris JR, Lippman ME, Morrow M & Hellman S (eds) Diseases of the Breast. Philadelphia, Lippincott-Raven, pp 629-647
19. Landis SH, Murray T, Bolden S, Wingo PA (1998) Cancer Statistics, 1998. CA Cancer J Clin 48:6-29
20. Tonin P, Weber B, Offit K et al (1996) Frequency of recurrent BRCA1 and BRCA2 mutations in Ashkenazi Jewish breast cancer families. Nature Med 2:1179-1183
21. Marcus JN, Page DL, Watson P, Narod SA, Lenoir GM, Lynch HT (1997) BRCA1 and BRCA2 hereditary breast carcinoma phenotypes. Cancer 80:543-546
22. Porter DE, Cohen BB, Wallace MR et al (1994) Breast cancer incidence, penetrance and survival in probable carriers of BRCA1 gene mutation in families linked to BRCA1 on chromosome 17q12-21. Br J Surg 81:1512-1515
23. Jóhannsson Ó, Ranstam J, Borg Å, Olsson H (1998) Survival of BRCA1 breast and ovarian cancer patients: A population based study from Southern Sweden. J Clin Oncol 16:397-404
24. Narod, S, Goldgar D, Cannon-Albright L et al (1995) Risk modifiers in carriers of BRCA1 mutations. Int J Cancer (Pred Oncol) 64:394-398
25. Ursin G, Henderson BE, Haile RW et al (1997) Does oral contraceptive use increase the risk of breast cancer in women with BRCA1/2 mutations more than other women? Cancer Res 57:3678-3681
26. Narod SA, Risch H, Moslehi R et al (1998) Oral contraceptives and the risk of hereditary ovarian cancer. N Engl J Med; 339: 424-8
27. Phelan CM, Rebbeck TR, Weber BL et al (1996) Ovarian cancer risk in BRCA1 carriers is modified by the *HRAS1* variable number of tandem repeat (VNTR) locus. Nature Genet 12:309-311
28. Malkin D (1993) The Li-Fraumeni syndrome. Principles and Practice of Oncology Updates 7:1-14
29. FitzGerald MG, Bean JM, Hegde SR et al (1997) Heterozygous ATM mutations do not contribute to early onset breast cancer. Nature Genet 15:307-310

30. Savitsky K, Bar-Shira A, Gilad S et al (1995) A single ataxia telangiectasia gene with a product similar to PI-3 kinase. Science 268:1749-1753
31. Athma P, Rappaport R, Swift M (1996) Molecular genotyping shows ataxia telangiectasia heterozygotes are predisposed to breast cancer. Cancer Genet Cytogenet 92:130-134
32. Starink TM, Van der Veen JPW, Arwert F et al (1986) The Cowden syndrome: a clinical and genetic study in 21 patients. Clin Genet 29:222-233
33. Nelen MR, Padberg GW, Peeters EAJ et al (1996) Localization of the gene for Cowden disease to chromosome 10q22-23. Nature Genet 13:114-116
34. Szabo CI, King M-C (1997) Invited editorial: population genetics of BRCA1 and BRCA2. Am J Hum Genet 60:1013-1020
35. Ford D, Easton DF, Peto J (1995) Estimates of the gene frequency of BRCA1 and its contribution to breast and ovarian cancer incidence. Am J Hum Genet 57:1457-1462
36. FitzGerald MG, MacDonald DJ, Krainer M et al (1996) Germ-line BRCA1 mutations in Jewish and non-Jewish women with early onset breast cancer. N Engl J Med 334:143-149
37. Muto MG, Cramer DW, Tangir J, Berkowitz R, Mok S (1996) Frequency of the BRCA1 185delAG mutation among Jewish women with ovarian cancer and matched population controls. Cancer Res 56:1250-1252
38. Abeliovich D, Kaduri L, Lerer I et al (1997) The founder mutations 185delAG and 5382insC in BRCA1 and 6174delT in BRCA2 appear in 60% of ovarian cancer and 30% of early-onset breast cancer patients among Ashkenazi Jewish women. Am J Hum Genet 60:505-514
39. Schubert EL, Mefford HC, Dann JL, Argonza RH, Hull J, King M-C (1997) BRCA1 and BRCA2 mutations in Ashkenazi Jewish families with breast and ovarian cancer. Genetic Testing 1:41-46
40. Parmigiani G, Berry DA, Aguilar O (1998) Determining carrier probabilities for breast cancer susceptibility genes BRCA1 and BRCA2. Am J Hum Genet 62:145-158
41. Frank TS, Manley SA, Olopade OI, et al. Sequence analysis of BRCA1 and BRCA2: correlation of mutations with family history and ovarian cancer risk. J Clin Oncol 1998; 16: 2417-25
42. Matloff ET, Peshkin BN (1998) Complexities in cancer genetic counseling: breast and ovarian cancer. Principles and Practice of Oncology Updates 12 (1):1-11
43. Croyle RT, Smith KR, Botkin JR, Baty B, Nash J (1997) Psychological responses to BRCA1 mutation testing: preliminary findings. Health Psychol 16:63-72
44. Lerman C, Narod S, Schulman K et al (1996) BRCA1 testing in families with hereditary breast-ovarian cancer: a prospective study of patient decision making and outcomes. JAMA 275:1885-1892
45. Burke W, Daly M, Garber J et al (1997) Recommendations for follow-up care of individuals with an inherited predisposition to cancer: II. BRCA1 and BRCA2. JAMA 277:997-1003
46. Hartmann L, Jenkins R, Schaid D, Yang P (1997) Prophylactic mastectomy (PM): preliminary retrospective cohort analysis. Proc Am Assoc Cancer Res 38:1123 (Abstract)
47. Ziegler LD, Kroll SS (1991) Primary breast cancer after prophylactic mastectomy. Am J Clin Oncol 14:451-454
48. Fisher B, Costantino JP, Wickerham DL, et al. Tamoxifen for prevention of breast cancer: report of the National Surgical Adjuvant Breast and Bowel Project P-I Study. J Natl. Cancer Inst 1998; 90: 1371-88

49. NIH Consensus Development Panel on Ovarian Cancer (1995) Ovarian cancer: screening, treatment and follow-up. JAMA 273:491-497

50. Piver MS, Jishi MF, Tsukada Y, Nava G (1993) Primary peritoneal carcinoma after prophylactic oophorectomy in women with a family history of ovarian cancer. Cancer 71:2751-2755

51. Struewing JF, Watson P, Easton DF, Ponder BA, Lynch HT, Tucker MA (1995) Prophylactic oophorectomy in inherited breast/ovarian cancer families. J Natl Cancer Inst Monogr 17:33-35

52. Vessey MP, Painter R (1995) Endometrial and ovarian cancer and oral contraceptives. Br J Cancer 71:1340-1342

53. Rosenberg L, Palmer JR, Zauber AG et al (1994) A case-control study of oral contraceptive use and invasive epithelial ovarian cancer. Am J Epidemiol 139:654-661

54. Brinton LA, Daling JR, Liff JM et al (1995) Oral contraceptives and breast cancer risk among younger women. J Natl Cancer Inst 87:827-835

55. Rosenberg L, Palmer JR, Rao S et al (1996) Case-control study of oral contraceptive use and risk of breast cancer. Am J Epidemiol 143:25-37

56. Collaborative Group on Hormonal Factors in Breast Cancer (1996) Breast cancer and hormonal contraceptives: collaborative reanalysis of individual data on 53 297 women with breast cancer and 100 239 women without breast cancer from 54 epidemiological studies. Lancet 347:1713-1727

57. Grady D, Rubin SM, Petitti DB et al(1992) Hormone therapy to prevent disease and prolong life in postmenopausal women. Ann Int Med 117:1016-1037

58. Colditz GA, Hankinson SE, Hunter DJ et al (1995) The use of estrogens and progestins and the risk of breast cancer in postmenopausal women. N Eng J Med 332:1589-1593

59. Statement of the American Society of Clinical Oncology (1996) genetic testing for cancer susceptibility. J Clin Oncol 14:1730-1736

60. McKinnon WC, Baty BJ, Bennett RL et al (1997) Predisposition genetic testing for late-onset disorders in adults: a position paper of the National Society of Genetic Counselors. JAMA 278:1217-1220

Acknowledgments: We gratefully acknowledge Lenora Johnson, MPH, CHES and Aba Bonney, BS for their invaluable assistance with manuscript preparation. We would also like to thank Caryn Lerman, PhD and Barbara Brogan, RN, MS for their thoughtful review of the manuscript.

Clinical Applications of Angiogenesis Inhibitors

I. J. Fidler, D. R. Bielenberg

Introduction

Most deaths from cancer result from the relentless growth of metastases that are resistant to conventional therapies [1]. Significant improvements in therapy of metastasis depend on a better understanding of the biology of the metastatic process which can provide a sound basis for the design of specific antimetastatic regimens. This chapter reviews recent data on the role of angiogenesis in metastasis and how its regulation may inhibit disseminated cancer.

The pathogenesis of cancer metastasis consists of a series of linked, sequential, and selective steps. Metastasis begins with the detachment of tumor cells from the primary neoplasm and the invasion of the surrounding stroma by single cells or a group of cells with increased motility and secretion of degradative enzymes. Once the invading cells penetrate the lymphatic or vascular channels, they may grow there or a single cell or clumps of cells may detach and be transported within the circulatory system. Tumor emboli must survive the host's immune and nonimmune defenses and the turbulence of the circulation, arrest in the capillary bed of receptive organs, extravasate into the organ parenchyma, proliferate, and establish a micrometastasis. Growth of these small tumor lesions requires the development of a vascular supply and continuous evasion of host defense cells. When the metastases grow, they can shed tumor cells into the circulation and thus produce metastasis of metastases [1].

In 1889, Paget proposed that metastasis was not random and occurred only when certain favored tumor cells (the "seed") interacted with certain specific organs (the "soil") [2]. A modern definition of the "seed and soil" hypothesis consists of three principles. First, neoplasms are biologically heterogeneous and contain subpopulations of cells with different metastatic properties [1]. Second, the process of metastasis is selective for cells that preexist in the parental neoplasm [3]. Third, the outcome of metastasis, as shown in human and rodent tumors, depends on multiple interactions of metastatic cells with homeostatic mechanisms shown to influence growth, vascularization, invasion, and drug sensitivity [4].

A crucial step in continuous growth of tumors and development of metastasis is the recruitment of new blood vessels in and around tumors [5]. A tumor mass that is <1 mm in diameter can receive oxygen and nutrients by diffusion. Any increase in tumor mass requires angiogenesis, i.e. the proliferation and morphogenesis of vascular endothelial cells [5-7]. The process of angiogenesis consists of multiple, sequential and interdependent steps. It begins with local degradation of the basement membrane surrounding capillaries, followed by invasion of the surrounding stroma by the underlying endothelial cells in the direction of the angiogenic stimulus. Endothelial cell migration is accompanied by the proliferation of endothelial cells at the leading edge of the migrating column. Endothelial cells then organize into three-dimensional structures to form new capillary tubes.

The onset of angiogenesis involves a change in the local equilibrium between positive and negative regulatory molecules [5-8]. Some of the major angiogenic factors include basic fibroblast growth factor (bFGF), vascular endothelial growth factor/vascular permeability factor (VEGF/VPF), interleukin 8 (IL-8), platelet-derived endothelial cell growth factor (PD-ECGF), platelet-derived growth factor (PDGF) and hepatocyte growth factor (HGF) [9-11].

Regulation of Angiogenic Factors by the Organ Environment

In many normal tissues, factors which inhibit angiogenesis predominate [6, 9, 11]. The switch from angiogenesis inhibiting to an angiogenesis stimulating phenotype has been studied in different models. For example, in cultured fibroblasts, the loss of wild-type allele of the p53 tumor suppressor gene coincides with the acquisition of angiogenic phenotype, and is the result of reduced production of thrombospondin-1 (TSP-1) [12]. The production of angiogenic molecules is regulated in part by cell-to-cell contact, i.e. cell density [13]. Human renal cell carcinoma (HRCC) cells express low levels of bFGF (both at mRNA and protein levels) under dense culture conditions compared to sparse cultures. Similar data were obtained in endothelial cells [13]. In contrast to the inverse correlation of cell density and bFGF expression, expression of VEGF is directly correlated with cell density in human colon carcinoma cell lines [14].

Expression of bFGF

Previous studies from our laboratory and others have demonstrated that the orthotopic implantation of human renal cell cancer (HRCC) cells and human colon cancer (HCC) cells is associated with extensive angiogenesis, invasion, and metastasis, whereas the ectopic implantation (subcutaneous) does not [1, 4].

The production of degradative enzymes is differentially regulated by the organ microenvironment. Highly metastatic human colon cancer (HCC) cells implanted in the cecum of nude mice produced high levels of type IV collagenase (gelatinase) and heparinase (heparin sulfate-specific endo-ß-D-glucuronidase) whereas the same cells implanted subcutaneously did not [15]. Ectopic tumors did not produce visceral metastases, while orthotopic tumors metastasized to lymph nodes and to the liver. A similar increase in gelatinase activity was found using an HRCC line injected into the kidney of nude mice as compared to the subcutis [16]. When HCC or HRCC cells were cocultured with skin fibroblasts, their production of type IV collagenase was inhibited. Collagenase levels were not inhibited when HCC cells were cocultured with colon or lung fibroblasts [17], and collagenase levels in HRCC cells were not inhibited by kidney fibroblasts [16]. Interferon-beta (IFN-ß) is produced by fibroblasts and differentiated epithelial cells in the skin. When HCC cells were incubated in serum-free medium containing IFN-ß, gelatinase activity was significantly reduced [16, 17], indicating that organ-specific fibroblasts can regulate an important step in angiogenesis, invasion, and metastasis.

Our laboratory has shown that expression of bFGF by tumor cells is also dependent on the site of implantation. When HRCC cells were implanted in different organ microenvironments in nude mice, the expression of bFGF was 10-20 times higher in those tumors implanted in the kidney than those implanted in the subcutaneous tissues [18]. The kidney tumors were more highly vascularized than tumors implanted in the subcutis. In sharp contrast, the expression of IFN-ß was high in epithelial cells and fibroblasts surrounding the subcutaneous tumors, whereas no IFN-ß was found in or around HRCC tumors growing in the kidney. The parental cell line and metastatic clone also differed in bFGF expression. The alteration in bFGF level by the site of implantation was due to adaptation to the organ microenvironment, as was demonstrated when the cells were reestablished in culture and the levels of bFGF returned to the previously *in vitro* concentration after 4 weeks [18].

Expression of bFGF in HRCC is cell density-dependent. By *in situ* mRNA hybridization (ISH) and northern blot analysis, we found an inverse correlation between increasing cell density and bFGF expression [13]. Fluorescence-activated cell sorting (FACS), immunohistochemistry and ELISA confirmed this finding at the protein level. Tumor cells harvested from dense cultures (low bFGF expression) and then plated under sparse conditions expressed high levels of bFGF. Similar data were obtained using endothelial cells. The effect was not mediated by soluble factors released into the culture medium. The *in vivo* manifestations of cell density-dependent regulation are likely to be found by differences in gene expression in the center of a tumor versus the periphery or leading edge [1].

The expression of bFGF in surgical specimens of HCC was determined by *in situ* hybridization (ISH) technique and northern blot analysis. ISH analysis revealed that the level of bFGF was significantly higher in Duke's stage C or D tumors than in Duke's stage B tumors. Northern blot hybridization did not detect mRNA transcripts for bFGF. However, analysis by ISH revealed that bFGF was overexpressed at the periphery of the tumor (leading edge), where cells were rapidly dividing. This observation confirms that tumors are heterogeneous for cells with various degrees of expression of invasion and metastasis-related genes and that a subpopulation of cells within a tumor can give rise to distant metastasis [19]. In a follow-up study with colon cancer patients, bFGF expression was found to be highest in primary tumors of patients who presented with metastatic disease [20]. This study identified patients who appeared to be free of metastasis at the time of initial surgery (Duke's stage B) yet developed distant metastasis at a later date; these patients had relatively high bFGF expression along with increased expression of other metastasis related genes especially at the invasive edge of the tumor [19, 20].

Expression of IL-8

The production of angiogenic molecules, e.g. VEGF, bFGF, and IL-8 by melanoma cells is regulated by complex interactions with keratinocytes in the skin [21]. Recent reports from our laboratory show that IL-8 is an important molecule in melanoma growth and progression. Constitutive expression of IL-8 directly correlated with the metastatic potential of human melanoma cells. Further, IL-8 induced proliferation, migration, and invasion of endothelial cells and, hence, neovascularization [22]. Several organ-derived cytokines (produced by inflammatory cells) are known to induce expression of IL-8 in normal and transformed cells [21].

Since IL-8 expression in melanocytes and melanoma cells can be induced by inflammatory signals, the question of whether specific organ microenvironments could influence the expression of IL-8 was analyzed. Melanoma cells were implanted into the subcutis, the spleen (to produce liver metastasis), and intravenously (to produce lung metastasis) of athymic nude mice. Subcutaneous tumors, lung lesions, and liver lesions expressed high, intermediate, and no IL-8 mRNA and protein, respectively [84]. Melanoma cells established from the tumors growing *in vivo* exhibited similar levels of IL-8 mRNA transcripts as continuously cultured cells, thus demonstrating that the differential expression of IL-8 was not due to the selection of a subpopulation of cells [23].

IL-8 expression can be upregulated by coculturing melanoma cells with keratinocytes (skin) and inhibited by coculturing melanoma cells with hepatocytes (liver). We also investigated the effects of two cytokines produced by keratinocytes (IL-1, IFN-ß) and two cytokines produced by hepatocytes (TGF-α, TGF-ß) on the regulation of IL-8 in human melanoma cells. IL-1 upregulated the expression of IL-8 in human melanoma cells at both the mRNA and protein levels in a dose- and time-dependent manner in the presence of *de novo* protein synthesis [24]. IFN-ß did not affect constitutive IL-8 mRNA and protein production in human melanoma cells, but it did block the induction of IL-8 by IL-1 [24]. TGF-ß inhibited the expression of IL-8, while TGF-α had no effect on IL-8 expression.

The expression of a common angiogenic molecule VEGF is increased in necrotic areas of human tumor as shown by *in situ* hybridization [25]. *In vitro* studies have confirmed that VEGF expression is increased in response to hypoxia, probably due to increased transcription and to increased mRNA stability [26]. Treatment of cells with IL-1, IL-6, IL-8, TGF-, PDGF, HGF and bFGF can increase expression of VEGF [27]. VEGF expression is also regulated by certain oncogenes (*src* and *ras*) and tumor suppressor genes like p53 [28].

The organ microenvironment also influences the expression of VEGF/VPF. Human gastric cancer cells were implanted into orthotopic (stomach) and ectopic (subcutaneous) organs of nude mice. Tumors in the stomach were highly vascularized, expressed high levels of VEGF, and grew more rapidly than the subcutaneous tumors. In addition, metastasis occurred only from the tumors implanted in the stomach [29].

Molecular Determinants of Angiogenesis in Cutaneous Hemangiomas of Infants

Infantile cutaneous hemangiomas represent a unique form of pathologic angiogenesis in which tumors grow rapidly in the first year of life (proliferative phase), followed by a slow regression during the next 5 years (involuting phase), and eventual involution or complete regression (involuted phase) by the age of 10-15 years. Treatment with systemic IFN-α has been shown to accelerate the involution of fatal hemangiomas [30]. We investigated whether the progression and involution of infantile cutaneous hemangiomas was associated with an imbalance between positive and negative regulators of angiogenesis and found that proliferating hemangiomas expressed high levels of bFGF and VEGF/VGF but not IFN-ß (mRNA and protein). The epidermis from normal individuals and the epidermis overlying involuted lesions or at sites distant to the proliferating hemangiomas was not hyperplastic and expressed bFGF, VEGF/VPF, and IFN-ß, suggesting that the proliferating hemangiomas may induce hyperplasia in the surrounding normal tissues which also produce bFGF and VEGF/VPF, but not IFN-ß (Bielenberg et al., unpublished data). This represents another example of the concept that neoplastic cells subvert and usurp host homeostatic mechanisms for their growth advantage.

To study the relationship between hemangiomas and the microenvironment, we studied epidermal hyperplasia and dermal angiogenesis and telangiectasia in mice subsequent to UV-B radiation. We found that UV-B irradiation induced production of bFGF in the keratinocytes of the epidermis, followed by the division of epidermal cells. Days 3-7 following UV-B irradiation showed marked hyperplasia and angiogenesis. The expression of VEGF/VPF was slightly increased by day 5. Most interestingly, the expression of IFN-ß in the epithelium decreased as the epidermis became increasingly hyperplastic but was again expressed as the hyperplasia and angiogenesis subsided. Whether expression of IFN-ß caused the eventual decrease in epidermal and endothelial cell proliferation remains unclear.

Lymphoid-mediated Angiogenesis

Angiogenesis is essential to homeostasis and its regulation by lymphoid cells, such as T-lymphocytes, macrophages, and mast cells is well recognized [31-37]. A local inflammatory reaction consisting of T-lymphocytes and macrophages is often associated with invasive cutaneous melanoma, and an intense inflammatory reaction is often associated with increased risk of metastasis, suggesting that angiogenesis induced by inflammation may contribute to melanoma progression and metastasis [36].

Immunological mechanisms involved in physiological angiogenesis occur subsequent to wound healing [37]. Systemic chemotherapy has been shown to retard the process of wound healing, possibly by decreased immune response; whether this is mediated by inhibition of angiogenesis is not clear [38]. We have investigated the role of tumor vascularization and its effect on tumor growth in immunosuppressed mice. The growth of weakly immunogenic B16 melanoma was retarded in myelosuppressed mice compared with control mice [39]. Further evidence implicating myelosuppression in the retardation of tumor growth and vascularity was obtained from doxorubicin (DXR)-pretreated animals injected with normal spleen cells one day before tumor challenge. Tumor growth in these mice was comparable to control mice [39]. Similar results were obtained in athymic mice suggesting that the tumor vascularization observed in DXR-treated mice reconstituted with normal spleenocytes was not mediated solely by T-lymphocytes. Since reconstitution with spleen cells enhanced vascularization of the B16 tumors, the results suggest that myelosuppressive chemotherapeutic drugs, e.g. DXR, can inhibit host-mediated vascularization and support the concept that developing tumors can usurp homeostatic mechanisms to their advantage [4].

The role of infiltrating cells in angiogenesis of human colon cancer has recently been reported [40]. High expression of PD-ECGF was found in infiltrating cells, mostly macrophages and lymphocytes, and very little expression of PD-ECGF in the cancer epithelium. The intensity of staining for PD-ECGF in infiltrating cells correlated with vessel counts suggesting the involvement of these cells in the angiogenesis of HCC.

The Role of Macrophages in Angiogenesis: Production of Angiostatin

Macrophages have been recognized as important angiogenesis effector cells for a number of years [34-37]. They may influence new capillary growth by several different mechanisms. First, macrophages produce in excess of 20 molecules that influence endothelial cell proliferation, migration and differentiation *in vitro*, and are potentially angiogenic *in vivo* [35]. A second mechanism by which macrophages might modulate angiogenesis is by modifying extracellular matrix (ECM). The composition of the ECM has been shown to influence endothelial cell shape and morphology dramatically, and may profoundly influence new capillary growth [41, 42]. Macrophages can influence the composition of the ECM either through the direct production of ECM components, or through the production of proteases, which effectively alter the structure and composition of the ECM [35-37]. Third, macrophages have been shown to produce substances that suppress angiogenesis, e.g. treatment of macrophages with a chemopreventive agent, retinoic acid, leads to production of an angiogenesis inhibitor, TSP-1 [43].

Recently we examined the mechanism of generation of angiostatin, an angiogenesis inhibitor isolated from plasma of mice bearing Lewis lung carcinoma (3LL) [44]. Our results demonstrate that the generation of angiostatin by the subcutaneous tumors requires the presence of macrophages and is directly correlated with their metalloelastase activity [45]. The addition of plasminogen to 3LL cells cultured in vitro did not result in generation of angiostatin, whereas the addition of plasminogen to cocultures of macrophages and 3LL cells did. Elastase activity in macrophages was up-regulated by the cytokine GM-CSF [46]. GM-CSF secreted by 3LL cells significantly enhanced the production of elastase by macrophages and hence the generation of angiostatin from plasminogen [45]. These data suggest that elastase released from tumor-infiltrating macrophages is responsible for the angiostatin production in this tumor model and the angio-inhibitory role of macrophages in neovascularization.

Most recently, we determined whether tumor cells consistently generating granulocyte-macrophage colony-stimulating factor (GM-CSF) can recruit and activate macrophages to generate angiostatin and hence inhibit the growth of distant metastasis. Two murine melanoma lines, B16-F10 (syngeneic to C57BL/6 mice) and K-1735 (syngeneic to C3H/HeN) were engineered to produce GM-CSF. High and low GM-CSF-producing clones were identified. Parental, low and high GM-CSF-producing cells were injected subcutaneously into syngeneic and into nude mice. Parental and low-producing cells produced rapidly-growing tumors, whereas the high GM-CSF-producing cells produced slow-growing tumors. Macrophage density inversely correlated with tumorigenicity and directly correlated with levels of steady-state macrophage metalloelastase mRNA. B16 and K-1735 subcutaneous tumors producing high levels of GM-CSF significantly suppressed lung metastasis of many murine tumors, but parental or low-producing tumors did not. The level of angiostatin in the serum directly correlated with the production of GM-CSF by the subcutaneous tumors. These data provide direct evidence that GM-CSF released from a primary tumor can upregulate metalloelastase expression in infiltrating macrophages which, in turn, leads to production of angiostatin and suppression of metastasis.

Microvessel Density and Tumor Progression

With few exceptions, benign neoplasms are sparsely vascularized and tend to grow slowly, whereas malignant neoplasms are highly vascular and fast-growing [1, 5-11]. The increase in vasculature also increases the probability that tumor cells will enter the circulation and possibly give rise to metastasis [47]. Immunohistochemical staining of breast cancer sections with antibodies against factor VIII, a protein expressed only on the surface of endothelial cells, allowed Weidner and colleagues to determine the density of microvessels [48, 49]. The number of microvessels in microscopic fields selected from the most vascular areas ('hot spots') of the sections correlated directly with metastasis and inversely with survival.

Most, but not all, recent studies have concluded that increased microvessel density in the areas of most intense neovascularization is a significant and independent prognostic indicator in early-stage breast cancer, melanoma, ovarian carcinoma, gastric carcinoma, and colon carcinoma, also supporting the conclusion that the angiogenesis index is a useful prognostic factor [48-51]. However, expectation that an angiogenesis index can identify all patients with occult metastatic disease or those with probable distant metastases may be unrealistic [52]. First, human tumors are heterogeneous and consist of subpopulations of cells with different biological properties [1]. Heterogeneity of angiogenic molecule expression has recently been documented in human renal carcinomas and human colon carcinomas [19, 20]. Second, the process of cancer metastasis is sequential and selective and consists of a series of interlinked independent steps [1]. To produce clinically relevant metastases, tumor cells must complete all the steps in the process. Tumor cells that can induce intense angiogenesis but cannot survive in the circulation or proliferate in distant organs will not produce metastases. Like all other steps in the metastatic cascade, angiogenesis is necessary but not sufficient for the pathogenesis of a metastasis. Third, although not all large angiogenic tumors can produce metastasis, inhibition of angiogenesis prevents the growth of tumor cells at both the primary and secondary sites, and thus can prevent the development of clinically relevant metastases.

Inhibition of Angiogenesis by Interferons

The IFN family consists of three major glycoproteins that exhibit species specificity: leukocyte-derived IFN-α, fibroblast-derived IFN-ß, and immune cell-produced IFN-γ. Although IFN-α and IFN-ß share a common receptor (the type I IFN receptor) and induce a similar pattern of cellular responses, certain cellular reactions can be stimulated only by IFN-ß, probably by the phosphorylation of a receptor-associated protein that is uniquely responsive to IFN-ß [53]. IFNs were originally discovered as antiviral agents [54], but subsequent studies revealed that IFNs regulate multiple biological activities such as cell growth, differentiation, oncogene expression, host immunity, and tumorigenicity [53]. A growing body of evidence demonstrates that IFNs are also important in regulating a number of steps in the angiogenic process. IFN has antiproliferative properties, especially on tumor cells [53], and this effect has also been demonstrated on endothelial cells *in vitro* [55]. IFN-α inhibited FGF-induced endothelial proliferation, and IFN-γ inhibited ECGF-induced endothelial proliferation [56]. IFN-α and IFN-γ were cytostatic to human dermal microvascular endothelial cells and human capillary endothelial cells [57]. The mechanisms by which IFNs exert their direct antiproliferative effects are not clearly understood, but they appear to lengthen all phases of the cell cycle and deplete essential metabolites such as ornithine decarboxylase.

Several lines of evidence suggest that IFN-ß and IFN-α can inhibit angiogenesis. The systemic administration of IFN-α2a or IFN-α2b has been shown to accelerate the regression of infantile hemangiomas [30], hemangioendothelioma [58], pulmonary hemangiomatosis [59], hemangiopericytoma [60], and Kaposi's sarcoma [61]. These findings stimulated us to investigate whether IFNs could modulate the expression of bFGF. IFN-α and IFN-ß but not IFN-γ downregulated the expression of bFGF mRNA and protein in HRCC. The incubation of human bladder, prostate, colon and breast carcinoma cells with non-cytostatic concentrations of IFN-α and IFN-ß also inhibited bFGF production. This effect was independent of the antiproliferative effect of IFNs. The downregulation of bFGF required long exposure of the cells to a low concentration of IFNs. Moreover, once IFN was withdrawn, cells resumed production of bFGF [62]. We recently confirmed that IFN can inhibit bFGF production in an *in vivo* model system. Systemic administration of human IFN-α decreased the *in vivo* expression of bFGF, decreased blood vessel density, and inhibited tumor growth of a human bladder carcinoma implanted orthotopically in nude mice [63]. Both *in vitro* and *in vivo*, the downregulation of bFGF required a long exposure of cells to low concentrations of IFNs. In addition, when IFN was withdrawn, cells resumed production of bFGF. These observations are consistent with the findings that the complete regression of fatal hemangioma required daily subcutaneous injections of low level IFN-α-2a over a course of 7 to 8 months [30].

The antiangiogenic effect of IFNs is not due to antiproliferative effects. IFN-α/ß inhibited endothelial cell and tumor cell migration [64]. Subcutaneous injection of IFN-α/ß adjacent to a wound delayed the healing process by inhibiting the proliferation, migration, and invasion of many cell types, including capillary buds, fibroblasts, and epithelium [65]. IFN-α/ß injected intratumorally or peritumorally into tumor cells resistant to the antiproliferative effects of IFN resulted in damaged tumor blood vessels which disrupted blood flow and led to ischemia and necrosis [66]. Murine IFN-α/ß inhibited vascularization of murine tumor cells, and human IFN-α/ß suppressed vascularization of human tumor cells in nude mice, thus demonstrating that IFN-α/ß can inhibit angiogenesis without a direct cytostatic effect on murine endothelial cells, possibly by suppressing tumor cell-produced angiogenic factors [67].

We have recently demonstrated that IFN-ß gene therapy can eradicate tumor cells of various histological origin and found that the sustained local production of murine IFN-ß could inhibit the tumorigenicity and metastasis of human and murine tumor cells implanted into nude mice [68, 69]. All human tumor cell lines transfected with the murine IFN-ß gene grew well *in vitro*, but none grew *in vivo*. IFN-ß transfected cells could prevent the outgrowth of parental or control-transfected cells when injected at the same site, but not when injected at distant sites, suggesting that IFN-ß promoted a local lysis of the bystander cells [68, 69]. Similar results were found when murine UV-2237m fibrosarcoma cells were infected with the murine IFN-ß gene using a retroviral vector. The IFN-ß transduced cells were sensitive to macrophage-mediated lysis. All transfected and transduced cells stimulated a high level of nitric oxide in murine macrophages which correlated with the vigorous antitumor activities [69].

We also determined whether the IFN-ß gene can be used to suppress angiogenesis, tumor growth, and metastasis of human prostate cancer cells growing in the prostate of nude mice. Highly metastatic human prostate cancer cells were engineered to constitutively produce murine IFN-ß subsequent to infection with a retroviral vector containing murine IFN-ß cDNA. Parental, control vector-transduced, and IFN-ß-transduced cells were injected into the prostate (orthotopic) or subcutis (ectopic) of nude mice. Control cells produced rapidly growing tumors and regional lymph node metastases, whereas IFN-ß-producing cells did not. IFN-ß-producing cells also suppressed the tumorigenicity of bystander non-transduced prostate cancer cells. Immunohistochemical staining revealed that IFN-ß-producing tumors were homogeneously infiltrated by macrophages, whereas control tumors contained fewer macrophages at their periphery. Most tumor cells in the control tumors were stained positive by an antibody to proliferative cell nuclear antigen; very few were positively stained by terminal deoxynucleotidyl transferase-mediated dUTP-biotin nick-end labeling. In sharp contrast, IFN-ß-producing tumors contained fewer dividing cells and many apoptotic cells. Staining with antibody against CD31 showed that control tumors contained more blood vessels than IFN-ß tumors. Collectively, the data suggest that the suppression of tumorigenicity and metastasis of IFN-ß-producing prostate cancer cells is due to inhibition of angiogenesis and activation of host effector cells.

Conclusions

Inhibition of angiogenesis presents an attractive target for therapy of metastases. To be effective, this form of therapy must overcome several obstacles. First, a single antiangiogenesis agent may have limited usefulness because vascular endothelial cells differ among different organs and may not respond to a specific agent. Second, homeostatic regulation of angiogenesis functions because both the endogenous stimulating and inhibiting molecules are produced continuously. It is therefore unlikely that the intermittent administration of "maximal tolerated dose" of anti-angiogenic agents will produce desirable effects. Third, antiangiogenic therapy may need to be delivered for several months because the half-life of endothelial cells is rather long (it may exceed 1500 days!). Fourth, since regression of neoplasms may occur only after months of continuous therapy, initial stabilization of neoplasms may predict eventual regression should be taken to signify potential success. The development of surrogate markers such as serum level of VEGF/VPF, bFGF, and IL-8 is therefore a crucial prognostic factor. In any event, the outcome of metastasis depends on the interaction of metastatic cells with homeostatic mechanisms that include angiogenesis. Therapy of metastasis, therefore, should be directed against both tumor cells, e.g. chemotherapy and host factors that favor tumor growth. Inhibition of angiogenesis provides an attractive mechanism to achieve this goal.

References

1. Fidler IJ (1990) Critical factors in the biology of human cancer metastasis: twenty-eighth G.H.A. Clowes Memorial Award Lecture. Cancer Res 50:6130-6138
2. Paget S (1989) The distribution of secondary growths in cancer of the breast. Lancet 1:571-573
3. Fidler IJ, Kripke ML (1977) Metastasis results from preexisting variant cells within a malignant tumor. Science 217:893-895
4. Fidler IJ (1995) Modulation of the organ microenvironment for treatment of cancer metastasis. J Natl Cancer Inst 87:1588-1592
5. Liotta LA, Steeg PS, Stetler-Stevenson WG (1991) Cancer metastasis and angiogenesis: an imbalance of positive and negative regulation. Cell 64:327-336
6. Auerbach W, Auerbach R (1994) Angiogenesis inhibition: a review. Pharmacol Ther 63:265-311
7. Folkman J (1995) Clinical applications of research on angiogenesis. N Engl J Med 333:1753-1763
8. Bouck N, Stellmach V, Hsu SC (1996) How tumors become angiogenic. Adv Cancer Res 69:135-174
9. Hanahan D, Folkman J (1996) Patterns and emerging mechanisms of the angiogenic switch during tumorigenesis. Cell 86:353-364
10. Folkman J, Klagsbrun M (1987) Angiogenic factors. Science 235:442-447
11. Dvorak HF (1986) Tumors: wounds that do not heal. N Engl J Med 315:1650-1659
12. Dameron KM, Volpert OV, Tainsky MA, Bouk N (1994) Control of angiogenesis in fibroblasts by p53 regulation of thrombospondin-1. Science 265:1502-1504
13. Singh RK, Llansa N, Bucana CD, Sanchez R, Koura A, Fidler IJ (1996) Cell density-dependent regulation of basic fibroblast growth factor expression in human renal cell carcinoma cells. Cell Growth Differen 7:397-404
14. Koura AN, Liu W, Kitadai Y, Radinsky R, Ellis LM (1996) Regulation of vascular endothelial growth factor expression in human colon carcinoma cells by cell density. Cancer Res 56:3891-3894
15. Nakajima M, Morikawa K, Fabra A, Bucana CD, Fidler IJ (1990) Influence of organ environment on extracellular matrix degradative activity and metastasis of human colon carcinoma cells. J Natl Cancer Inst 82:1890-1898
16. Gohji K, Fidler IJ, Tsan R et al (1994) Human recombinant interferons beta and gamma decrease gelatinase production and invasion by human KG-2 renal carcinoma cells. Int J Cancer 58:380-384
17. Fabra A, Nakajima M, Bucana CD, Fidler IJ (1992) Modulation of the invasive phenotype of human colon carcinoma cells by organ specific fibroblasts of nude mice. Differentiation 52:101-110
18. Singh RK, Bucana CD, Gutman M, Fan D, Wilson MR, Fidler IJ (1994) Organ site-dependent expression of basic fibroblast growth factor in human renal cell carcinoma cells. Am J Pathol 145:365-374

19. Kitadai Y, Ellis LM, Takahashi Y et al (1995) Multiparametric in situ mRNA hybridization analysis to detect metastasis-related genes in surgical specimens of human colon carcinoma. Clin Cancer Res 1:1095-1102

20. Kitadai Y, Ellis LM, Tucker SL et al (1996) Multiparametric in situ mRNA hybridization analysis to predict disease recurrence in patients with colon carcinoma. Am J Pathol 149:1541-1551

21. Herlyn M (1990) Human melanoma: development and progression. Cancer Metastasis Rev 9:101-109

22. Singh RK, Gutman M, Radinsky R, Bucana CD, Fidler IJ (1994) Expression of interleukin-8 correlates with the metastatic potential of human melanoma cells in nude mice. Cancer Res 54:3242-3247

23. Gutman M, Singh RK, Xie K, Bucana CD, Fidler IJ (1995) Regulation of IL-8 expression in human melanoma cells by the organ environment. Cancer Res 55:2470-2475

24. Singh RK, Gutman M, Llansa N, Fidler IJ (1996) Interferon-β prevents the upregulation of interleukin-8 expression in human melanoma cells. J Interferon Cytokine Res 16:577-584

25. Brown LF, Berse B, Jackman RW et al (1993) Expression of vascular permeability factor (vascular endothelial growth factor) and its receptors in adenocarcinomas of the gastrointestinal tract. Cancer Res 53:4727-4735

26. Shweiki D, Itin A, Stoffer D, Keshet E (1992) Vascular endothelial growth factor induced by hypoxia may mediate hypoxia-initiated angiogenesis. Nature 359:843-845

27. Levy AP, Levy NS, Wegner S, Goldberg MA (1995) Transcriptional regulation of the rat vascular endothelial growth factor gene by hypoxia. J Biol Chem 270:13333-13340

28. Rak J, Filmus J, Finkenzeller G, Grugel S, Marme D, Kerbel RS (1995) Oncogenes as inducers of tumor angiogenesis. Cancer Metastasis Rev 14:263-277

29. Takahashi Y, Mai M, Wilson MR, Kitadai Y, Bucana CD, Ellis LM (1996) Site-dependent expression of vascular endothelial growth factor, angiogenesis and proliferation in human gastric carcinoma. Int J Oncol 8:701-705

30. Ezekowitz RAB, Mulliken JB, Folkman J (1992) Interferon alfa-2a therapy for life-threatening hemangiomas of infancy. N Engl J Med 326:1456-1463

31. Sidky YA, Auerbach R (1976) Lymphocyte-induced angiogenesis in tumor-bearing mice. Science 192:1237-1238

32. Meininger CJ, Zetter BR (1992) Mast cells and angiogenesis. Semin Cancer Biol 3:73-79

33. Fidler IJ, Gersten DM, Kripke ML (1979) Influence of immune status on the metastasis of three murine fibrosarcomas of different immunogenicities. Cancer Res 39:3816-3821

34. Polverini P, Cotran R, Gimbrone N, Unanue E (1977) Activated macrophages induce vascular proliferation. Nature 269:804-805

35. Leek RD, Harris AL, Lewis CE (1994) Cytokine networks in solid human tumors: regulation of angiogenesis. J Leukoc Biol 56:423-435

36. Brocker EG, Rechenbeld C, Hamm H, Ruiter DJ, Sorg C (1992) Macrophages in melanocytic naevi. Arch Dermatol Res 284:127-131

37. Sunderkotter C, Steinbrink K, Goebeler M, Bhardwaj R, Sorg C (1994) Macrophages and angiogenesis. J Leukoc Biol 55:410-422

38. Noh R, Karp GI, Devereaux DF (1991) The effect of doxorubicin and mitoxanthrone on wound healing. Cancer Chemother Pharmacol 29:141-144

39. Gutman M, Singh RK, Yoon S, Xie K, Bucana CD, Fidler IJ (1994) Leukocyte-induced angiogenesis and subcutaneous growth of B16 melanoma. Cancer Biother 9:163-170
40. Takahashi Y, Bucana CD, Liu W et al (1996) Platelet-derived endothelial cell growth factor in human colon cancer angiogenesis: role of infiltrating cells. J Natl Cancer Inst 88:1146-1151
41. Polverini PJ (1996) How the extracellular matrix and macrophages contribute to angiogenesis-dependent diseases. Eur J Cancer 32A:2430-2437
42. Ingber D (1991) Extracellular matrix and cell shape: potential control points for inhibition of angiogenesis. J Cell Biochem 47:236-241
43. Lingen MW, Polverini PJ, Bouck N (1996) Retinoic acid induces cells cultured from oral squamous cell carcinomas to become antiangiogenic. Am J Pathol 149:247-258
44. O'Reilly MS, Holmgren L, Shing Y et al (1994) Angiostatin: a novel angiogenesis inhibitor that mediates the suppression of metastases by a Lewis lung carcinoma. Cell 79:315-328
45. Dong Z, Kumar R, Yang X, Fidler IJ (1997) Macrophage-derived metalloelastase is responsible for the generation of angiostatin in Lewis lung carcinoma. Cell 88:801-810
46. Kumar R, Dong Z, Fidler IJ (1996) Differential regulation of metalloelastase activity in murine peritoneal macrophages by GM-CSF and M-CSF. J Immunol 157:5104-5111
47. Liotta LA, Kleinerman J, Saidel GM (1974) Quantitative relationships of intravascular tumor cells, tumor vessels, and pulmonary metastases following tumor implantation. Cancer Res 34:997-1003
48. Weidner N, Semple JP, Welch WR et al (1992) Tumor angiogenesis: a new significant and independent prognostic indicator in early-stage breast carcinoma. J Natl Cancer Inst 84:1875-1887
49. Weidner N, Carroll PR, Flax J, Flumenfeld W, Folkman J (1993) Tumor angiogenesis correlates with metastasis in invasive prostate carcinoma. Am J Pathol 143:401-409 401-408
50. Graham CH, Rivers J, Kerbel RS, Stankiewicz KS, White WL (1994) Extent of vascularization as a prognostic indicator in thin (<0.76 mm) malignant melanomas. Am J Pathol 147:33-41
51. Hollingsworth HC, Kohn EC, Steinberg SM, Rothenberg ML, Meriono MJ (1995) Tumor angiogenesis in advanced stage ovarian carcinoma. Am J Pathol 147:33-41
52. Ellis LM, Fidler IJ (1995) Angiogenesis and breast cancer metastasis. Lancet 346:388-389
53. Uze G, Lutgalla G, Morgensen KE (1995) α and β interferons and their receptor and their friends and relations. J Interferon Cytokine Res 15:3-26
54. Gresser I (1989) Antitumor effects of interferon. Acta Oncol 28:347-353
55. Gutterman JU (1994) Cytokine therapeutics: lessons from interferon α. Proc Natl Acad Sci 91:1198-1205
56. Heyns AP, Eldor A, Vlodavsky I, Kaiser N, Fridman R, Panet A (1985) The antiproliferative effect of interferon and the mitogenic activity of growth factors are independent cell cycle events. Exp Cell Res 161:297-306
57. Hicks C, Breit SN, Penny R (1989) Response of microvascular endothelial cells to biological response modifiers. Immunol Cell Biol 67:271-277
58. Orchard PJ, Smith CM, Woods WG, Day DL, Dehner LP, Shapiro R (1989) Treatment of hemangioendotheliomas with alpha interferon. Lancet 2:565-567

59. White CW, Sondheimer HM, Crouch EC, Wilson H, Fan LL (1989) Treatment of pulmonary hemangiomatosis with recombinant interferon-alpha2a. N Eng J Med 320:1197-1200
60. Ohlms LA, Jones DT, McGill TJI, Healy GB (1994) Interferon-α-2A therapy for airway hemangiomas. Ann Otol Rhinol Laryngol 103:1-8
61. Groopman JE, Gottlieb MS, Goodman J et al (1984) Recombinant alpha-2 interferon therapy for Kaposi's sarcoma associated with the acquired immunodeficiency syndrome. Ann Intern Med 100:671-676
62. Singh RK, Gutman M, Bucana CD, Sanchez R, Llansa N, Fidler IJ (1995) Interferons alpha and beta downregulate the expression of basic fibroblast growth factor in human carcinomas. Proc Natl Acad Sci USA 92:4562-4566
63. Dinney CPN, Bielenberg DR, Reich R et al (1998) Inhibition of basic fibroblast growth factor expression, angiogenesis, and growth of human bladder carcinoma in mice by systemic interferon-alpha administration. Cancer Res 58:808-814
64. Brouty-Boye D, Zetter BR (1980) Inhibition of cell motility by interferon. Science 208:516-518
65. Stout AJ, Gresser I, Thompson WD (1992) Inhibition of wound healing in mice by local interferon-α/β injection. Int J Exp Pathol 74:79-85
66. Dvorak HF, Gresser I (1989) Microvascular injury in pathogenesis of interferon-induced necrosis of subcutaneous tumors in mice. J Natl Cancer Inst 81:497-502
67. Sidky YA, Borden EC (1987) Inhibition of angiogenesis by interferons: effects on tumor- and lymphocyte-induced vascular responses. Cancer Res 47:5155-5161
68. Xie K, Bielenberg D, Huang S et al (1997) Abrogation of tumorigenicity and metastasis of murine and human tumor cells by transfection with the murine interferon-beta gene: possible role of nitric oxide. Clin. Cancer Res 3:2283-2294
69. Dong Z, Juang S-H, Kumar R et al (1998) Suppression of tumorigenicity and metastasis in murine UV-2237 fibrosarcoma cells by infection with a retroviral vector harboring the interferon-beta gene. Cancer Immunol Immunother 46:137-146

Part III
Lung Cancer

Current Management and New Leads in Small Cell Lung Cancer

F. A. Greco, J. D. Hainsworth

Current Standard Therapy

The introduction of the cisplatin/etoposide combination chemotherapy in the early 1980's, was the last important improvement in the therapy for patients with small cell lung cancer. Since then further progress in the treatment of small cell lung cancer has been minimal. The outcome of treatment is highly dependent on initial disease stage and performance status. Median survival durations are usually 7 to 10 months in patients with extensive stage disease, and 15 to 20 months in patients with limited stage disease [1-3]. Patients with poor performance status and/or advanced age do worse. Combination chemotherapy is the cornerstone of therapy. In patients with limited stage disease concurrent thoracic radiation therapy produces a modest survival advantage [4]. Although platinum plus etoposide is now generally accepted as superior chemotherapy, the literature has no citations of large direct randomized comparisons versus other regimens. The relative effectiveness, ease of administration, and lack of common severe toxicity, particularly to heart and lungs, when used concurrently with radiotherapy, explains in part the popularity of the platinum plus etoposide regimen.

We have learned that, despite a very high relapse rate, no further therapy beyond remission induction (with 4-6 courses) has improved survival. Further research regarding "maintenance" therapy or "continued therapy during remission" is critical, but the standard approach currently is to stop therapy after 4-6 courses of induction chemotherapy.

There is as yet no evidence that high dose chemotherapy (with or without stem cell transplantation) or alternating "non-cross resistant" chemotherapy improves survival. Furthermore, prophylactic whole brain radiotherapy does not improve survival when used with our best chemotherapy, but does significantly reduce the incidence of clinical brain metastasis.

The expected results of optimum therapy for patients with small cell lung cancer are illustrated in Table 1. Patients with limited stage disease have a high overall response rate (> 85%) with complete response rate in 40-60%. Median survivals in large series of good performance status patients have ranged from 15 to 20 months, with 40% of patients surviving two years, but only 10-20% five years after diagnosis. Results of therapy in patients with extensive stage disease are considerably worse. The complete response rate is only 15-25%, with median survival of 8 to 10 months, two year survival of approximately 10-20% and five year survival of 1-2%.

At present, comparable treatment results have been reported with a number of combination chemotherapy regimens but with few direct randomized comparisons. Commonly-used regimens include platinum (cisplatin or carboplatin)/etoposide; cyclophosphamide/doxorubicin/ etoposide (CAE); and ifosfamide/cisplatin or carboplatin/etoposide (ICE). In extensive stage patients, ifosfamide-based regimens, with cisplatin or carboplatin and etoposide, may have a modest therapeutic advantage, but are more toxic. In limited stage disease, the cisplatin/etoposide regimen has replaced previous cyclophosphamide/doxorubicin-based regimens, due to the favorable toxicity profile when administered concurrently with radiation therapy.

Although the efficacy of several combination regimens appears about the same, substantial differences in toxicity have been documented. In particular, the relatively favorable toxicity profile of carboplatin has favored it in combination regimens. Only one randomized trial has directly addressed this issue. In this a study, the combination of cisplatin ($50mg/m^2$ days 1 and 2) and etoposide ($100mg/m^2$ days 1-3) was compared to carboplatin ($300mg/m^2$) and etoposide ($100mg/m^2$ days 1-3) [5]. One hundred forty-seven patients were enrolled in this study and the efficacy of the two regimens was equivalent as judged by response rates, median survival, and two-year survival. However, the carboplatin/etopo-

Table 1. Small cell lung cancer: outcome with optimal therapy

	Limited stage	Extensive stage
Complete response	40-60%	15-25%
Median survival (months)	15-20	8-10
Two-year survival	40%	10-20%
Five-year survival	10-20%	1-2%

side regimen produced substantially less toxicity including sepsis, nausea and vomiting, mucositis, nephrotoxicity, and neurotoxicity. These results, taken together with the results of numerous phase II trials in small cell lung cancer and consistent findings in randomized trials in other malignancies (i.e. equivalent efficacy and decreased toxicity of carboplatin compared to cisplatin), favors the use of the carboplatin/etoposide regimen rather than cisplatin/etoposide in patients with extensive stage small cell lung cancer. Since large randomized trials have not been conducted with carboplatin/etoposide plus radiation therapy in limited stage disease, some oncologists may wish to retain the cisplatin/etoposide regimen in this subset of patients. However, there is little reason to suspect that the efficacy of treatment would be jeopardized by the substitution of carboplatin in this setting. Table 2 summarizes suggested "standard" regimens for current therapy of small cell lung cancer.

New Therapeutic Leads

Despite the fact that therapy has changed very little in the past decade, there are currently reasons for encouragement. Two major areas of investigation are likely to improve therapy for patients with small cell lung cancer in the near future.

Table 2. Standard regimens

- Carboplatin AUC 6.0 IV day 1
  Etoposide 80-100mg/m^2 IV days 1, 2, 3

- Cisplatin 60-80mg/m^2 IV day 1
  Etoposide 80-100mg/m^2 IV days 1, 2, 3

- Cyclophosphamide 1000mg/m^2 day 1
  Doxorubicin 45mg/m^2 IV day 1
  Etoposide 80-100mg/m^2 IV days 1, 2, 3

- Ifosfamide 4-5mg/m^2 total dose day 1 or days 1 to 5
  Etoposide 60mg/m^2 days 1, 2, 3

- Carboplatin AUC=5 day 1 or Cisplatin 60mg/m^2 day 1

The first major area of investigation which produces important therapeutic leads is based on a better understanding of the biology of small cell
lung cancer. This area will not be detailed here but has been reviewed by
others recently [1, 6]. Over the next several years, it is likely that mech-
anistically-based therapy will prove to be not only more effective than
previous therapy, but much less toxic. However, at this time, these treatments represent only an exciting potential. They are not yet feasible or
practical and very few clinical trials are currently active. Nonetheless,
this area of investigation deserves a very high priority for further development.

The second general area has been the development and introduction of
several new cytotoxic agents (paclitaxel, docetaxel, gemcitabine, vinorelbine, topotecan, irinotecan). These drugs are currently on the market for
several indications and presently very little data are available concerning
small cell lung cancer. However, multiple phase II trials have been done
or are in progress, and phase III trials are likely to promptly follow. It is
ironic that these same new agents have been studied considerably more
in patients with non-small cell lung cancer and all show noteable activity.
The most likely prospect for immediate improvement in therapy for small
cell patients involves further study and definition of the value of these
new cytotoxic agents. Table 3 illustrates the available phase II data of
these newer agents in patients with both previously untreated and previously treated tumors [7-13]. Paclitaxel has thus far been studied more
than any of the other agents and these data will be reviewed further here.

The single agent activity of paclitaxel has been investigated in previously untreated patients and in refractory patients. Prior to the general
availability of paclitaxel, two phase II trials investigated the efficacy of
this drug as first-line treatment of extensive stage patients. Ettinger et

Table 3. New agents in small-cell lung cancer [7-13]

	Response rate	
	Previously untreated	Previously treated
Paclitaxel	52%	29%
Docetaxel	25%	13%
Topotecan	27%	10%
Gemcitabine	27%	–
Vinorelbine	27%	16%
Irinotecan	50%	41%

al. [7] used a paclitaxel dose of $250mg/m^2$ by 24-hour infusion in a group of 36 patients. Eleven partial responses were observed and three other patients probably also had a partial response, but the required confirmatory scans after four weeks of remission were not performed. Kirschling et al. [8] obtained a response rate of 62% in a group of 37 patients, using an identical dose and schedule of paclitaxel. Due to the limited availability of the drug at that time, patients in both trials were switched to standard regimens after only four doses of paclitaxel; the response duration or survival cannot be ascertained from these trials. In both studies, subsequent treatment with a platinum/etoposide regimen produced additional responses, suggesting incomplete cross-resistance between paclitaxel and these agents.

Results of a phase II study in previously treated patients has also been reported by Smit et al. [13]. All 24 patients in this phase II trial had received at least one previous chemotherapy regimen, and all had developed progressive disease within three months of receiving previous chemotherapy. Seven patients (29%) had partial responses to paclitaxel ($175mg/m^2$, 3-hour infusion). The duration of response was brief in most patients (median 108 days, range 64 to 243 days), but suggested activity in refractory tumors.

On the basis of these data, paclitaxel has single agent activity comparable to that of the best agents in the treatment of small cell lung cancer. The results are particularly impressive in patients with refractory small cell lung cancer, since most reported response rates with single agents or combination regimens have been less than 15% in this group of patients. These single agent studies provide strong rationale for the continued development of paclitaxel and its incorporation into combination chemotherapy regimens. This is also true for the other new agents, but at present the majority of these combination data are with paclitaxel.

Information regarding the use of paclitaxel in combination regimens is also limited to several phase II studies. Many of these studies have been reported only in preliminary form, with scanty survival data. In most studies, paclitaxel has been combined either with a platinum agent or with a combination of platinum/etoposide. However, other novel combinations are now being investigated, in which paclitaxel is combined with other new agents (e.g. vinorelbine, topotecan), and these results are eagerly awaited.

The largest experience with this three-drug regimen has been reported by our group [14,15]. In our initial trial, the following regimen was used: paclitaxel $135mg/m^2$ by 1-hour IV infusion, day 1; carboplatin AUC 5.0

IV, day 1; etoposide 50mg alternating with 100mg PO, days 1-10, repeated every 21 days for four courses. Patients with limited stage disease received concurrent radiation therapy to a total of 45Gy (single daily dose, 1.8Gy/day) beginning with the third course of chemotherapy. This therapy proved highly efficacious and was well tolerated in a group of 38 patients, with response rates in limited and extensive stage disease of 93% and 65%, respectively, and median survivals of 17 months (limited stage) and 7 months (extensive stage).

This regimen was extremely well tolerated, and based on emerging data with the paclitaxel/carboplatin combination in non-small cell lung cancer, a subsequent second phase II study was performed using higher doses. The paclitaxel dose was increased from 135mg/m^2 to 200mg/m^2, the carboplatin dose increased from AUC 5.0 to AUC 6.0, and the etoposide dose remained unchanged. Limited stage patients received radiation therapy as in the first study. A total of 79 patients were treated with this higher dose regimen, which again proved efficacious and well tolerated. Table 4 summarizes and compares results using these two sequential regimens. Myelosuppression was more severe with the higher dose regimen. Grade III/IV leukopenia was observed in 71% of patients (38% of courses) with the higher dose regimen as compared to 24% of patients (11% of courses) with the lower dose regimen. Complications related to myelosuppression remained relatively infrequent, and the frequency of hospitalization for neutropenia and fever did not increase with the higher dose regimen. Other non-hematologic toxicities were also not significantly different with the higher dose regimen.

These sequential studies do not allow definitive comparisons of treatment efficacy, but improved efficacy was suggested with the higher dose regimen. Median survival with extensive disease was significantly better (10 months vs. 7 months, p = .008). In limited stage patients, median survival was somewhat prolonged (20 months vs. 17 months), but was not statistically significant.

The results demonstrate that a full dose of paclitaxel can be added as a third drug to a carboplatin/etoposide regimen while preserving an acceptable toxicity profile. With this regimen, the median survival, one-year survival, and actuarial two-year survival for patients with either limited or extensive stage small cell lung cancer are similar to the best reported results using other combination chemotherapy regimens.

Reck et al. [16] have studied the same three-drug combination, using lower doses of all three drugs (paclitaxel 135mg/m^2, 3-hour IV infusion, day 1; carboplatin AUC 5.0, day 1; etoposide 50mg PO days 2-8). They

Table 4. Paclitaxel/carboplatin/oral etoposide in small-cell lung cancer [15]

	Lower Dose Regimen		Higher Dose Regimen	
	Number	%	Number	%
Number of evaluable patients	38		79	
Efficacy				
• Complete responses				
Limited stage	6/15	40	29/41	71
Extensive stage	4/23	17	8/38	21
• Objective responses				
Limited stage	14/15	93	40/41	98
Extensive stage	15/23	65	32/38	84
• Median survival (months)				
Limited stage	17		20	
Extensive stage	7		10	
Toxicity				
• Hospitalization, neutropenia/ fever	15	39 (11% of courses)	25	32 (9% of courses)
• Grade 3/4 leukopenia	9	24	36	71
• Treatment-related death	1	3	2	3
• Grade 3/4 esophagitis	6	16	18	23

observed an overall response rate of 77% (25% complete responses) in an interim analysis of the first 61 patients treated. Survival data have not yet been reported.

A phase I trial evaluating the addition of paclitaxel to a cisplatin/etoposide regimen was recently completed by Kelly et al. [17]. The recommended doses of the three drugs determined by this Phase I study were: paclitaxel 175mg/m^2, 3-hour IV infusion, day 1; cisplatin 80mg/m^2 IV, day 1; etoposide 80mg/m^2 IV, days 1-3. This regimen used G-CSF (5μg/kg/day, beginning day 4 until WBC >10,000/μL). In a group of 23 patients, an 82% response rate was observed, with a median survival of ten months. This three-drug regimen is currently being further evaluated in a phase II trial by the Southwest Oncology Group.

Preliminary results of three phase II trials of paclitaxel plus either cisplatin or carboplatin have been reported [18-20]. The response rates are high, but only one trial reported a median survival of nine months in a group of extensive stage patients. Additional data are required regarding these two-drug combinations, since the impact of eliminating etoposide from first-line treatment is not known.

Several other small trials have studied other novel combinations. The combination of topotecan ($1.0mg/m^2$ IV, days 1-5) and paclitaxel ($135mg/m^2$, 24-hour IV infusion, day 5) every three weeks was reported by Jett et al. [21]. This treatment required the use of G-CSF. In a small group of extensive stage patients, a 92% response rate was reported. The median survival in this group was 12 months, with 25% actuarial two-year survival. Confirmation of these results in larger numbers of patients is warrented.

The activity of the paclitaxel/topotecan was also suggested by our recently completed phase I trial evaluating the three-drug combination of paclitaxel/carboplatin/topotecan. Seven of ten previously treated small cell lung cancer patients had objective responses [22].

The combination of vinorelbine and paclitaxel has been evaluated in a phase I study in patients with previously treated small cell lung cancer [23]. The doses found tolerable were: paclitaxel $180mg/m^2$ (3-hour infusion), day 1; vinorelbine $30mg/m^2$ IV on day 1; cycles repeated every 21 days. The cumulative dose of vinorelbine was considerably lower than with most standard weekly schedules, but seven of 22 evaluable patients (32%) had objective responses. All patients had received previous treatment.

The possibility of improving treatment results by adding paclitaxel to a platinum/etoposide combination has been of interest. Two groups are now conducting randomized trials to directly address the role of paclitaxel in the treatment of small cell lung cancer. An ongoing trial is being performed at the Sarah Cannon Cancer Center and in the Response Oncology Network. The three-drug combination of paclitaxel/carboplatin/oral etoposide is being compared to a standard carboplatin/etoposide regimen. At present, 150 patients have entered this trial. A planned CALGB/Intergroup trial will also address this issue. Paclitaxel/cisplatin/etoposide will be compared to cisplatin/etoposide. Results of these trials will determine whether the addition of paclitaxel to current standard regimens improves the results of treatment for small cell lung cancer.

The development of the other newer agents is also ongoing, and should remain a priority. The combination of paclitaxel and topotecan is active, and the development of tolerable regimens containing these two drugs is being pursued by several investigators. The evaluation of other new, active drugs (e.g. gemcitabine, irinotecan, docetaxel and vinorelbine) in combination may produce valuable new treatment options. If truly non-cross resistant, active regimens are found with several of these new drugs, a re-evaluation of treatment with alternating chemotherapy regimens would be reasonable. In addition to new drug combinations, further exploration of new administration schedules of the taxanes (e.g. weekly dosing) may optimize therapeutic efficacy.

After many years of relative pessimism regarding opportunities for therapeutic improvements in small cell lung cancer, the current availability of several new agents with novel mechanisms of action represent an exciting potential. After a relatively slow start, interest in evaluating these new agents in the treatment of small cell is increasing, and these results will be available in the near future.

References

1. Comis RL, Friedland DM, Good BC (1998): Small cell lung cancer: A perspective on the past and a preview of the future. Oncology 12 (Suppl 2):44-50
2. Turrisi AT (1998) Integrating thoracic radiotherapy in the treatment of limited stage small cell lung cancer. Oncology 12 (Suppl 2):15-18
3. Ihde DC, Pass HI, Glatstein E (1997) Cancer of the lung: Small cell lung cancer. In: DeVita VT Jr, Hellman S, Rosenberg SA (eds) Cancer: Principles and Practice of Oncology. 5th ed, Lippincott-Raven, Philadelphia, pp 911-949
4. Wande P, Payne D (1992) Does thoracic irradiation improve survival and local control in limited-stage small cell carcinoma of the lung? A meta-analysis. J Clin Oncol 10:890-895
5. Kosmidis PA, Samantas E, Fountzilas G et al (1994) Cisplatin/etoposide versus carboplatin/etoposide chemotherapy and irradiation in small cell lung cancer: A randomized phase III study. Semin Oncol 21 (Suppl 3):23-30
6. Johnson BE, Kelley MJ (1998) Autocrine growth factors and neuroendocrine markers in the development of small cell lung cancer. Oncology 12 (Suppl 2):11-14
7. Ettinger DS, Finkelstein DM, Sarma RP et al (1995) Phase II study of paclitaxel in patients with extensive disease small cell lung cancer: an Eastern Cooperative Group study. J Clin Oncol 13:1430-1435
8. Kirschling RJ, Jurg SH, Jett JR (1994) A phase II trial of Taxol and G-CSF in previously untreated patients with extensive stage small cell lung cancer. Proc Am Soc Clin Oncol (Abstr) 13:326
9. Cormier Y, Eisenhauer E, Muldal A et al (1994) Gemcitabine is an active new agent in previously untreated extensive small cell lung cancer: a study of the National Cancer Institute of Canada Clinical Treatment Group. Ann Oncol 5:283-285
10. Perez-Soler R, Glisson BS, Lee JS et al (1995) Phase II study of topotecan in patients with small cell lung cancer refractory to etoposide. Proc Am Soc Clin Oncol (Abstr)14:355
11. Masuda N, Fukuoka M, Kusumaki Y et al (1992) CPT-11: A new derivative of camptothecin for the treatment of refractory or relapsed small cell lung cancer. J Clin Oncol 10:1225-1229

12. Jassem J, Karnicka-Mindkowska H, van Pottelsberghe CH et al (1993) Phase II study of vinorelbine (navelbine) in previously treated small cell lung cancer patients. Eur J Cancer 29:1720-1722
13. Smit EF, Fokkema E, Biesma B et al (1998) A phase II study of paclitaxel in heavily pretreated patients with small cell lung cancer. Br J Cancer 77(2):347-351
14. Hainsworth JD, Stroup SL, Greco FA (1996) Paclitaxel, carboplatin, and extended schedule etoposide in the treatment of small cell lung carcinoma. Cancer 77:2458-2463
15. Hainsworth JD, Gray JR, Stroup SL et al (1997) Paclitaxel, carboplatin, and extended-schedule etoposide in the treatment of small cell lung cancer: comparison of sequential phase II trials using different dose intensities. J Clin Oncol 15:3464-3470
16. Reck M, Jagos V, Kaukel E et al (1997) Chemotherapy of limited stage small cell lung cancer with carboplatin, paclitaxel and oral etoposide: a phase II trial. Lung Cancer 18 (Suppl 1):31 (Abstr)
17. Kelly K, Wood ME, Bunn PA Jr (1997) A phase I study of cisplatin, etoposide, and paclitaxel (PET) in small cell lung cancer (SCLC). Lung Cancer 18 (Suppl 1):28 (Abstr)
18. Faoro C, Wolf M, Schroder M et al (1997) Paclitaxel/cisplatin chemotherapy in extensive stage small cell lung cancer. Lung Cancer 18 (Suppl 1):51 (Abstr)
19. Deppermann KM, Kurzeja A, Lichey J et al (1997) Paclitaxel and carboplatin in advanced SCLC: A phase II study. Lung Cancer 18 (Suppl 1):46 (Abstr)
20. Nair S, Marschke R, Grill J et al (1997) A phase II study of paclitaxel (Taxol) and cisplatin (CDDP) in the treatment of extensive stage small cell lung cancer. Proc Am Soc Clin Oncol 16:454A (Abstr)
21. Jett JR, Day R, Levitt M et al (1997) Topotecan and paclitaxel in extensive stage small cell lung cancer (ED-SCLC) in patients without prior therapy. Lung Cancer 18 (Suppl 1):13 (Abstr)
22. Raefsky EL, Hainsworth JD, Burris HA et al (1988) Phase I trial of topotecan, paclitaxel, and carboplatin in patients with advanced refractory malignancies. Proc Am Soc Clin Oncol (In press)
23. Jaffaioli RV, Faccini G, Tortoriello A et al (1997) Phase I study of vinorelbine and paclitaxel in small cell lung cancer. Cancer Chemother Pharmacol 41:86-90

Progress in Lung Cancer Surgery

G. MOTTA

Introduction

The turning point of modern surgery for lung cancer treatment can be identified around the beginning of the 80s, when the general thoracic surgery already mature to pave the way to the present advances, was initially meeting the novel organisation of surgical minds inspired by the New International System for Staging Lung Cancer [1]. The System was firstly presented by Clifton F. Mountain in 1985, during the IV IASLC World Congress on lung cancer in Toronto. At that time the surgical attitude was generally inclined to resect lung cancers radically whenever technically possible, according to the diffuse belief that "resectability is a state of mind" and "the decision whether to resect a particular neoplasm often depends on the respective surgeon's philosophy more than on objective facts"! [2]. Indeed, the great experience previously acquired on the field of World War II, the ensuing establishment of modern general thoracic surgery with the direct filiation of cardiac and vascular ones, and the meaningful results already obtained on the threshold of the 80s in terms of prolonged survival after lung resection (27-40% 5 yr) and of lowered operative mortality (-10%) [3-5], would have then really allowed thoracic surgeons to think in such a way!

The new rationale for staging lung cancer by grouping patients in key stages according to TNM and the end results after surgery, represented a new cultural tool helping the surgeon not only to recognise the disease better, but also to provide a better surgical procedure. It has represented, indeed, a step forward of the mind over the hands!

The staging system based now upon a large body of statistically accrued data, has even become the universal language for formally presenting the disease and comparing the results, as well as the sound method to analytically study the clinical courses after surgery or, even, after medical treatment protocols.

Nevertheless, in spite of such a large amount of demonstrated advantages, criticism of the staging rationale and proposals of minor changes or full revisions, have since the beginning been pushed forward. This situation, playfully defined by J.R Jett as an attempt at "… casting aspersions on the merits of some aspect of the staging system…" [6], has recently pressed Mountain to operate a substantial revision of the System [7] and to offer a new lymph node map (Fig.2) [8].

According to present revision, the stage groups have become eight, the survival rates have all been recalculated offering better analytical responses, while actually getting further statistical support from parent studies [9,10]. In more detail, the descriptor T4 now includes those satellite tumor nodule(s) lying within the ipsilateral primary tumor-lobe, and the subgroup T3N0 is pushed back to the stage IIB, according to the consistency of survival rates with the subgroup T2N1, stage IIB. As far as the new lymph node map, station No. 4 is confirmed as mediastinal one according to the Naruke map (Fig. 1), but differently named as "Lower Paratracheal Nodes".

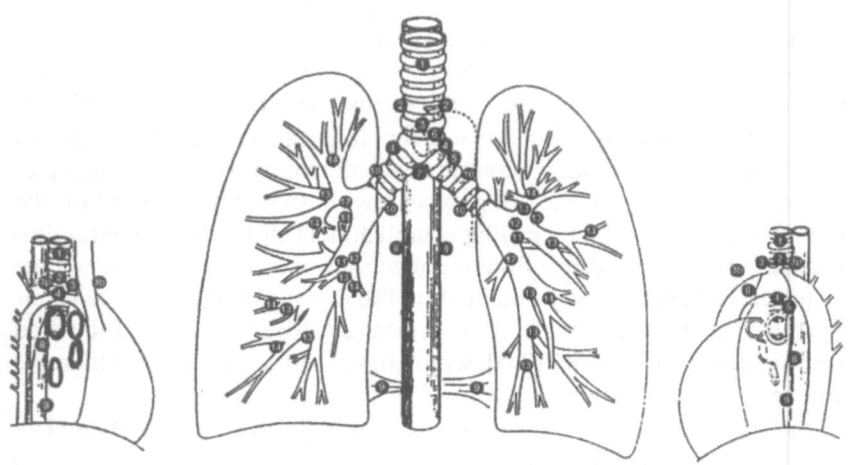

The Naruke Lymph Node Map

#1 Superior mediastinal or highest mediastinal	**#8 Paraesophageal (below carina)**
#2 Paratracheal	**#9 Pulmonary ligament**
#3 Pretracheal, retrotracheal or posteriomediastinal (#3p), and anterior mediastinal (#3a)	**#10 Hilar**
	#11 Interlobar
	#12 Lobar ---- upper lobe middle lobe and lower lobe
#4 Tracheobronchial	
#5 Subaortic or Botallo's	**#13 Segmental**
#6 Paraortic (ascending aorta)	**#14 Subsegmental**
#7 Subcarinal	

Fig. 1. Naruke lymph node map

Regional Nodal Stations For Lung Cancer Staging

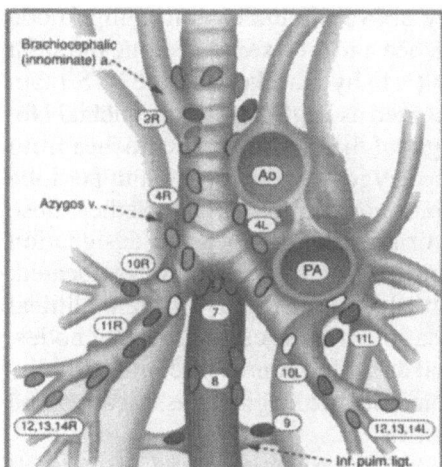

Superior Mediastinal Nodes

● 1 Highest Mediastinal

● 2 Upper Paratracheal

● 3 Pre-vascular and Retrotracheal

● 4 Lower Paratracheal
(including Azygos Nodes)

N_2 = single digit, ipsilateral
N_3 = single digit, contralateral or supraclavicular

Aortic Nodes

● 5 Subaortic (A-P window)

● 6 Para-aortic (ascending
aorta or phrenic)

Inferior Mediastinal Nodes

● 7 Subcarinal

● 8 Paraesophageal
(below carina)

● 9 Pulmonary Ligament

N_1 Nodes

○ 10 Hilar

● 11 Interlobar

● 12 Lobar

● 13 Segmental

● 14 Subsegmental

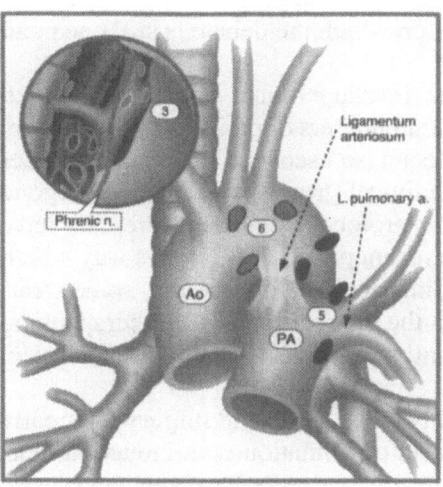

(Mountain/Dresler modifications from Naruke/ATS-LCSG Map)

© 1997 Reprints are permissible for educational use only

Provided as an educational service by
Bristol-Myers Squibb Oncology.

Fig. 2. Mountain new lymph node map

Station No. 4, right, has represented a true matter of concern simply because in another even more widely expanded lymph node map, the one supported by the American Thoracic Society (ATS) (Fig. 3), the same group of nodes already defined by Naruke as mediastinal (N2), No. 4, "tracheobronchial", located "in the obtuse angle level with and beneath the azygos vein", were not considered as mediastinal. Furthermore, No. 4 station is located immediately above the underlying lymph node groups which are just distal to the trachea and are extended along the stem bronchi and defined as No.10, Hilar (N1) by Naruke. On the ATS map, both these regions of nodes were designed as Right Tracheobronchial No. 10 R, and defined as "nodes to the right of the midline of the trachea from the level of the cephalic border of the azygos vein to the right upper lobe bronchus". There was, for long time, no mention as to whether these nodes were to be considered as N1 or N2 and there was no designation for "Hilar" nodes. The designation N2 for those superiorly located, appeared only years later. Obviously, due to the rather different clinical prospects linked to the different allocation of these close groups of nodes, one can easily imagine how equivocal and what source of continued misunderstanding such an issue was, from both the staging classification and the prognostic previsions after treatment.

Nevertheless, despite the conceptual improvements and Mountain's complete revision, the issue concerning the staging of lung cancer still appears as a real cultural challenge, on which the debate is still open and a final agreement pending.

On the other hand, besides the formal clinical application which requires controlled groups, significant numbers of patients and long-term follow up, the staging system has been also used as a statistical shoulder for those still numerically limited clinical groups who have undergone new surgical or combined treatment protocols, and therefore they have begun the clinical course in a more recent past. Through this way which allows consideration of only their intermediate end points, some treatment protocols have already gained the recognition of true therapeutical advances as well as clearly representing progress in the field of surgical oncology of the lung.

Surgical results with early staged NSCLC, extended surgery for locally advanced NSCLC, surgery alone or in combination with induction therapy for N2 mediastinal disease and surgical approach to lung metastases, belong by right to this category of present surgical achievements.

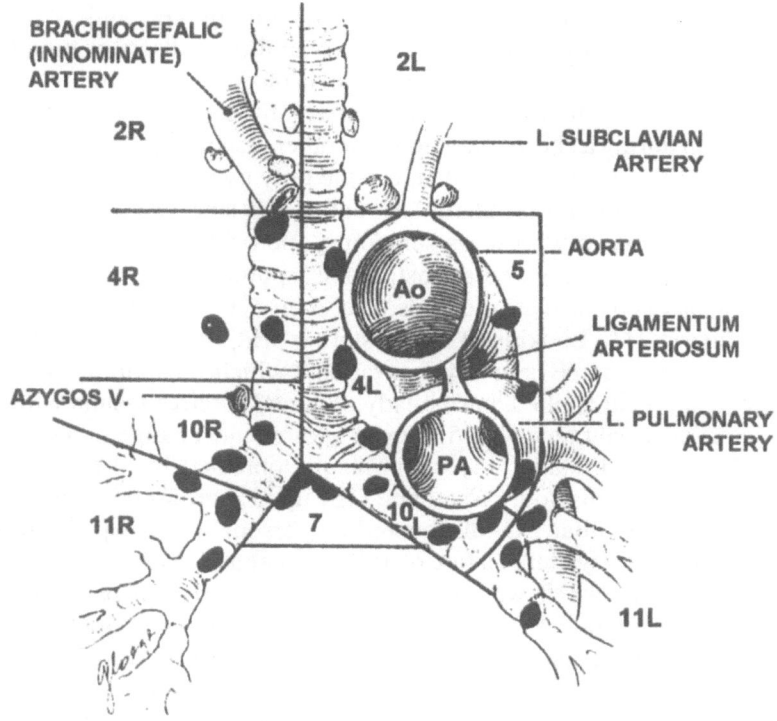

The ATS Lymph Node Map

Fig. 3. ATS lymph node map

Surgical Results with Early Staged NSCLC

A part from some subtle and even worthwhile remarks made by epidemiologists [11,12] and the negative experience with previous mass surveys programms [13], when dealing with the old and somewhat controversial problem of screening for lung cancer, we must not deny the clinical evidence that patients affected by early stage lung cancer have the greatest chance for cure. Accordingly, any effort to positively cope with this task trying to discover lung cancer as early as possible, mainly when it is still roentgenographically occult, has to be taken in due consideration. Based on the assumption that the overall survival for patients with pathologic stage I is of 67% (range 55 to 72) according to the ISS database [7], any clinical reported result which exceeds the maximum survival peak of 72%, has to be appropriately highlighted and possibly followed-up. It is also evident that the probability to discover tumor in an early stage and even still asymptomatic, is closely connected with the ability to anticipate the diagnosis. Nowadays, the lucky event of finding a coin lesion during a chest X-ray done for other reasons, or the yield from a more involving mass survey plan, are the only two real possibilities to cope positively with this problem. Presently, only some Japanese groups are actively engaged with mass-screening upon selected population at recognised risk, by using as diagnostic tools, sputum cytology, fiberoptic bronchoscopy and correlate methods, and, more recently, the mobile spiral volumetric TC. Looking at the western world, only an authoritative north-American source is presently available which, in spite of the limited screening plan applied, has already obtained positive results with an increase of survival rate up to 45%, even without any change in the treatment plan for each stage [14]. The results obtained by the Japanese groups are interesting too. Watanabe [15] upon a group of 27 patients affected by "early hilar LC" discovered by personal check-up and mass screening as well, registered a rate of 100% 5 year and 91,7% 10 year survival after surgery, which was mainly represented by tissue-sparing bronchoplastic procedures. Fujimura [16] upon 198 cases of peripheral "Rx occult bronchogenic squamous cell carcinoma" discovered by mass screening, obtained a rate of 90% 5 year survival after surgical resection by using radical segmentectomy. Sano [17] upon a group of 208 patients affected by peripheral early stage I tumors with an overall 5 year survival of 70% after resection, found a significant difference in survival among the mass screening group of patients who showed a rate of 87,9% and the group discovered by a personal check-up, where this rate was much lower (46,9%). Shimizu [18] over a group of 41 cases of "minute peripheral primary pulmonary carcinoma" detected by mass screening survey, obtained a meaningful 5 year survival rate of 89,4%.

On the other hand, the positive experience of the above mentioned North-American Group backed by Geno Saccommanno, and based upon a case-by-case sputum cytology examination as the first check, has clearly demonstrated the clinical usefulness and the cost-effectiveness of an even limited screening plan tailored to a community Hospital, responsible for a population at risk due to high incidence of heavy smokers and uranium miners.

Extended Surgery for Locally Advanced NSCLC

Extended Surgery for Apical Invasive Lung Cancer

Apical invasive lung cancer with or without Pancoast's syndrome according to the anterior location of some of them, belongs to Stage III in relation to its advanced peripheral T (T3-4), coupled or not with an ipsilateral mediastinal lymphatic spread (N2) [19]. Stage IIIA includes the "still operable" T3 N1-2 M0 tumors, while the involvement of the vertebral body (T4- Stage IIIB) by those apical tumors which are more posteriorly located, decides the assignment to the true Pancoast's tumor class as well as their conventional level of inoperability. A unique thoracic and arm irradiated pain, the Horner's syndrome, the destruction of bone and the atrophy of hand muscles represent the established clinical scene of Pancoast's syndrome. On the other hand, the other apical invasive but not Pancoast's tumors since they are anteriorly located right above the anterior side of the thoracic outlet, show specific symptoms ultimately based on phrenic nerve palsy, shoulder pain and venous dilatation in the limb, through the involvement of the subclavian vein.

The initial radio-surgical approach tried by Shaw et al. in 1961 [20] had basically contributed not only to provide a sound treatment protocol but also to improve the knowledge of these tumors until then considered of unclear origin and far from any cure. The 31% 5-year (44% in patients without nodal involvement), the 26% 10-year and the 22% 15-year survivals reported by Paulson in 1985 [24], still represent a therapeutic cornerstone.

Afterwards, the surgical contributions by Miller [22], Attar [23] and Stanford [24] in the 70s and those by Wright [25], Shaian [26] and De Meester [27] collected in the 80s, further expanded the clinical experience obtaining a 5 year survival rate of 32% ± 3.3 with a range from 27 to 42%. What is interesting to say is that, at that time, they were facing the so-called whole symptom inclusive "superior pulmonary sulcus syndrome", where a clear difference between symptoms of more "anterior" or "posterior" origin was not considered at all.

In more recent years, the contribution of Dartevelle [28] was of great importance in this field for two main reasons: the use of a new transcervical-thoracic route for the handling of all tumors invading the cervical structures of thoracic outlet better, and the definite anatomo-surgical classification of apical tumors in two main groups, according to their more anterior or posterior location within the apical area, above the thoracic outlet. Through such basic contribution a true new sight has been opened in the "misty" area traditionally named "superior pulmonary sulcus". Moreover, the radical resection of apical tumors en-bloc with chest wall and posteriorly till the hemivertebrectomy in a few highly selected cases, has gained in the hands of the French group chaired by Dartevelle, an overall 5 year survival of 34,5% with a median follow-up time of 2,5 years and a mean survival of 18 months, over a selected group of 55 patients [29].

In a parallel study presented by Niwa and Masaoka in 1993 [30], a similar anterior approach was followed with a smaller group of 8 patients affected by apical tumors more anteriorly located. In spite of the favourable surgical approach and the ensuing positive short-term results, all eight patients died from recurrence 4 months to 3 years after surgery.

More recently, Grunenwald from the Institute Mountsouris, Paris [31], has applied the transmanubrial osteomuscolar sparing approach in 6 patients, obtaining an excellent exposure of thoracic outlet, while sparing the osteomuscolar component of the cervical and shoulder articulations, thus avoiding the functional and cosmetic consequences of clavicle resection. The same author also performed [32] a total vertebrectomy for an en-bloc resection of lung cancer invading the spine, thus demonstrating the feasibility of the procedure, and the positive clinical result which one could obtain by this more advanced surgical step.

The Extended Lobectomy with Bronchial Reanastomosis for Ostial Bronchial Tumors with Mediastinal Proximity

This matter regards those central tumors which are located in or next to the lobar bronchial orifices and whose complete resection would require a pneumonectomy, if one wants to follow the dictates of conventional surgery. On the contrary, using the more refined procedure of extended lobectomy with bronchial reanastomosis (Bronchoplastic Lobectomies - BLs), it is possible to remove en-bloc the lobe together with its bronchial junction and a sleeve or a wedge of the contiguous main bronchus wall, while sparing one or two still healthy lobes. The extent of main bronchus wall to be removed is ruled by the size and location of tumor as well as by the mode of bronchial reanastomosis. The operation is systematically concluded by reanastomising the opposite free bronchial cut edges, namely the main bronchus stump on one side and the intermediate or lower bronchus stump on the other, so recovering one or two still healthy lobes, whose bronchial stem has been proximally interrupted as it is included in the resectional area. Moreover, BLs are again indicated for radically resecting those peripheral tumors which have disclosed positive nodes (N1) infiltrating the foot of the corresponding lobar bronchus. Such special extended lobectomies correlate well with the criteria of oncological clearance being complete resections and, at the same time, conservative procedures by right. On the other hand, pneumonectomy is the obliged procedure for approaching these tumors when one decides to follow the conventional surgery. Moreover, since they are true conservative procedures able to spare lobes, BLs recognise variable indication criteria, according to the cardiac and pulmonary reserve of patients undergoing lung resection. Therefore, in case of ventilatory insufficiency the indication can be either *relative,* when the value of FEV1 presents less than -25% of the predicted, or *absolute* when this value goes under -45%. On the other hand, BLs can be *electively* performed upon patients in good physical condition whenever technically possible, provided that a qualified surgical standard can be assured.

Personal Contribution

Since the first bronchoplastic procedure performed by Allison in 1952 [33] and in line with the following worldwide experience (Table. 1) [34-41], we have performed, starting from the early 80s, 70 BLs among a group of 107 tracheobronchoplastic procedures also including tracheal pipe, carena and tracheobronchial angle. BLs have been performed according to the three well established modes of "upper sleeve lobectomy", "upper wedge-bronchial lobectomy" and "lower bilobectomy and upper lobe turn up bronchoplasty", which are recognised to offer the best oncological clearance [42]. At times, some changes have been made to these basic procedures, dealing with the completeness of resection as well as the property of restored airway.

Upper Sleeve Lobectomy (Fig. 4)

For tumor located along the upper bronchial orifice, a sleeve of about 2 cm of mainstem bronchus is resected en-bloc with the upper lobe. The proximal stump is reanastomized to intermediate bronchus while the middle and lower bronchus are saved.

Upper Wedge-Bronchial Lobectomy (Fig. 5)

The upper lobe is resected together with a "wedge" of mainstem bronchus. The bronchial "wedge" is tailored larger proximally to give the

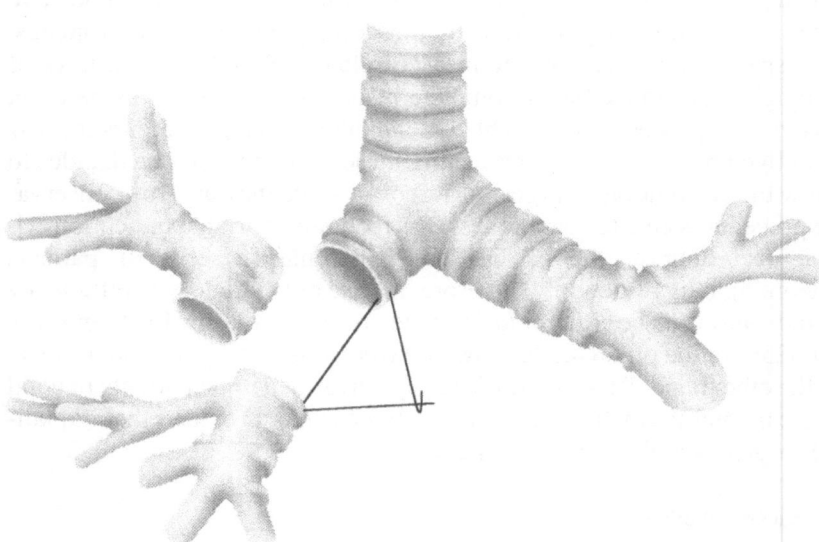

Fig. 4. Upper sleeve lobectomy

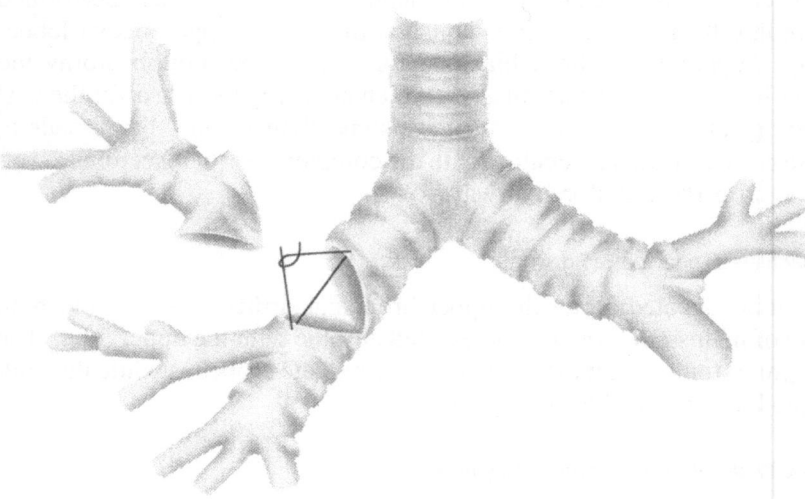

Fig. 5. Upper wedge-bronchial lobectomy

Table 1. Previous experience in bronchoplastic lobectomies

Authors		Pts.	Survival	
			5 yr	10 yr
Allison [33]	1952			
Mac Hale [34]	1966	59	26%	
Paulson [35]	1970	54	39%	
Rees [36]	1970	46	35%	
Vogt-Moykopf [37]	1986	48	35%	
Faber [38]	1987	118	33%	22%
Watanabe [39]	1990	75	45%	
Van Den Bosch [40]	1991	145	49%	37%
Deslauriers [41]	1993	142	46%	33%

greatest clearance around the bronchial junction. On the opposite side, the resection remains incomplete, since a strip of mainstem bronchial wall is left in place. Therefore, this "wedge" bronchial lobectomy is a less heavy procedure than the previous "sleeve" one, since the bronchial tree is not completely interrupted.

Lower Bilobectomy and Upper Lobe "Turn Up" Bronchoplasty (Fig. 6)

This procedure is applied in tumors of the intermediate or lower lobar bronchus which show the tendency to grow towards the medial wall of the mainstem bronchus. The surgical clearance assured by such distal extended bilobectomy (uni on the left) will involve the intermediate bronchus (only the lower on the left), together with the upper bronchial spur and the medial wall of the mainstem bronchus, reaching proximally the tracheobronchial angle and the related lymph node stations. This results in an oncological benefit of more than 1,5 centimetres extended proximally, along the medial side of main stem wall. The upper lobe to be spared is then turned medially and upwards anticlockwise over the hinge of its residual proximal upper bronchial rim. The bronchial orifice, properly tailored diagonally, is now able to fit together with the opposite mainstem stump and there be reanastomized. The re-implanted upper lobe now results to be more medially located with the major bronchial axis pointing straight down.

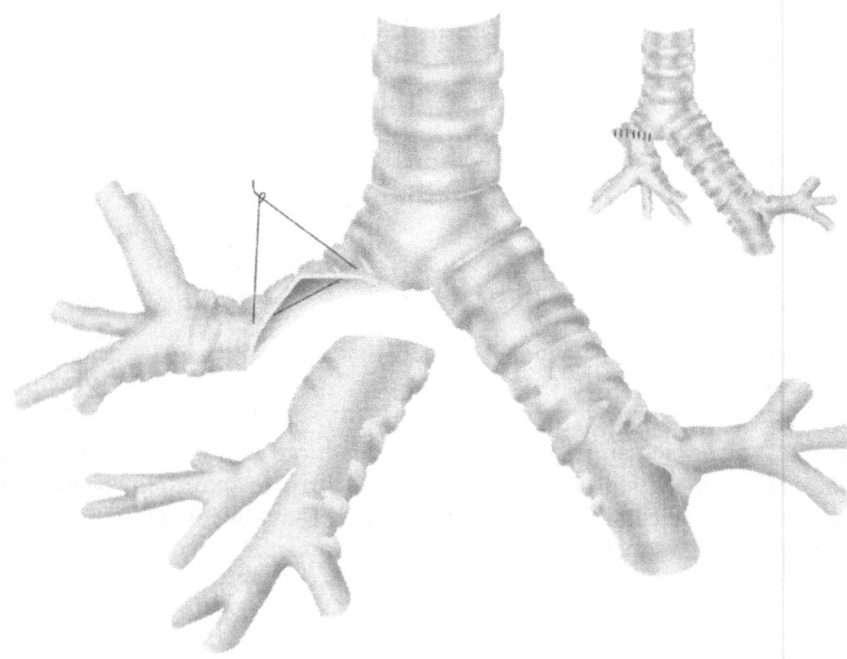

Fig. 6. Lower bilobectomy and upper lobe "turn up" bronchoplasty

Results and considerations

In the whole group of 70 patients with 66 males and 4 females (mean age 62 years with a range of 18-77) the 5 and 10 year actuarial survival, calculated by the Kaplan Meier's method, was respectively of 29 and 26%. In stage I, the 5 year and 10 year survival was a constant 41%, while it was of 42 and 35% in stage II and of 10% in stage IIIA. No patient in stage IIIB survived over 18 months. Tumor size appeared as a prognostic factor in multivariate analysis which recognizes also mediastinal proximity as a joined negative factor. Accordingly, in stage I and II, a subgroup of T2N0-1 tumors with a maximum diameter of over 5 cm (range 5,5-12 cm) (17 cases) showing a 5 year survival of 7%, was overstaged to T3 stage IIIA. Following such further selection, stage I 5 year and 10 year survival raised to a constant 75% rate (11 cases), the survival of stage II raised to 70% and 57%, respectively (10 cases), while the 5 year survival of stage IIIA (42 cases) was 8%. Mediastinal lymphoadenectomy, routinely performed, revealed 22 patients as N0 (32%), 30 as N1 (43%) and

18 (25%) as N2. five and ten-year survival was 36% in N0 group, while it was 40% and 36% in N1, and 0 in N2 group.

Bronchoplastic lobectomies, initially indicated for patients with severe ventilatory insufficiency (absolute indication), have been recently applied on an elective basis, without the pressure of an impaired pulmonary function [43]. The specific risks of BLs (positive margin, leak of suture lines, tardive bronchostenosis and recurrence) have to be deeply considered when one is dealing with such a kind of refined surgery [44]. Moreover the challenge of a risky completion pneumonectomy has to be also expected. BLs appeared curative for stage I and stage II patients with 5 year survival of 75% and 70% when these groups were stripped of the tumors of over 5 cm in their maximum diameter (overstaged as T3 stage IIIA according to the low survival and mediastinal proximity) [45, 46].

Moreover, the postoperative respiratory performance is clearly better and mortality less when compared with pneumonectomy [41].

In conclusion, BLs are curative for stage I and II tumors located in the ostial area of upper lobe bronchus or in the intermediate or lower bronchus. In such selected cases, BLs can really avoid pneumonectomy, while the related long-term survival is fully comparable to that of simple lobectomies. BLs alone, instead, as well as any other single treatment for locally advanced lung cancer, cannot be considered curative for stage IIIA central hilar tumors, in spite of the radicality of resection and the complete node dissection. Mediastinal proximity, the frequent N2 disease (25%) and the high number of large sized tumors (24%), appear really to play a relevant role in negatively affecting the survival of stage IIIA centrally located tumors (5 year survival: 8%).

Nevertheless, when dealing with the newer Inductive Multimodal Treatment for stage IIIA-N2 tumors, BLs, as a surgical share of such combined protocols, appear again as the best surgical option for all ostial-bronchial tumors, despite their actual progression. In such cases, as complete resections and tissue/function saving procedures, BLs, by assuring a better respiratory performance, could basically improve not only the quality but also the lenght of life in such a prognostically compromised group of patients.

Surgery Alone or in Combination with Induction Chemo (RT) Therapy for N2 Mediastinal Disease

N2 mediastinal disease has been for long time a widely debated matter from both diagnostic and therapeutical point of view, and the related treatment options have largely fluctuated in close connection with a continued search for a better strategy [47-49]. The assessment of mediastinal involvement in terms of imaging, level of stations interested, number of single lymph nodes involved and their structural changes, actually due to an expected infiltration, is the matter of concern. On the other hand, N2 mediastinal disease has meant for many years the exclusion from surgery, in line with previously settled clinical directions, of those patients complaining a clinical manifest N2 disease and, meanwhile, the sound obligation for the surgeon to recognise in the clinical setting through an involved work-up, as many patients as possible not to be denied surgery [47]. In such a concern, a subgroup with "more limited" mediastinal lymphatic invasion was identified as "clinically unsuspected N2" cases, just because, while actually escaping clinical staging, they are destined to be discovered only during thoracotomy. This subgroup enjoys a better prognostic expectation compared to the former one which, due to the clinical evidence of the mediastinal lymph node(s) involvement, would have usually been excluded from the benefit of surgery, since the related 5 year survival rate is very poor (< 9%).

The "clinical unsuspected, or unrecognised or unforeseen N2 disease" has been given great attention by a number of qualified surgical groups and, consequently, the general impact on survival of patients with N2 disease discovered at thoracotomy and undergoing complete resection, has been, on the whole, reconsidered.

Goldstraw [50] in a group of 578 patients who underwent thoracotomy because they were thought not to have N2 disease based on clinical staging, found that 149 cases were, in fact, positive for N2 at the routine surgical staging through a complete mediastinal lymph node dissection. In 127 of these latter cases (85%), a complete resection was performed with a resulting 5 year actuarial survival rate of 20,1%. Squamous cell and the involvement of one nodal station were the most important factors in survival, while neither the extent of resection nor the involvement of any specific nodal station influenced long-term survival. As for the value of intrathoracic staging, despite a negative rigorous preoperative investigation, the routine mediastinal lymph node dissection demonstrated a mediastinal positivity in 26% (149/578) of the total group of patients.

Upon a group of 115 patients with clinical N2 surgically explored by Watanabe [51], 53 of them underwent a complete resection with an overall survival of 20%. Moreover, in 47 patients whose ipsilateral N2 was not recognised before the operation, the overall 5 year survival was again of 20%, while the rate was 33%, when only the curatively resected cases were considered. Martini [52] reports a 5 year survival of 30% with a group of 151 completely resected patients complaining an ipsilateral N2 disease. De Leyn [53] upon a group of 103 patients with "unsuspected N2" discovered at thoracotomy, registered a 22% 5 year survival after complete resection. He concluded that resection is justified in patients with "unforeseen N2 disease", provided that a rigorous clinical staging of the mediastinum even by cervical mediastinoscopy or anterior mediastinotomy is performed. Such an approach will assure a high rate of resectability by excluding any form of major mediastinal lymph node involvement and allowing, instead, the disease to be discovered only at thoracotomy.

As a matter of fact, the above mentioned results obtained by completely resecting the limited N2 disease, have clearly demonstrated that this approach is to be followed, even if the end points in survival cannot be considered statistically significant when compared with the historical control of 15% obtained by Naruke [54], with the systematic dissection of mediastinal lymph node stations.

This rather steady situation met a substantial change with the development of Induction Chemo-Surgical Treatment Protocols which were, from the beginning, preferentially addressed against the associated N2 disease (STAGE 0 IIIA - T1-3 N2). These protocols were aimed basically at "downstaging" tumors by preoperative chemo or chemo+RT and, so, making unresectable tumors resectable, by reducing the volume and/or the local extension. Takita [55] first tried this approach in 1979, then Faber in 1989 [56] and Martini in 1993 [57]. These initial results collecting median survival rates of respectively 14.5, 22.1 (36.6 in resected patients) and 19 months (27 in resected patients), contributed to create a firm scientific background to the whole subject. It is interesting to note that the expected gradual progression of this research was dramatically boosted to a worldwide expansion by 1994, when Roth and Rosell [58, 59] published the impressive results of their own randomized studies. Roth [58] obtained a median survival of more than five times in the preoperative chemotherapy group (64 months) compared with the 11 months of the surgery alone group. Rosell [59] registered a median survival of 26 months in the group receiving chemotherapy prior surgery, while the other arm of the protocol receiving surgery plus radiotherapy showed a median survival of only eight months.

What is interesting to note is that these results have never been repeated, even if similar research plans have grown very active and in great number since then.

Presently, besides a diffuse inclined attention towards such Inductive Treatment Protocols for NSCLC [60, 61], a number of controlled studies are already in progress and, among them, the ones worthy of mention are those chaired respectively by Rush [62], Sugarbaker [63] and Mathisen [64]. The intermediate end points in survival of these protocols appear interesting, even if still far from the results of the previously mentioned couple of unique studies.

On the other hand, the chapter of Induction Therapy for Locally Advanced NSCLC represents now one of the most frequently requested subjects in discussion of the medical conferences on thoracic oncology, worldwide.

The Surgical Approach to Lung Metastases

The sound hypothesis of a surgical approach to the secondary (metastatic) lung tumors, as irregularly tried through the 60s and 70s, was for a long time skeptically considered [65-68].

The following great expansion of the "basic" knowledge on tumor progression at the end of the 70s [69-71], helped collaterally to widen this narrow horizon, offering to the surgeon's attention, the stimulating theory of the "metastatic stepwise cascade". According to this, some organs like the liver, lung and brain were thought to act as a preferential key site, where the initial metastasis from a primary solid tumor could be allowed to stay quiescent for a variable length of time, before initiating the final step of systemic diffusion. Therefore, the idea "to be still in time", in spite of the already started but still possibly limited progression of the tumor into the preferential organ, fostered the surgical interest and, accordingly, an increasing number of surgeons and institutions (Table. 2) were involved, during the 80s, with the advanced project of directly removing metastases from the lung.

With the beginning of the 90s the problem was fully taken on by two well known European groups, namely the one at Brompton, London, and the other one at Thoraxklinik, Heidelberg. Through their contribution, the whole clinical matter was then organised better and sound guidelines for a definite surgical approach to the lung metastatic disease were settled. First of all, the concept of pulmonary metastasectomy was closely linked to that of the intent of cure [72]. Accordingly, any attempt of palliation was excluded from this advanced surgical approach, which is aimed at removing, by one or more conservative operations, all the pulmonary metastases, uni or even bilaterally located. Goldstraw [72] firstly

Table 2. Previous experience in pulmonary metastasectomies

Institutions	Authors	Pts
MSKCC, New York	Cahan, Martini, 1973-79	473
STANF, Stanford	Girisky, 1978	12
MINN, Minneapolis	Morrow, 1980	116
RPMI, Buffalo	Takita, 1981	234
IOWAC, Iowa	Wright, 1982	142
UTMDACC, Houston	Mountain, 1984	443
DANAF, Boston	Goorin, 1984	93
NCI, Bethesda	Putnam, 1984	80
MARILA, Paris	Regnard, Merlier, 1985	324
MAYO, Rochester	Mansell, Jett, 1986	110
SJUCHIRH, Memphis	Meier, 1987	39
UCLA, Los Angeles	Wong, 1988	47
SMODAVJE, Montreal	Brister, 1988	27

reported 311 pulmonary metastasectomies which have met the request of a complete resection, upon a group of 243 patients. The overall 5 year survival rate according to the histotype was 84% (± 7%) for teratomas, 51% (± 12%) for sarcomas and 35% (± 12%) for carcinomas. Afterwards, in a slightly more expanded group at patients (No. 276), the same author [73] has evaluated the intriguing problem of relapsing metastases after metastasectomy, with 63 patients (23%) who required a second metastasectomy, 12 (4%) who required a third and 2 who had four metastasectomies. As to the main factors of prognosis in this special surgical ambit, survival resulted directly related to the size of the largest growth excised at the first metastasectomy as well as to the histology of the primary tumor. The multivariate analysis, instead, showed that only the histology was predictive. On the other hand it was demonstrated that [74], at the thoracotomy, in about 40% of patients, uni or bilateral adjunctive metastases are discovered, in spite of a careful preoperative diagnostic work up. Moreover, since the bilateral consecutive thoracotomy is associated with a risk of a secondary inoperability, it was pointed out that the median thoracotomy through a sternotomy represents the best option for a simultaneous bilateral approach to the lungs. According to these guidelines, Vogt-Moykopf et al. [75], with 843 thoracotomies in 729 lung metastatic patients, reported a probability of survival at 3 and 5 year of 43 and 33%, respectively. The 30-day mortality rate was 2,8% and the radicality of the operation, regardless of the primary tumor, was the most significant prognostic factor. The 5 and 10 year survival rates according to the location of the tumor, were respectively 31 and 28% for breast cancers; 62% for carcinomas of the testis; 40 and 17% for colorectal carcinomas; 21 and 9% for osteosarcomas, and 22 and 10% for soft-tissue sarcomas.

Subsequently, apart from the continued flow of new clinical experiences [76-81] supporting the above mentioned data, some concerns have emerged. First of all, Aberg [82] underlined the diluting effect of the "selection mechanism" upon the statistical consistency of survival after surgery, while Temeck et al. [83] signalled the need to find definite prognostic factors allowing the right indication to metastasectomy as well as the clearer definition of its therapeutical limits. Frost [84] concluded that, while there may be some merit to pulmonary metastasectomy in highly selected patients, aggressive pulmonary metastasectomy does not seem justified by the available data.

A definite answer to such a problem seems to have been offered by the recent analysis based on the data of the Intl. Registry of Pulmonary Metastases, which was opened at London Brompton Hospital at the end of 1996 [85]. The Registry already includes more than 5, 000 operated cases collected worldwide, and 4, 572 of which (88%) have undergone a complete surgical resection. According to the analysis, the actuarial survival after complete metastasectomy was 36% at 5 year, 26% at 10 year with a median of 35 months. Again, among complete resections, the five-year survival was 33% for patients with an interval of 0 to 11 months and 45% for those with a disease-free interval of more than 36 months. Furthermore, the survival rate was 43% when the lesion was single, while 27% when there were four or more. In the end, the multivariate analysis showed a better prognosis for patients with germ cell tumors, disease-free intervals of 36 months or more, and a single metastasis. In conclusion, as a safe and potentially curative procedure, lung metastasectomy can be now rationally offered to the formal surgical armamentarium.

References

1. Mountain C. F (1986) A New International Staging for Lung Cancer. Chest 89:2255-2335
2. Weissberg D. (1981) Extended Resections of locally Advanced Stage III Lung Cancer. Thor Cardiovasc Surg 29:238-241
3. Abbey Smith R. (1981) Evaluation of the Long-Term Results of Surgery for Bronchial Carcinoma. J Thor Cardiovasc Surg 82 (3):325-33
4. Brewer L. A (1977) Pattern of Survival in Lung Cancer. Chest 71 (5):644-650
5. Paulson D. L (1976) Long-term Survival after Resection for Bronchogenic Carcinoma. Ann Surg 184 (3):324-332
6. Jett J. R (1997) What's New in Staging of Lung Cancer? Chest 11 (6):1486-1487

7. Mountain C. F (1997) Revisions in the International System for Staging Lung Cancer. Chest 111:1710-1717
8. Mountain C. F, Dresler M (1997) Regional Lymph Node Classification for Lung Cancer Staging. Chest 11:1718-1723
9. Padilla J, Penalver J. C, Sales C, Calvo V, Morcillo A, Paris F (1995) Stage I Lung Cancer, T1 and T2 Tumour should be grouped in the same Stage? Proc 3rd European Conf ESTS, Lausanne
10. Buelzebruck H, Krysa E, Bauer E, Probst G, Drings P, Vogt-Moykopf I (1991) Validation of the TNM Classification (4th edn) for Lung Cancer: First Results of a prospective study of 1086 patients with surgical treatment. Eur J Cardio-Thor Surg 4:356-362
11. Friberg S (1997) 5-Year Cure Rate: Yet Another Myth. J Surg Oncol 65:73-75
12. Spratt J. S (1997) Commentary to the "Myth of 5-year Cure Rate". J Surg Oncol 65:75
13. Smart C. R (1997) Limitations of the Randomized Trial for the Early Detection of Cancer. Cancer 79 (9):1740-1746
14. Bechtel J. J, Kelley W. R, Petty T. L, Patz D. S, Saccommanno G (1994) Outcome of 51 Patients with Roentgenografically Occult Lung Cancer Detected by Sputum Cytologic Testing: A Community Hospital Program. Arch Inter Med 154:975-980
15. Watanabe Y, Shimizu J, Oda M, Iwa T, Takashima T et al (1991) Early Hilar Lung Cancer: Its Clinical Aspect. J Surg Oncol 48:75-80
16. Fujimura S, Endo C, Saito Y et al (1997) Radical Segmentectomy for Roentgenographically Occult Bronchogenic Squamous Cell Carcinoma. Lung Cancer 18 (51) 399:103 (8th World Conference on Lung Cancer, Dublin)
17. Sano I, Nakamura Y, Itoyanagy N et al (1997) A Clinical Study of p-Stage I Lung Cancer. Lung Cancer 18 (51) 425:110 (8th World Conference on Lung cancer. Dublin)
18. Shimizu H, Aoe M, Mukaida T et al (1997) Clinico-Pathological Study of Resected Peripheral Small Pulmonary Carcinomas - Twenty Years Experience. Lung Cancer 18 (51) 397:103 (8th World Conference on Lung Cancer, Dublin)
19. Motta G, Nahum M. A, Testa T, Spinelli E, Gasparo A, de Bernardis E (1996) Resection for Peripheral Higher Stage Lung Tumor. A Compared Italian Cumulative Experience. Ann Ital Chir LXVII 3:381-385
20. Shaw R. R, Paulson D. L, Kee JL Jr (1961) Treatment of Superior Sulcus Tumor by Irradiation Followed by Resection. Ann Surg 1:29-39
21. Paulson D. L (1985) The "Superior Sulcus" Lesion. In: Delarue N. C, Eschapasse H (eds) International Trends in General Thoracic Surgery. Vol 1:Lung Cancer. W. B Saunders, Philadelphia, pp 121-131
22. Miller J. I, Mansour K. A, Hatcher C. R (1979) Carcinoma of the Superior Pulmonary Sulcus. Ann Thorac Surg 28:44-47
23. Attar S, Miller J. E, Satterfield J, et al (1979) Pancoast's Tumour: Irradiation or Surgery? Ann Thorac Surg 28:578-586
24. Stanford W, Barnes R. P, Tucker A. R (1979) Influence of Staging in Superior Sulcus (Pancoast) Tumours of the Lung. Ann Thorac Surg 29:406-409
25. Wright C. D, Moncure A. C, Shepard J. O, Wilkins E. W, Mathisen D. J Jr, Grillo H. C (1987) Superior Sulcus Lung Tumours. J Thorac Cardiovasc Surg 43:32-38
26. Shaian D. M, Neptune W. B, Ellis F. H Jr (1987) Pancoast Tumours: Improved Survival with Preoperative and Postoperative Radiotherapy. Ann Thorac Surg 43:32-38
27. De Meester T. R, Albertucci M, Dawson P. J, Montener S. M (1989) Management of Tumour adherent to the Vertebral Column. J Thorac Cardiovasc Surg 97:373-378

28. Dartevelle P, Chapelier A, Macchiarini P et al (1993) Anterior Transcervical Approach for Radical Resection of Lung Tumors Invading the Thoracic Inlet. J Thor Cardiovasc Surg 105:1025-1034
29. Dartevelle P. G (1997) Extended Operations for the Treatment of Lung Cancer. Ann Thor Surg 63:12-19
30. Niwa H, Masaoka A et al (1993) Surgical Therapy for Apical Invasive Lung Cancer: Different Approaches According to Tumor Location. Lung Cancer 10:63-71
31. Grunewald D, Spaggiari L (1996) Transmanubrial Osteomuscular Sparing Approach for Apical Chest Tumors. Ann Thorac Surg 61:723-726
32. Grunewald D, Mazel C, Girard P, Berthiot G, Dromer C, Baldeyrou P (1996) Total Vertebrectomy for En Bloc Resection of Lung Cancer Invading the Spine. Ann Thorac Surg 61:723-726
33. Allison P. R (1959) Meeting of the Association of Thoracic Surgeons. Jones PH, Ann R Coll Surg Engl 25:20
34. Mac Hale S. J (1966) Carcinoma of the Bronchus: Survival Following Conservative Resection. Thorax 21:343
35. Paulson D. L, Urschel H. C Jr, Mc Namara J. J, Shaw R. R (1970) Bronchoplastic Procedures for Bronchogenic Carcinoma. J Thor Cardiovasc Surg 59 (1):38-48
36. Rees G. M, Paneth M (1970) Lobectomy with Sleeve Resection in the Treatment of Bronchial Tumours. Thorax 25:160
37. Woght-Moykopf I, Fritz T. H, Meier G, Bulzebruck H, Daskos G (1986) Bronchoplastic and Angioplastic Operation in Bronchial Carcinoma: Long Term Results of a Retrospective Analysis from 1973 to 1983. Int Surg 71:211-220
38. Faber L. P (1987) Results of Surgical Treatment of Stage III Lung Carcinoma with Carinal Proximity. The Role of Sleeve Lobectomy versus Pneumonectomy and the Role of Sleeve Pneumonectomy. Surg Clin North Am 67:1001-1014
39. Watanabe Y, Shimizu J et al (1990) Results in 104 Patients Undergoing Bronchoplastic Procedures for Bronchial Lesions. Ann Thorac Surg 50:607-614
40. Van Schil P. E, Brutel de la Rivière A, Knaepen P. J, Van Swieten H. A, Defauw J. J, Van den Bosch J. M (1991) TNM Staging and Long-Term Follow-up after Sleeve Resection for Bronchogenic Tumors. Ann Thor Surg 52:1096-1101
41. Deslaurier J, Mehran R. J, Guimont C, Brisson J (1993) Staging and Management of Lung Cancer: Sleeve Resection. World J Surg 17:712-718
42. Motta G (1997) Tracheobronchoplastic Procedures for Centrally Located Lung Cancer. Proc 7th Intl Cong on Anticancer Treatment, Paris, Abstract No. 181
43. Krishna K, Duurkens V, Verijbergen F. F, Huysmans H. A, Knaepen P. J (1994) Pulmonary Function after Sleeve Lobectomy. Ann Thorac Surg 57:1302-1304
44. Kawahara K, Akamina S (1994) Management of Anastomotic Complications after Sleeve Lobectomy for Lung Cancer. Ann Thorac Surg 57:1529-1533
45. Motta G, Nahum M. A, Beatini M (1993) Bronchoplasty versus Carinoplasty: the Oncological Value of Two Methods. Lung Cancer 9:213-220
46. Motta G, Nahum M. A, Testa T, Spinelli E, Gasparo A, de Bernardis E, Carbone E (1996) Size and Mediastinal Proximity as Joined Factors Enconding T3-Status. The experience of Genoa. Proc Intl Workshop on Intrathoracic Staging, Royal Brompton Hospital, London, Oct 28-29
47. Shields T. W (1990) The Significance of Ipsilateral Mediastinal Lymp Node Metastasis (N2 Disease) in Non-Small Cell Carcinoma of the Lung. J Thorac Cardiovasc Surg 99:48-53

48. Pearson F. G, De Larne N. C, Ilves R, Todd T. R. J, Cooper J. D (1982) Significance of Positive Superior Mediastinal Nodes Identified at Mediastinoscopy in Patients with Resectable Cancer of the Lung. J Thor Cardiovasc Surg 83:1-11

49. Mountain C et al (1992) Lung Cancer: a Handbook for Staging and Imaging. CP Young Co Ed, Houston, USA, 35

50. Goldstraw P, Mannam G. C, Kaplan D. K, Michail P (1994) Surgical Management of Non-Small Cell Lung Cancer with Ipsilateral Mediastinal Node Metastasis (N2 Disease). J Thorac Cardiovasc Surg 107:19-28

51. Watanabe Y, Shimizu J, Oda M et al (1991) Aggressive Surgical Intervention in N2 Non-Small Cell Cancer of the Lung. Ann Thorac Surg 51:253-261

52. Martini N, Flehinger B. J (1987) The Role of Surgery in N2 Lung Cancer. Surg Clin North Am 67:1037-1049

53. De Leyn P, Schoonooghe P, Deneffe G, Van Raemdonck D, Coosemans W, Vansteenkiste J, Lerut T (1996) Surgery for Non-Small Cell Lung Cancer with Unsuspected Metastasis to Ipsilateral Mediastinal or Subcarinal Nodes (N2 Disease). Eur J Cardio-Thorac Surg 10:649-655

54. Naruke T, Goya T, Tsuchiya R, Suemasu K (1988) Prognosis and Survival in Resected Lung Carcinoma Based on the New International Staging System. J Thor Cardiovasc Surg 96:440-447

55. Takita H, Hollinshead A. C, Rizzo D. J (1979) Treatment of Inoperable Lung Carcinoma: A Combined Modality Approach. Ann Thorac Surg 28:363-368

56. Faber L. P, Kittle C. F, Warren W. H (1989) Preoperative Chemotherapy and Irradiation for Stage III Non-Small Cell Lung Cancer. Ann Thorac Surg 47:669-677

57. Martini N, Kris M. G, Flehinger B. J (1994) Preoperative Chemotherapy for Stage III (N2) Lung Cancer: The Sloan-Kettering Experience with 136 Patients. Ann Thorac Surg 55:1365-1374

58. Roth J. A, Fossella F, Komaki R et al (1994) A Randomized Trial Comparing Perioperative Chemotherapy and Surgery with Surgery Alone in Resectable Stage IIIA Non-Small Cell Lung Cancer. J Natl Cancer Inst 86:673-680

59. Rosell R, Gomez-Codina J, Camps C, Maestre J, Padille J, Cantò A, Mate J. L, Li S, Roig J (1994) A Randomized Trial Comparing Pre-operative Chemotherapy Plus Surgery with Surgery Alone in Patients with Non-Small Cell Lung Cancer. NEJM 330:153-158

60. Martini N (1994) Surgical Options for Patients with Mediastinal Node Involvement. Lung Cancer 11 (Suppl. 2):43-44

61. Ginsberg R. J (1994) Surgical Treatment in Locally Advanced Lung Cancer. Lung Cancer 11 (Suppl. 2):144-145

62. Rusch V. W, Albain K. S, Crwley J. J et al (1994) Neodjuvant Therapy: a Novel and Effective Treatment for Stage IIIb Non-Small Cell Lung Cancer. Southwest Oncology Group. Ann Thorac Surg 58:290-294

63. Sugarbaker D. J, Herndon J, Kolman L. J et al (1995) Results of Cancer and Leukemia Group B Protocol 8935. J Thorac Cardiovasc Surg 109:473-485

64. Mathisen D. J, Wain J. C, Wright C, Choi A, Carey R, Hilgenbreg A, Grossbard M, Lynch T, Grillo H (1996) Assessment of Preoperative Accelerated Radiotherapy and Chemotherapy in Stage IIIA (N2) Non-Small Cell Lung Cancer. J Thorac Cardiovasc Surg 111:123-133

65. Cahan W. G, Castro El B (1975) Significance of a Solitary Lung Shadow in Patients with Breast Cancer. Ann Surg 181 (2):137-143

66. Gromet M. A, Ominsky S. H, Epstein W. L, Blois M (1979) The Thorax as the Initial Site for Systemic Relapse in Malignant Melanoma. Cancer 44:776-784

67. Kinsey D. L (1960) An Experimental Study of Preferential Metastasis. Cancer 13 (4):674-676
68. Tarin D (1971) Tissue Interaction in Carcinogenesis. N. Y, pp 274-283
69. Fidler I. J (1976) Patterns of Tumor Cell Arrest and Development. In:Weiss L (ed) Fundamental Aspect of Metastasis. Amsterdam, North Holland, pp 275
70. Viadana E, Bross I. J. D, Pickren K. W (1978) Cascade spread of Blood-Borne Metastases in Solid and Nonsolid Cancers of Humans. In:Weiss L, Gilbert H. A (eds) Pulmonary Metastasis. Hall, Boston, pp 142-167
71. Nicolson G. L, Poste G (1983) Tumor Implantation and Invasion at Metastatic Sites. Int Rev Exp Pathol 25:77-181
72. Goldstraw P (1994) Surgery of Pulmonary Metastases. In: Motta G (ed) Lung Cancer: Frontiers in Science and Treatment. Grafica LP, Genoa (I), pp 47-504
73. Robert J, Ambrogi V, Mermillod B, Dahabareh D, Goldstraw P (1995) Factors Influencing Long-Term Survival after Lung Metastasectomy. Proc 3rd European Conference ESTS, Lausanne Abstr No 61
74. Vogt-Moykopf I, Meyer G (1986) Surgical Technique in Operations on Pulmonary Metastases. Thorac Cardiovasc Surgeon 34:125-132
75. Vogt-Moykopf I, Buelzebruck H, Krysa S, Kruschinsky H, Schirren J (1994) Surgery of Pulmonary Metastases Techniques, Results and Perspectives. In: Motta G (ed) Lung Cancer: Frontiers in Science and Treatment. Grafica LP, Genoa (I), 483-495
76. Cerfolio R. J, Allen M. S, Deschamps C et al (1994) Pulmonary Resection of Metastatic Renal Cell Carcinoma. Ann Thor Surg 57:332-344
77. Shimizu J, Oda M, Hayashi Y et al (1995) Results of Surgical Treatment of Pulmonary Metastases. J Surg Onc 58:57-62
78. Van Geel A. N, Pastorino U, Jauch K. W et al (1996) Surgical Treatment of Lung Metastases. Cancer 77 (4):675-682
79. Okumura S, Kondo H, Tsuboi M et al (1996) Pulmonary Resection for Metastatic Colorectal Cancer: Experiences with 159 Patients. J Thorac Cardiovasc Surg 112:867-874
80. Girard P, Spaggiari L, Baldeyrou P et al (1997) Should the Number of Pulmonary Metastases Influence the Surgical Decision? Eur J Cardio-Thor Surg 12:385-392
81. Fourquier P, Regnard JF, Rea S et al (1997) Lung Metastases of Renal cell Carcinoma: Results of Surgical Resection. Eur J Cardio-Thor Surg 11:17-21
82. Aberg T (1997) Selection Mechanisms as Major Determinants of Survival after Pulmonary Metastasectomy. Ann Thor Surg 63:611-612
83. Temeck B. K, Wexler L. H, Steimberg S. M et al (1995) Metastasectomy for Sarcomatous Pediatric Histologies: Results and Prognostic Factors. Ann Thor Surg 59:1385-1390
84. Frost D. B (1995) Pulmonary Metastasectomy for Soft Tissue Sarcomas: Is it Justified? J Surg Onc 59:110-115
85. Pastorino U, Buyse M, Friedel G et al (1997) Long-Term Results of Lung Metastasectomy: Prognostic Analyses Based on 5200 Cases. J Thor Cardiovasc Surg 113:37-49

New Drug Combinations in NSCLC: Progress in Cancer Therapy

A. F. Soriano, P. A. Bunn Jr

Introduction

Lung cancer is the leading cause of cancer mortality in both men and women in the United States, accounting for 29% of all cancer deaths in 1997. The estimated number of new cases of lung cancer in 1997 was 178,000 with an estimated 160,400 lung cancer deaths [1]. Lung cancer is the third most common cancer in the United States behind prostate and breast cancer, but more Americans will die from this dreaded disease than from breast cancer, prostate cancer and colorectal cancer combined because of the low 14% cure rate [1]. This low cure rate can be ascribed almost exclusively to the high propensity for metastatic spread, the lack of effective screening measures and the inability of systemic therapy to cure metastatic spread.

The majority of patients present with inoperable stage III disease (40%) or stage IV disease (32%) [2]. Patients with stage IV disease are rarely cured. A small minority of patients, about 10-15%, with advanced regional disease stage III with either small cell lung cancer (SCLC) or non-small cell lung cancer (NSCLC) may be cured with intensive combined modality approaches. Because most patients develop systemic disease, chemotherapy will be indicated for a high percentage of patients. Prior agents included alkylating agents and antimetabolites, which produced response rates below 15% in NSCLC patients and did not improve survival [3]. As a result, the role of chemotherapy in advanced NSCLC was viewed with pessimism.

The first chemotherapeutic agent that was shown to improve survival in advanced NSCLC patients was cisplatin. As a single agent, cisplatin produced response rates in 20% or less of the patients [4]. During the 1980's, a number of randomized trials compared cisplatin based chemotherapy combinations to best supportive care. All of the studies showed superior survival with the cisplatin therapy but this difference was statistically significant in only some of the trials. A meta-analysis was performed and showed a highly statistically significant survival advantage for patients receiving cisplatin-based therapy compared to those receiving best supportive care (BSC). For stage III NSCLC, the meta-analysis also evaluated cisplatin-based therapy combined with radiotherapy compared to radiotherapy alone, and surgery alone compared to surgery followed by cisplatin-based chemotherapy in operable stages of NSCLC. Survival was improved in these stages of lung cancer as well [3]. In stage IV, cisplatin-based therapy significantly improved median survival by about 2 months with a 10% (from 10-15% to 20-25%) increase in the percent of patients alive at one year. In stage III, survival improvement was about 4 months at the median and 5 year survival was improved by 4-10%. In earlier stage disease, the hazard rate of death was reduced by 13% leading to a 5% improvement in the 5 year survival.

Cisplatin based regimens also improved quality of life and palliated symptoms [3, 5, 6]. Randomized trials compared quality of life, as assessed by patients, in subjects receiving chemotherapy or best supportive care in stage IV NSCLC and chemotherapy or radiotherapy in stage III NSCLC [3]. Sixty-six percent of stage IV patients and 78% of stage III experienced relief of their lung cancer related symptoms even though objective responses occurred in only about 25% of stage IV NSCLC patients and 50-60% with stage III disease [6].

During the 1990's, five new drugs were shown to produce response and survival which was equivalent or superior to that achieved with cisplatin [7]. These agents included the taxanes, paclitaxel and docetaxel; a vinca alkaloid, vinorelbine; an antimetabolite, gemcitabine, and a topoisomerase I inhibitor, irinotecan (CPT-11). These agents alone and in combination with platinum agents have shown better activity than any agent previously available and have improved the survival and quality of life of NSCLC patients.

New Single Agents in NSCLC

Vinorelbine

In the 1990's, the first new drug to be studied and approved by the FDA for NSCLC was vinorelbine, a novel vinca alkaloid which produced response rates ranging from 14% to 29% with a median survival of about 32 weeks [8]. Two randomized trials showed an average response rate of 20%, a median survival of 30 weeks and a one year survival rate of 25% for single agent vinorelbine [9,10] (see Table 2). In the European study,

Table 1. Staging classification of lung cance

Primary Tumor (T)
Tx - Primary tumor cannot be assessed, or tumor proven by the presence of malignant cells in sputum or bronchial washings but not visualized by imaging or bronchoscopy
T0 - No evidence of primary tumor
Tis - Carcinoma *in situ*
T1 - Tumor that is 3.0 cm or less in greatest diameter, surrounded by lung or visceral pleura, and without evidence of invasion more proximal than the lobar bronchus (i.e., not in the main bronchus)
T2 - Tumor with any of the following features of size or extent:
More than 3.0 cm in greatest dimension
Involving the main bronchus, 2.0 cm or more distal to the carina
Invading the visceral pleura
Associated with atelectasis or obstructive pneumonitis that extends to the hilar region but does not involve the entire lung
T3 - Tumor of any size with direct extension to the chest wall (including superior sulcus tumors), diaphragm, mediastinal pleura, parietal pericardium; tumor in the main bronchus less than 2.0 cm distal to the carina but without involvement of the carina; associated atelectasis or obstructive pneumonitis of the entire lung
T4 - Tumor of any size that invades any of the following: mediastinum, heart, great vessels, trachea, esophagus, vertebral body, carina; or tumor with a malignant pleural or pericardial effusion, or with satellite tumor nodule(s) within the ipsilateral primary-tumor lobe of the lung

Nodal Involvement (N)
NX - Regional lymph nodes cannot be assessed
N0 - No regional lymph node metastasis
N1 - Metastasis in ipsilateral peribronchial and/or ipsilateral hilar lymph nodes, including direct extension
N2 - Metastasis in ipsilateral mediastinal and/or subcarinal lymph nodes
N3 - Metastasis in contralateral mediastinal, contralateral hilar, ipsilateral or contralateral scalene, or supraclavicular lymph nodes

Distant Metastasis (M)
MX -Presence of distant metastasis cannot be assessed
M0 -No distant metastasis
M1 -Distant metastasis (beyond the ipsilateral supraclavicular nodes)

STAGING	TNM	5 Yrs Survival Rate (%)	
		Clinical stage	Pathologic stage
Stage 0	Tis, N0, M0	-	-
Stage IA	T1, N0, M0	61	67
Stage IB	T2, N0, M0	38	57
Stage IIA	T1, N1, M0	34	55
Stage IIB	T2, N1, M0	24	39
	T3, N0, M0	22	38
Stage IIIA	T3, N1, M0	9	25
	T1-3, N2, M0	13	23
Stage IIIB	T4, any N, M0	7	< 5
	Any T, N3, M0	3	
Stage IV	Any T, any N, M1	1	< 1

(Modified from Mountain CF. [2])

single agent vinorelbine was compared to the standard 2-drug combination of vindesine + cisplatin and the new regimen of vinorelbine + cisplatin. Single agent vinorelbine produced an objective response of 14%, a median survival of 31 weeks and a one-year survival rate of 25% compared to 19% objective response, median survival of 32 weeks and 1-year survival rate of 27% for the combination of cisplatin and vindesine and 30% objective response, a median survival of 40 weeks and a 1-year survival rate of 35% for the combination of cisplatin and vinorelbine [9]. Vinorelbine alone was shown to be less toxic than either of the two drug combinations. In the United States study comparing vinorelbine to the combination of 5 FU and leucovorin, single agent vinorelbine was shown to be superior to the combination of 5 FU and leucovorin with a median survival of 29 weeks and a 1-year survival rate of 25% compared to 22 weeks and 16% in the % 5 FU arm [10]. In patients who progressed on prior platinum-based chemotherapy, vinorelbine was shown to have an overall response rate of 5% in three European studies [11,12,13], the first two show no response in 32 patients and the third show 2 partial responses in 10 evaluable patients.

In four studies, vinorelbine at doses ranging from 25 mg/m^2 to 30 mg/m^2 given on a weekly basis resulted in an average response rate of about 30%, median survival of 9-10 months and, in one study, a one-year survival rate of 38% [14-17]. A randomized phase III trial comparing vinorelbine plus best supportive care (BSC) to BSC alone in patients aged 70 years or more in advanced NSCLC showed an improved survival in the group receiving single agent vinorelbine [18]. An overall response rate of 20% was noted with a median survival of 27 weeks and a one year survival rate of 27% compared to 21 weeks and 5% for BSC.

Paclitaxel

Paclitaxel was the second of these new agents introduced in the 1990's and approved by the FDA (for ovarian and breast cancers and more recently for lung cancer). Initial studies using a long, 24-hour infusion schedule produced an overall response rate of 22% in 49 patients evaluated [19, 20]. Subsequent studies using one- to three-hour infusion schedules produced a response rate of 21%, nearly identical to the studies using the 24-hour schedule [21, 22]. A summary of both long (24-hour) and short (1-3-hour) paclitaxel infusions confirmed both the high response rate (average 26% among 10 studies), long median survival (average 37.3 weeks among 6 studies) and a high one-year survival rate

Table 2. Randomized trials of new drug combinations

Study Group	Treatment Regimen	No. of Patients	Response Rate (%)	Median Survival (mos)	1 Yr Survival (%)
LeChevalier et al. [9]	V 30 mg/m² weekly	206	14	7.2	30
	CDDP 120 mg/m² D1 and D29 V 30 mg/m² weekly	206	30	9.2	35
	CDDP 120 mg/m² D1 and D29 Vds 3 mg/m²/wk x 6 wks	200	19	7.4	27
Wozniak et al. [40]	CDDP 100 mg/m² every 3 wks V 25 mg/m² weekly x 3	206	26	8	36
	CDDP 100 mg/m² every 4 wks	209	12	6	20
Bonomi et al. [41]	P 135 mg/m² IV over 24 h CDDP 75 mg/m² D1	201	27	9.6	37
	P 250 mg/m² IV over 24 h + GCSF CDDP 75 mg/m² D1	196	32	10	40
	E 100 mg/m² IV D1-3 CDDP 75 mg/m² D1	200	12	7.7	31
Giaccone et al. [47]	P 175 mg/m² IV over 3 h CDDP 80 mg/m² D1	155	41	9.7	43
	Ten 100 mg/m² D 1,3,5 C 80 mg/m² D1	162	28	9.9	41
Gatzemeier et al. [48]	P 175 mg/m² D1 over 3h Cisplatin 80 mg/m² D1 every 3 wks	207	26	8.1	30
	CDDP 100 mg/m² D1 q 3 wks	207	17	8.6	36
Belani et al. [51]	P 225 mg/m² D1 over 3h C AUC 6 D1 every 3 wks	190	23	7.7	32
	CDDP 75 mg/m² D1 E 100 mg/m² D1-3 every 3 wks	179	14	9.1	37
Sandler et al. [60]	Gem 1000 mg/m² D1, D8 and D15 CDDP 100 mg/m² D1	155	32	9.1	39
	CDDP 100 mg/m²	154	10	7.6	28
Crino et al. [61]	G 1000 mg/m² D1,8,15 CDDP 100 mg/m² D2 every 4 wks	155	38	8.6	33
	M 6 mg/m² D1 I 3 gm/m² D1 CDDP 100 mg/m² D2 every 4 wks	152	26	9.6	34

CDDP, cisplatin; V, vinorelbine; Vds, vindesine; P, paclitaxel; E, etoposide; Ten, tenoposide; C, carboplatin; Gem, gemcitabine; M, mitomycin C; I, ifosfamide (average 41% among 7 studies) [7]. These single agent results were superior to those reported for most cisplatin combination studies.

A phase II study using weekly paclitaxel (175 mg/m²/wk) for 6 to 8 weeks in chemo-naïve advanced NSCLC showed an overall response rate of 56%, duration of response of 6.5 months and a one year survival rate of 53% [23]. A study of weekly paclitaxel in patients with stage IV or recurrent NSCLC showed a response rate of 30%, median survival of about 200 days and a one year survival of 42.5% [24]. While these are the best results reported to date, additional studies will be required before this more costly, less convenient approach is more widely adopted.

As second line therapy in platinum refractory or resistant patients, paclitaxel has only modest activity. A study at MD Anderson in 40 patients who failed platinum therapy showed that paclitaxel, given at a dose of 175 mg/m² over 24 hours, produced only one partial response in 37 evaluable patients (3%), with median survival of 17.5 weeks and one year survival of 16% [25]. Another study using paclitaxel at 200 mg/m² or 250 mg/m² (depending on whether the subject received prior radiotherapy) showed a response rate of 14% and median survival of 17 weeks in 14 evaluable patients [26]. However, a study by Hainsworth [27] in 30 patients who failed one or two prior chemotherapy regimens (26 with platinum based and 4 with other front line regimens) showed a 38% response rate (6 of 16) in the 200 mg/m² group compared to 0% in the 135 mg/m² group.

Docetaxel

Docetaxel, the other taxane which is active in NSCLC, has been approved by the FDA for breast cancer but not yet for lung cancer. In 8 studies of 300 patients, docetaxel produced an overall response rate of 26%, similar to the 26% rate reported in the paclitaxel studies. Median survival ranged from 27 to 48 weeks (average 41 weeks) and one year survival ranged from 41% to 71% (average 52%) [7]. A recent multicenter study in France, in 72 evaluable patients with locally advanced or metastatic NSCLC, showed a 32% partial response, median survival of 44 weeks and one year survival of 45% [28].

Docetaxel was studied in doses ranging from 60 mg/m² to 100 mg/m². The higher doses were associated with more toxicity, especially grade 4 myelosuppression (about 80% of patients) and fluid accumulation. The efficacy results showed response rates of 29% for the 100 mg/m² dose and 23% for the 60 mg/m² dose. No published randomized trials have compared the two dose regimens to determine whether the excess toxicity of the higher dose is justified by improved response or survival.

As salvage therapy in patients who progressed on prior platinum-based chemotherapy, docetaxel was found to be effective. Three trials involving a total of 168 patients, showed an average response rate of about 16% with a median survival greater than 8 months and a one year survival rate of about 34% [29, 30]. This was superior to other single agents or combination agents used as second line. A randomized study comparing docetaxel at 75 mg/m^2 or 100 mg/m^2 to vinorelbine or ifosfamide has completed accrual and results should be available soon [31].

Gemcitabine

Previous antimetabolites had minimal activity in NSCLC. A US study comparing vinorelbine to the combination of cisplatin, 5 FU and leucovorin showed the response rate of the 5 FU and leucovorin combination to be only 8% with a median survival of 5.5 months and a one year survival rate of 12% [10]. Gemcitabine is a novel deoxycytidine analog that is structurally related to cytosine arabinoside. A summary of phase II trials in 572 patients showed an overall response rate of 21%, a median survival of 40.6 weeks and a one year survival rate of 39% [7]. Gemcitabine was remarkably well-tolerated, with few toxicities other than myelosuppression. Two randomized studies compared single agent gemcitabine to the combination of cisplatin and etoposide [32, 33]. Single agent gemcitabine had equivalent efficacy with less toxicity compared to the two drug combination of etoposide and cisplatin, showing an average response rate of about 18%, median survival of 31 weeks and a one year survival rate of 32%. Quality of life analysis favored single agent gemcitabine.

As salvage therapy, gemcitabine as single agent was also effective. Two studies in patients previously treated with a platinum containing regimen showed an average partial response of 19% with a median duration of response of about 21 weeks [34, 35].

Gemcitab line was equally effective in elderly patients. In a study involving 329 patients, the overall response rate between patients < 70 years old and older than 70 years was similar (19% vs. 25%). Toxicity was also similar between both groups of patients [36].

Irinotecan

Irinotecan (CPT-11) is a semisynthetic derivative of camptothecin that was originally isolated from the stemwood of the Chinese tree *camptotheca acuminata*. Irinotecan produced an average response rate of 27% in 5 studies involving 138 patients with advanced NSCLC [7]. Median survival was about 35 weeks. No one year data were reported. Although irinotecan showed good second line activity in SCLC patients, several Japanese studies showed conflicting results [37-39]. The first study showed no response in 26 previously treated patients and the latter two showed a 14% response (3 of 22). No details were however given of the prior therapy.

Conclusions

These studies suggest that each new agent is superior to cisplatin alone (median and one year survival of 26 weeks and 12%) and comparable to cisplatin + etoposide combinations (median and one year survival of 32 weeks and 31%) [40, 41]. These agents are as efficacious with considerably less toxicity. As second line therapy, vinorelbine, docetaxel (and perhaps paclitaxel) and gemcitabine produce responses in $\geq 10\%$ of patients. Vinorelbine and gemcitabine are also effective in elderly patients with similar response rates compared to the younger population.

Combination Chemotherapy with New Agents in Advanced NSCLC

Because of the impressive results of these new single agents, attempts were made to combine these drugs with older agents including cisplatin and carboplatin. Carboplatin has been shown to be as effective as cisplatin in NSCLC and is considerably more convenient and less toxic [42]. Thus, it seemed logical to combine a new agent with carboplatin also. In each instance, the combination of any of these new agents with either cisplatin or carboplatin led to higher response rates than with either agent alone. Median and one year survival rates were also generally higher. Each new agent in combination with a platinum analog shall be discussed separately.

Vinorelbine + Cisplatin or Carboplatin

Several phase II studies of vinorelbine combined with cisplatin showed higher response rates than reported with single agent vinorelbine. The combination of vinorelbine and cisplatin produced an average objective response of 41%, a median survival of 44 weeks and a one year survival rate of 45% in several phase II studies [7]. Two randomized studies comparing the combination to either vinorelbine or cisplatin alone were subsequently initiated [9, 40] (see Table 2). The US study showed a higher response rate (26% vs. 12%), median survival (30 vs. 26 weeks), and one and two year survival (36% vs. 20%, and 12% vs. 6%) for the combination [40]. The French study showed similar results, response rate (30% vs. 14%), median survival (40 vs. 31 weeks) and one year survival (35% vs 30%) [9]. The Southwest Oncology Group (SWOG) recently conducted a phase III randomized trial in which cisplatin and vinorelbine was compared to paclitaxel and carboplatin (Table 3). The trial recently finished accrual and the results will be available in the next year.

In 4 phase II studies, the combination of vinorelbine and carboplatin produced response rates ranging from 10% to 40% with an average of 25% with median survival about 10.8 months [43-46]. One study documented a one year survival rate of 37% [43].

Table 3. Ongoing randomized phase III studies

Study Group	Control Arm	Experimental Arm
ECOG	Paclitaxel + Cisplatin	Paclitaxel + Carboplatin Vs Gemcitabine + Cisplatin Vs Docetaxel + Cisplatin
SWOG	Cisplatin + Vinorelbine	Paclitaxel + Carboplatin
CALGB	Paclitaxel	Paclitaxel + Carboplatin

Paclitaxel + Cisplatin or Carboplatin

A 24 hour infusion of paclitaxel was used in initial combination studies with cisplatin. Scheduling was extremely important since the infusion of cisplatin prior to paclitaxel resulted in considerable myelotoxicity. This was thought to be due to modulation effect of cisplatin on cytochrome p450 enzymes resulting in decreased plasma clearance of paclitaxel. When a short infusion paclitaxel schedule was used, the sequence was less important. A summary of phase II studies of paclitaxel and cisplatin showed response rates ranging from 31 to 56% with an average of 42% [7]. This response rate was higher than those observed for either drug alone. The survival was however only slightly superior to paclitaxel alone (median survival of 44 weeks and one year survival of 38%). Two randomized studies were subsequently initiated [41, 47] (see Table 2). The ECOG study comparing two doses of paclitaxel (135 mg/m^2 or 250 mg/m^2 with G-CSF infused over 24 hours with cisplatin (75 mg/m^2) to the combination of cisplatin and etoposide showed significantly higher response rates (27 or 32% vs. 12%), longer median (41 or 43 weeks vs. 32 weeks) and one year survival rates (37% or 40% vs. 31%) for the paclitaxel combinations [41]. Severe neutropenia occurred with similar frequency in each of the arms, but thrombocytopenia and neuropathy were more frequent in the higher dose paclitaxel arm. The EORTC comparing a 3 hour infusion of paclitaxel with cisplatin to the combination of teniposide and cisplatin reported a significantly higher response rate for the paclitaxel combination (41% vs. 28%) [47]. The median and one year survival was similar in both arms (9.7 mos vs. 9.9 mos, and 43% vs. 41%). The toxicity was much lower and quality of life was superior in the paclitaxel arm. A recent randomized trial comparing cisplatin and paclitaxel to cisplatin alone confirmed the higher response rate of the paclitaxel combination (26% vs. 17%), but median and one year survival rates were similar in both arms (8.1 vs. 8.6 mos and 30% vs. 36%, respectively) [48].

The combination of paclitaxel and carboplatin produced response rates of about 46%, median survivals of about 39 weeks and one year survival rates of 40-45% in several studies [7]. Some of the studies used the 24 hour paclitaxel schedule while others used the more convenient 1-3 hour infusion schedule. No difference was noted with either schedule in regards to response rates and survival although no randomized comparative trials have been completed to date. Both thrombocytopenia and peripheral neuropathy were less frequent with this combination compared to the paclitaxel-cisplatin combination. Three recent phase II studies of 1 hour infusion paclitaxel with carboplatin showed an overall response rate of 37% in 201 evaluable patients [49, 50]. Median survival ranged from 8 to 11 months and one year survival was about 44%. Less myelosuppression was noted in the 1 hour infusion studies but more neurotoxicity was found. A more recent randomized trial comparing carboplatin and paclitaxel to cisplatin and etoposide showed a higher response rate in the paclitaxel arm (23% vs. 14%), but median and one year survival were slightly inferior (7.7 mos vs. 9.1 mos, and 32% vs. 37%) [51].

A German phase II study evaluated weekly administration of both paclitaxel and carboplatin in stage IV NSCLC patients. Escalating dose levels of paclitaxel from 90 mg/m^2/wk/6wks to 150 mg/m^2/6wks combined with carboplatin (AUC 2) were evaluated. Of the first twelve patients, six partial remissions were observed (50%) with minimal pronounced adverse effects [52]. More studies are required before this regimen can be adapted into clinical practice.

Docetaxel + Cisplatin or Carboplatin

The combination of docetaxel with cisplatin was also evaluated in advanced NSCLC patients. Phase II studies of the combination showed an average response rate of 35% and a median survival of 39 weeks in 5 studies involving 255 patients [7]. A study in Greece in 52 chemo-naïve patients with stage IIIB and IV NSCLC showed an overall response rate of 45% (1 CR and 23 PR) with a median survival of 11 months and a one year survival rate of 48% [53]. Based on these results, a randomized trial comparing this combination regimen to other new regimens has been initiated and is currently ongoing (see Table 3). Another study using alternating full doses of docetaxel (100 mg/m^2 cycle 1, 3, 5) and cisplatin (120 mg/m^2 cycle 2,4 and 100 mg/m^2 on cycle 6) showed a response rate of 33%, a median duration of response of 4 months and a median survival of 8.8 months [54]. Because of the high frequency of grade 4 myelosuppression that resulted with concurrent therapy, a French study evaluated the sequential administration of docetaxel followed by cisplatin-vindesine. Four cycles of docetaxel were given at a dose of 100 mg/m^2 q 3 weeks followed by 4 cycles of cisplatin (120 mg/m^2 D1 q 3 wks) and vindesine (3 mg/m^2 D1 weekly), then followed by three more cycles of docetaxel. Two PR were noted in ten evaluable patients (20%) [55].

The combination of doxetaxel and carboplatin was also evaluated. A multicenter phase II study evaluated the combination of docetaxel (80 mg/m^2) and carboplatin (AUC 6) in patients with stage IIIB and IV NSCLC. Of 10 evaluable patients, 5 partial responses were observed [56]. Median and one year survival data have not been reported. Another study with docetaxel (80 mg/m^2 D1) and carboplatin (AUC 6 D1) every 3 weeks showed a 48.1% response rate (1 CR/12PR) in 27 evaluable patients [57]. Weekly studies of docetaxel with carboplatin are also in progress. These studies are still in the initial phases and it's too early to make a decision regarding their effectiveness.

Gemcitabine + Cisplatin or Carboplatin

In vivo and *in vitro* assays have shown considerable synergy between cisplatin and gemcitabine [58]. A summary of phase II studies showed an overall response rate of 47% [7]. In five studies, median survival averaged about 48 weeks with an average one year survival rate of 48%. A randomized trial in Spain comparing the combination of gemcitabine and cisplatin to cisplatin and etoposide resulted in higher response rates (41% vs. 21%), median survival (35 weeks vs. 29 weeks) and one year survival rate (30% vs. 24%) in the gemcitabine arm [59]. A large multicenter study comparing gemcitabine with cisplatin to cisplatin alone also showed a higher response rate (32% vs. 10%), median survival (9.1 mos vs. 7.6 mos) and one year survival rate (39% vs. 28%) for the combination [60] (see Table 2). A third randomized trial comparing cisplatin and gemcitabine to mitomycin, ifosfamide and cisplatin (MIC) showed a higher response rate in the gemcitabine arm (38% vs. 26%) but median and one year survival was similar (8.6 mos vs. 9.6 mos and 33% vs. 34%) [61] (Table 2). The combination of gemcitabine and cisplatin is also one of the experimental arms in the ECOG study (Table 3).

Trials involving the combination of gemcitabine and carboplatin have also been initiated and are ongoing. One phase I study using gemcitabine at 1000 mg/m^2 on D1, 8 and 15 in a 28 day cycle with escalating doses of carboplatin starting from an AUC of 4 showed a 33% response rate in 12 evaluable patients and median survival of 45 weeks [62]. A phase II study of carboplatin (AUC 5 D1) and gemcitabine (1000mg/m^2 D1, 8, 15) every 4 weeks was terminated early after only 7 patients were entered because of severe thrombocytopenia. No objective responses were noted in these pateints [63].

Irinotecan + Cisplatin

The combination of irinotecan and cisplatin produced a response rate of 44% among 185 patients, with a median survival of 36 weeks in the only study providing survival data [7]. No survival results have yet been published. No combinations of irinotecan and carboplatin have been reported. Studies with irinotecan and a platinum analog are very few, and thus it is difficult to make an accurate assessment of its efficacy.

Conclusions

The combination of a new agent with either cisplatin or carboplatin produces response rates ranging from 35% to 47% with median and one year survivals of 36-48 weeks and 43%, respectively. This is significantly superior to the prior standard of cisplatin and etoposide as well as to best supportive care [64] (Table 4). It remains to be defined which combination is superior since no study has compared these agents together. The results of the randomized trials in SWOG, ECOG and CALGB will be eagerly awaited.

Table 4. New combinations compared to BSC and cisplatin alone

Drug combination	Response Rate (%)	Median Survival (mos)	1 Yr survival (%)
BSC [64]	-	3.9	10
Cisplatin alone	12	6	20
[40, 48, 60]	17	8.6	36
	10	7.6	28
Etoposide + Cisplatin	12	7.7	31
[41, 51]	14	9.1	37
Paclitaxel + Cisplatin	41	9.7	43
[47, 48]	26	8.1	30
Vinorelbine + Cisplatin	30	9.2	35
[9, 40]	26	8	36
Gemcitabine + Cisplatin	41	8.1	30
[59, 61]	38	8.6	33

Combinations with Two Single Agents

Since these five new agents are at least as effective as cisplatin, it seemed worthwhile to evaluate their efficacy in combination. A summary of these phase I/II studies is shown in Table 5.

Paclitaxel + Gemcitabine or Vinorelbine

Paclitaxel was evaluated in combination with both gemcitabine or vinorelbine. One phase II study of paclitaxel and gemcitabine evaluated patients who had failed prior cisplatin-based therapy. The study used the combination of paclitaxel (175 mg/m^2 D8) with gemcitabine (900 mg/m^2 D1 and 8) in patients who had failed first line docetaxel or cisplatin-based therapy. An overall response rate of 18% (1CR and 8 PR) and median survival of 8 months in 49 evaluable patients was reported [65]. Median survival was 11 months with a one year survival rate of 37%. No study in chemo-naïve patients has been reported.

A phase I dose finding study combined paclitaxel (1 hr infusion) concurrently with vinorelbine in chemo-naïve stage IIB/IV patients. Objective responses were observed in all levels 4/17 (24%) [66]. As second line therapy, the combination of paclitaxel and vinorelbine resulted in a 21% response rate (3/14), a median survival of 165 days and a one year survival rate of 26.7% with four patients surviving longer than one year from the initiation of treatment [67].

Docetaxel + Gemcitabine or Vinorelbine

The combination of docetaxel (100 mg/m^2 D 8) and gemcitabine (900 mg/m^2 D1 and 8) showed a 33.9% overall response rate with 19 partial responses in 52 patients with advanced NSCLC [68]. Median survival was 8.5 months and one year survival was 42%.

A phase I/II study of docetaxel 50 mg/m^2 and vinorelbine 15 to 45 mg/m^2 every 2 weeks demonstrated a partial response rate of 37% in 19 patients evaluated [69]. Median survival was 9 months and predicted one year survival was 35% A multicenter phase II study of 39 patients previously untreated locally advanced showed the combination of vinorelbine (20 mg/m^2 D1 and D5) followed by docetaxel (75 mg/m^2 on D1) to have a 27% partial response [70]. Dose limiting toxicity was grade 4 neutropenia which occurred in 85% of the patients. A subsequent study using G-CSF following vinorelbine (25 mg/m^2) and docetaxel (100 mg/m^2) every 3 weeks showed a partial response of 41% in 37 evaluable patients with median survival of 4 months. The occurrence of grade 3 or 4 neutropenia decreased to 49%, with 24% developing febrile neutropenia [71].

Gemcitabine and Vinorelbine

A phase II study of gemcitabine (1200 mg/m^2 D1,8) and vinorelbine (30 mg/m^2 D1,8) every 3 weeks showed a 36% response rate (3 CR/ 16PR) in 52 evaluable patients and a clinical benefit response (improvement in PS, > 10% weight gain and decrease in pain medication requirements) in 56% of the patients [72]. A phase I/II study with gemcitabine (1000-1250 mg/m^2) and vinorelbine (25-30 mg/m^2) D1 and 8 every 3 weeks showed a 43.3% response rate in 30 evaluable patients [73]. The Finnish Lung Cancer Group evaluated gemcitabine 1200 mg/m^2 and vinorelbine 35 mg/m^2 D1 and 15 every 4 weeks in 27 patients. Of the 7 assessable, one complete and 3 partial responses were noted [74]. Another study with gemcitabine (1000 mg/m^2 and vinorelbine 25 mg/m^2 D1 and 8 every 3 weeks showed an overall response rate of 27% with 3 partial responses [75].

Table 5. Phase I/II trials of new agents in combination

Author	Dosing Regimen	No. of Patients	Response Rate (%)	Median Survival (mos)	1 Yr Survival Rate (%)
Georgoulias et al. [65]	G (900 mg/m^2 D1,8) + P (175 mg/m^2 D8) q 3 wks	49	18	11	37
Breton et al. [66]	P (100-135 mg/m^2 D1) + V (20-25 mg/m^2 D1,5) q 3 wks	17	24	NR	NR
Chang et al. [67]	P (175 mg/m^2 D2) + V (25 mg/m^2 D1,2) q 3 wks	14	21	5.5	26.7
Georgoulias et al. [68]	G (900 mg/m^2 D1,8) + D (100 mg/m^2 D8) q 3 wks	56 (52 evaluable)	33.9	8.5	42
Miller et al. [69]	D (50 mg/m^2 D1,8) + V (15-45 mg/m^2 D1,8) q 2 wks	19	37	9	35
Trillet-Lenoir et al. [70]	D (75 mg/m^2 D1) + V (20 mg/m^2 D1,5) q 3 wks	39 (26 evaluable)	27	NR	NR
Kourousis et al. [71]	D (100 mg/m^2 D1) + V (25 mg/m^2 D1) + GCSF (5 ug/kg SQ D4-15) q 3 wks	43 (37 evaluable)	41	NR	NR
Lorusso et al. [72]	G 1200 mg/m^2 D1 and D8 + V 30 mg/m^2 D1 and D8 every 3 wks	52	36	NR	NR
Esteban et al. [73]	G 1000-1250 mg/m^2 D1,8 + V 25-30 mg/m^2 D1, 8 every 3 wks	30	43.3	NR	NR
Isokangas et al. [74]	G 1200 mg/m^2 D1 and D15 V 35 mg/m^2 D1 and D15	27(7 evaluable)	57	NR	NR
Lilenbaum et al. [75]	G 1000 mg/m^2 D1 and D8 + V 25 mg/m^2 D1 and D8 every 3 wks	11	27	NR	BR
Kudoh et al. [76]	I (40-60 mg/m^2 D1,8,15) + D (30-50 mg/m^2 D2) q 4 wks	26	32	NR	NR

Abbreviations: G, Gemcitabine; P, Paclitaxel; V, Vinorelbine; D, Docetaxel; I, Irinotecan ; NR, Not reported

Docetaxel and Irinotecan

A Japanese phase I/II study combining docetaxel (dose escalation starting at 30 mg/m^2) and irinotecan (starting from 40 mg/m^2) in advanced NSCLC with no prior therapy showed an overall response rate of 29% in 17 patients (5 PR) [76].

Non-platinum containing regimens combining new agents appear to be effective with response rates comparable to single agents in combination with either cisplatin or carboplatin. It is however too early to decide since these trials are mostly phase I. Randomized studies comparing the combination of a new agent with either cisplatin or carboplatin to two new agents are thus needed.

Triple Combinations With Two New Agents

If the two drug combination with new agents is superior to single agents, can a third agent added to an effective two drug combination be more effective? Several studies evaluating new 3 drug combinations are summarized in Table 6.

Paclitaxel and Gemcitabine with a Platinum Agent

The combination of paclitaxel, gemcitabine and a platinum agent was evaluated in 4 phase I/II studies. Two studies used carboplatin and the latter two used cisplatin (see Table 6). A phase I/II study at the University of Colorado Cancer Center evaluated the combination of carboplatin (AUC of 6 or 5) and paclitaxel (175 mg/m^2 over 3 hours) with escalating doses of gemcitabine [77]. After the first 14 patients, the dose of carboplatin was reduced to an AUC of 5 because of thrombocytopenia in later courses. Gemcitabine was administered on day 1 and 8 starting at a dose of 600 mg/m^2 with increasing increments of 100 mg/m^2. Of the first 37 patients, no patients developed febrile neutropenia. Median survival for all patients was 9.5 months with 39% alive at one year. A study at the Sarah Cannon Cancer Center using the same combination [carboplatin (AUC 6 D1), paclitaxel (200 mg/m^2 over 1 hr D1) and gemcitabine (800 mg/m^2 escalating D1 and 8) every 21 days] showed an overall response rate of 48%, median survival of 9.4 months and one year survival of 45% in 77 patients [78]. A third study combined cisplatin (50 mg/m^2 D1, 8), gemcitabine (1000 mg/m^2 D1, 8) and paclitaxel (50 mg/m^2 escalating) in both naïve and pretreated patients [79]. An overall response rate of 46% was noted with a 30% response seen in pretreated patients. The fourth study looking at a biweekly regimen of cisplatin (60 mg/m^2) gemcitabine (800 mg/m^2) and paclitaxel (100 mg/m^2) reported an overall response rate of 52% in 33 evaluable patients (3 CR/14 PR) [80]. Myelosuppression was however significant with treatment being postponed in 86% for one week secondary to neutropenia. This combination appears to have similar efficacy to the combination of a new agent with a platinum analog and is also tolerable. The studies are still too early to evaluate long term survival. If shown to be more effective, randomized studies comparing this triple combination to the standard two drug combination are warranted.

Paclitaxel and Vinorelbine with a Platinum Agent

The combination of paclitaxel, vinorelbine and carboplatin has been evaluated in several studies. A phase I study involved carboplatin, paclitaxel and vinorelbine. A partial response rate of 68% was noted in 19 evaluable patients [81]. A phase II study with carboplatin (AUC 6), paclitaxel (200 mg/m^2) and vinorelbine (22.5 mg/m^2) is in progress.

Gemcitabine and Vinorelbine with a Platinum Agent

Three studies evaluated the combination of gemcitabine, vinorelbine and cisplatin. A phase II study with gemcitabine (1000 mg/m^2), vinorelbine (25 mg/m^2) and cisplatin (50 mg/m^2) on D1 and D8 in 73 patients, showed an overall response rate of 62% and median survival of more than 14 months at a median follow-up of 8 months in 53 evaluable patients [82]. The second study with 83 patients combining gemcitabine (1000 mg/m^2 D1,15), vinorelbine (25 mg/m^2 D1,15) and cisplatin (100 mg/m^2 D1) every 4 weeks showed a 46% response rate (3 CR/ 25 PR) in 61 assessable patients [83]. Median survival was 11 months. A third study in 46 patients, combining gemcitabine (800 mg/m^2), vinorelbine 25 mg/m^2) and cisplatin (30 mg/m^2) D1, 8 and 15 every 4 weeks showed a 32.5% response rate with 2 CR and 12 PR [84].

Docetaxel and Vinorelbine with a Platinum Agent

Two phase II studies were conducted, one in Canada and the other in Greece. In the Canadian study, 46 chemo-naïve patients with stage IIIB and IV NSCLC received docetaxel (100 mg/m^2 D1), alternating with cisplatin (100 mg/m^2 D21), along with vinorelbine 30 mg/m^2 on D21, 28, 35 in a 6 week cycle. An overall response rate of 39% was noted (1 CR and 17 PR) [85]. In the Greek study, 19 previously untreated patients received

Table 6. Triple drug combination in advanced NSCLC

Author Patients	Dosing Regimen	No. of Pts	Response rate (%)	Median Survival (mos)	1 Yr Survival (%)
Kelly K. [77]	C (AUC 6 – 5 D1) + P (175 mg/ m^2 D1) + G (600-1000 mg/m^2 D1, 8) q 3 wks	37	32	9.5	39
Hainsworth et al. [78]	C (AUC 6) + P (200 mg/m^2 D1) + G (800 mg/m^2 escalating)	77	48	9.5	45
Frasci et al. [79]	CDDP 50 mg/m^2 D1 and 8 G 1000 mg/m^2 D1 and 8 T 50 mg/m^2 escalating	37	46	NR	NR
Greco et al. [81]	C (AUC 6) + P (200 mg/m^2) + V (22.5 mg/m^2)	19	68	NR	NR
Comella et al. [82]	CDDP (50 mg/m^2 D1,8) + G (1000 mg/m^2 D1, 8) + V (25 mg/ m^2 D1,8)	73	62	14+	NR
Gonzalez-Baron et al. [83]	G 1000 mg/m^2 D1 and D15 V 25 mg/m^2 D1 and D15 CDDP 100 mg/m^2 D1 every 4 wks	83 (61 evaluable)	46	11	NR
Dorta et al. [84]	CDDP 30 mg/m^2 D1, 8, 15 G 800 mg/m^2 D1, D8 and D15 V 25 mg/m^2 D1, D8 and D15 every 4 wks	46 (43 evaluable)	32.5	NR	NR
Viallet et al. [85]	D (100 mg/m^2 D1) + CDDP (100 mg/m^2 D21) + V (30 mg/m^2 D21, 28, 35) q 6 wks	46	39	NR	NR
Georgoulias et al. [86]	D (100 mg/m^2 D1) + CDDP (100 mg/m^2 D21) + V (30 mg/m^2 D21, 28, 35)	19	33	NR	NR
Masters et al. [87]	P (100 mg/m^2) + V (25 mg/m^2 D1,2,3) + I (1.6 mg/m^2 D1,2,3)	56	18	NR	NR
Comella et al. [89]	C (250 mg/m^2 D1) + CDDP (30 mg/m^2 D2,3) + E (100 mg/m^2 D1-3) + V (30 mg/m^2 D1) q 4 wks	55	25	6.2	NR
	CDDP (40 mg/m^2 D1-3) + E (100 mg/m^2 D1-3) q 4 wks	57	28	7.1	NR

Abbreviations: C, Carboplatin; P, Paclitaxel; G, Gemcitabine; V, Vinorelbine; D, Doc-etaxel; CDDP, Cisplatin; I, Ifosfamide; M, Mitomycin ; NR, Not reported cisplatin (80 mg/m^2 on D1), docetaxel 100 mg/m^2 D8 and vinorelbine 30 mg/m^2 D1 and D8. All patients received G-CSF from day 2 to day 7. One CR and 2PR for an overall response rate of 33% was noted [86].

Paclitaxel, Vinorelbine and Ifosfamide

A non-platinum containing regimen with escalating vinorelbine D1, 2, 3 and ifosfamide D1, 2, 3 and paclitaxel D2 in a 21 days cycle showed a 18% response rate with 10/56 achieving a PR. However, nearly all patients experienced grade 3/4 neutropenia and about 25% febrile neutropenia. Addition of a third drug such as an alkylating agent adds toxicity without benefit [87]. Another study of gemcitabine (1000 mg/m^2 or 1250 mg/m^2 D1, 8), vinorelbine (25 mg/m^2 D1, 8) and ifosfamide (3 mg/m^2 D1) every 3 weeks showed a 52.4% response rate (1 CR/10 Pr) in 21 evaluable patients [88].

The combination of two new agents with a platinum agent appears to be as efficacious as two drug combinations with similar response and one year survival rates. It is too early to assess if the addition of a third agent will translate to a longer survival, and a randomized trial comparing a three drug combination to the standard two drug regimen is warranted.

Triple Combination with One New Agent

Multiple studies have combined a new agent with a platinum agent plus either etoposide, mitomycin or ifosfamide [89-95]. Response rates ranged from 30% to as high as 67%. Median survival rates were similar to the two drug combination using a new agent and toxicity was higher. A randomized phase II trial comparing the combination of vinorelbine, etoposide and cisplatin/carboplatin to a cisplatin and etoposide regimen showed no significant difference between the two arms [89] (Table 6). A higher response rate was seen in the cisplatin-etoposide arm (28%) compared to the triple combination arm (25%). Median survival was also slightly longer in the two drug arm (7.1 mos vs, 6.2 mos). The addition of vinorelbine did not result in an added benefit in this study.

Triple combinations using only one new agent do not appear to add a significant benefit, but only toxicity. Thus, studies of three drug combinations should include at least two new agents.

Cost of New Agents

Compared to the 16 or 17 week median survival of patients who received best supportive care, patients treated with new agents alone or in combination have median survival of about 39-48 weeks, a gain of about 26 weeks. Chemotherapy, especially new agents, is expensive. Because they prolong survival, the costs per year of life gained can be determined and compared to other medical therapies. In a Canadian study, the survival benefit of 8 weeks in favor of patients receiving CAP chemotherapy was associated with an economic saving of Canadian $949.49 when compared to best supportive care [96]. This translated into savings of $6,171 per year of life gained. The VP arm, etoposide and high dose inpatient cisplatin, resulted in a mean survival benefit of 12.8 weeks and an increased cost of $3,637 per patient, translating to $14,777 per added year of life. The VP arm resulted in both increased costs and increased survival when compared to BSC. It was, therefore, less economically favorable than CAP but the costs associated with its use were still acceptable when compared with the benefits. Evans [97], using a model of lung cancer diagnosis and treatment by disease stage and cell type, examined the cost-effectiveness of common chemotherapy regimens compared to BSC. Cisplatin and etoposide saved $1,461 per case relative to supportive care. Newer chemotherapeutic regimens were compared to etoposide and cisplatin as the standard regimen. Cisplatin and vinorelbine cost $8,566/life year saved ; gemcitabine and cisplatin $10,963, and paclitaxel and cisplatin $12,116. Thus, the cost of chemotherapy for advanced NSCLC, though expensive, is well within the range of other accepted medical therapies and will be lowered considerably when generic agents become available.

Treatment of stage IIIB NSCLC

For locally advanced stage IIIB disease, studies before 1990 suggested that radiotherapy was the primary therapy, alleviating symptoms and producing a 5-10% survival benefit after 5 years. Median survival was, however, only 9-10 months. Subsequent studies in the late 80's and early 90's showed a survival advantage when chemotherapy was combined with radiotherapy. Several studies are summarized in Table 7. Meta-analyses confirmed the added benefit of cisplatin-based chemotherapy to radiotherapy [3, 98]. A meta-analysis of 14 randomized trials of combination therapy and radiotherapy alone in locally advanced, unresectable NSCLC showed that the combination of chemotherapy and radiotherapy reduced the risk for death by 12% at 1 year, 13% by 2 years and 17% by 3 years [98]. This corresponds to a mean gain in life expectancy of about 2 months from 10.3 months to 12.0 months by the end of 3 years. When considered separately, trials of concurrent and sequential chemotherapy yielded similar treatment effects. The addition of chemotherapy to radiotherapy was associated with a 10% to 20% decrease in the risk for death. The absolute benefit is relatively small, however, and should be balanced against the increased toxicity associated with the addition of chemotherapy. The addition of chemotherapy to radiotherapy also resulted in an improved quality of life [5].

Three trials cited above used the sequential approach of chemotherapy followed by definitive radiotherapy [99-102] (see Table 7). The CALGB, comparing two cycles of cisplatin and vinblastine induction followed by chest irradiation, to chest irradiation alone, showed a median survival of 13.8 months for the combined modality group compared to 9.7 months for the radiotherapy group alone [99]. Survival rates at 2 and 3 years were also significantly better (26% in 2 years and 23% in 3 years compared to 13% at 2 years and 11% at 3 years). The long-term survival remained greater for the combined modality group even after more than 7 years of follow-up (5 year survival rate of 17% vs. 6%) [100]. The RTOG compared induction chemotherapy of cisplatin and vinblastine followed by standard radiotherapy to standard radiotherapy alone and to twice-daily radiotherapy. Median and one year survival after combined modality therapy was 13.8 months and 60% compared to 11.4 months and 46% for the standard radiotherapy arm, and 12.3 months and 51% for the hyperfractionated arm [101]. A subsequent French study, using three monthly cycles of vindesine, cyclophosphamide, cisplatin and lomustine (VCPC) prior to radiotherapy compared to radiotherapy alone showed a significant improvement in median survival (12 months vs. 10 months) and a lower rate of distant metastases at 2 years (43% vs. 64%) [102].

In an effort to take advantage of radiosensitizing properties of cisplatin chemotherapy, several studies gave concurrent chemotherapy daily or weekly along with radiotherapy. The EORTC, comparing split course radiation therapy to split course radiation therapy combined with cisplatin, given either weekly or daily, showed a median survival of 13 months vs. 12 months for the combined modality arms and a 2 year survival rate of 26% compared to 13% [103] (see Table 7). Also noted was an improved local control in the daily cisplatin/radiotherapy group suggesting that this schedule results in maximal radiation enhancement. The combined modality arms had a significantly reduced local failure rate

Table 7. Randomized trials of sequential or concurrent chemotherapy and radiation therapy vs. radiation therapy alone

Study Group	No. of PatientS	Type	CT+RT Schedule	Median Survival (CT+RT/RT)	2 Yr Survival (CT+RT/RT) (%)
Dillman et al. [99]	155	Sequential	P/Vbx2à60 Gy/6wks	13.8/9.7	26 / 13
Sause et al. [101]	452	Sequential	P/Vbx2à60 Gy/6wks	13.8/11.4	30 / 19
LeChevalier et al. [102]	353	Sequential	VCPCx3à65 Gy/ 5.5wksàVCPCx3	12/10	21 / 14
Schaake-Koning et al. [103]	308	Concurrent	P + 30Gy/2wks + 25 Gy/ 2wks(split)	13/12	26 / 13
Jeremic et al. [105]	131	Concurrent	CBDCA+VP16+69.9 Gy/ 1.2 Gy BID/5wks	22/14	23 / 9 (4 yr)
Takada et al. [106]*	314	Concurrent	MVP+28 Gy/3wksà28 Gy/3wks	16.5	37
		Sequential	MVPà56 Gy	13.3	25.6

Abbreviations: P/Vb:cisplatin 100 mg/m^2, vinblastine 5 mg/m^2; VCPC:vindesine 1.5 mg/m^2 D1,2, lomustine 50 mg/m^2 D3, cyclophosphamide 200 mg/m^2 D2 and 4; P:30 mg/m^2 every wk x 4 or 6 mg/m^2 every day x 20; CBDCA+VP16:carboplatin 50 mg/m^2 and VP16 50 mg daily; MVP:mitomycin 8 mg/m^2 d1 and 29, vinblastine 3 mg/m^2 D1, 8, 29, 36 and cisplatin 80 mg/m^2 D1 and 29.
*Randomized trial of concurrent vs. sequential

suggesting that there was a radiosensitizing effect, but there was no effect on distant relapse. This study did not administer any full dose chemotherapy before or after radiotherapy. Jeremic et al. [104] compared hyperfractionated radiotherapy with or without concurrent chemotherapy with carboplatin (high and low dose) and etoposide. This study showed a substantially longer median survival and higher 3 year survival rate for the chemotherapy groups (13 months, 16% in the high dose carboplatin arm vs. 18 months, 23% in the low dose carboplatin arm vs. 8 months and 6.6% in the radiation arm). There was a higher incidence of acute and/or late high grade toxicity in the combined groups but no patient died of treatment-related toxicity. A subsequent study compared low dose carboplatin (50 mg) and etoposide (50 mg) with hyperfractionated radiotherapy to radiotherapy alone. Median survival was 22 months and a 4 year survival rate was 23% for the combined group compared to 14 months and 9% for the radiation arm alone [105] (see Table 7).

The optimum approach of combining the two modalities remains unclear. The meta-analysis showed similar treatment effects [98]. However, a Japanese study comparing concurrent vs. sequential thoracic radiotherapy in combination with mitomycin, vindesine and cisplatin in unresectable stage III NSCLC showed a significantly better response and survival in the concurrent chemoradiotherapy arm compared to the sequential arm (84% overall response, 16.5 months median survival and 3 year survival of 27% compared to 66.4%, 13.3 months and 12.5%, respectively) [106] (Table 7).

New Agents combined with XRT in Inoperable stage IIIA/B

Multiple studies have suggested that paclitaxel, docetaxel, gemcitabine and irinotecan have radiosensitizing properties [107-109]. Phase I and II studies combining these agents with radiotherapy are mostly preliminary. A summary of some of these trials are shown in Table 8.

Paclitaxel +/- Cisplatin/Carboplatin + XRT

Paclitaxel was given in various schedules: every 3 weeks, weekly, biweekly or daily, alone or in combination with a platinum agent with concurrent radiotherapy. Three studies gave induction chemotherapy for 2 to 3 cycles followed by concurrent chemotherapy every 3 weeks and radiotherapy. Langer et al. [110] administered 2 cycles of paclitaxel (175-225 mg/m^2 over 3 hrs) and carboplatin (AUC 7.5) followed by carboplatin (AUC 3.75-5) and paclitaxel (67.5-175 mg/m^2) every 3 weeks with concurrent TRT (60 Gy/30 fx/5days/wk). The major response after the combined modality therapy was 59% in 16 evaluable patients with a one year survival rate of 62% for the first 21 patients accrued. A Finnish study administered the combination of paclitaxel (135 mg/m^2 over 1h D1) and carboplatin (200 mg/m^2 D2) every 3 weeks for 3 cycles as induction therapy followed by thoracic radiation (56 Gy, 2 Gy/fx) along with cisplatin (30 mg/m^2) and paclitaxel (30 mg/m^2) given 2 to 4 hours prior to XRT on days 1, 2, 3 of cycles 4 and 5 [111]. An overall response rate of 8% was achieved after the combined treatment with 19% achieving a complete response median survival was 17 months with an estimated 2yr survival rate of 36%. Seven patients developed severe radiation pneumonitis and two developed severe neutropenia during the combined therapy portion. Greco et al. [112] administered paclitaxel (135 mg/m^2 D1), cisplatin (60 mg/m^2 D2) and etoposide (100 mg/m^2 D1, 2, 3) for two cycles followed by radiation therapy (60 Gy in 30 fractions) in conjunction with 2 additional courses of paclitaxel (135 mg/m^2 D1), cisplatin (5 mg/m^2 D2-10) and etoposide (25 mg/m^2 D1-10) in 33 patients. At completion of therapy, 82% had an objective response, median survival was greater than 14 months and one year survival was 65%.

Weekly paclitaxel regimens with concurrent radiotherapy were also initiated. A phase II study of weekly paclitaxel (60 mg/m^2/wk for 6 wks) with concurrent radiation therapy (2 Gy 5 days/wk for 6 wks) showed an overall response rate of 86% (3 CR, 22 PR) in 29 evaluable patients. Median survival was 20 months and one, two, and three year-survival rates of ware 60.6%, 33.3% and 18.2% respectively [113]. Esophagitis was the principal toxicity, with grade 3 or 4 occuring in 11 patients (37%). A phase II study of weekly paclitaxel (50 mg/m^2/wk/7 wks) combined with carboplatin (AUC 2) and concurrent thoracic RT (60 Gy/2Gy/fx over 6 wks) followed by 2 cycles of paclitaxel (200 mg/m^2) and carboplatin (AUC 6) showed an overall response rate of 75.3% (6 CR and 22 PR) in 31 evaluable patients with a median survival of 20.5 months and one and two years-survival rates of 56.3% and 38.3% respectively [114]. Principal toxicity was esophagitis grade 3 and 4, developing in 15% and 30%, respectively. A phase II study combining weekly carboplatin (100mg/m^2) and paclitaxel (45 mg/m^2 over 3 hours) with thoracic radiation (1.8 Gy fractions 5 times/wk for 6-7 wks to total of 60-65 Gy) showed 1 year, 2 year and 3 year actuarial survival rates of 63%, 54% and 54%, respectively [115]. The combination of paclitaxel (50 mg/m^2/wk/6 wks) and carboplatin (AUC 2) plus concurrent hyperfractionated chest irradiation (1.2 Gy twice daily for total dose of 69.6 Gy) followed by two cycles of carboplatin (AUC 6) and paclitaxel (200 mg/m^2) in unresectable stage IIIA and IIIB NSCLC demonstrated an overall response rate of 77.2% (1 CR and 16 PR) among the 22 patients evaluable for response [116]. A phase I study combining weekly paclitaxel (45 mg/m^2/wk) and cisplatin (35 mg/m^2/wk) with concurrent radiotherapy (1.2 Gy twice daily x 5d/wk x 5 wks for total dose of 60 Gy) in locally advanced NSCLC showed an overall response rate of 60% (2 CR and 13 PR) [117]. Median survival was 16 months with an estimated one year survival rate of 66%.

Other schedules of paclitaxel have also been attempted. A phase I study of concurrent thoracic irradiation and biweekly paclitaxel (escalating doses from 25 mg/m^2/d twice weekly) noted an overall response of 80% in 25 patients [118]. A phase I/II study combining daily paclitaxel (30 mg/m^2/d for 4 days) followed by cisplatin (100 mg/m^2 on day 5) and GCSF with uninterrupted twice a day irradiation showed an overall response of 100% (2 CR and 5 PR) in 7 patients [119]. A phase I study of daily paclitaxel (escalating from 2.5 mg/fx to 10 mg/fx over 1 hour) prior to thoracic radiotherapy (68 Gy in 34 fractions) after two induction cycles of carboplatin (AUC of 6) and paclitaxel (200 mg/m^2 over 3 hours) every 3 weeks showed a 75% objective response in 12 evaluable patients [120].

Docetaxel, Gemcitabine, Vinorelbine and Irinotecan + XRT

Studies combining the other new agents with radiotherapy have also been initiated. A Greek phase I/II study combining weekly docetaxel (escalating from 20 mg/m^2/wk) with accelerated chest radiotherapy (64 Gy in 5 weeks with concomitant boost technique) in 30 patients with stage IIIB/IV NSCLC showed overall response rate of 77% with 8 patients achieving a complete response [121]. Eighteen patients were resistant to prior cisplatin-based or adriamycin-based chemotherapy. Severe lymphocytopenia was invariably observed in all patients and acute radiation esophagitis grade 3 was noted in 6 of 30 patients, requiring interruption of treatment for 1-2 weeks.

Standard doses of gemcitabine (800 to 100 mg/m^2/wk) given concurrently with chest radiotherapy resulted in severe normal tissue toxicity to the esophagus and lungs and in one study, four of the first eight patients died from the toxicity [122]. Subsequent studies with gemcitabine are starting at low doses such as 200 mg/m^2/wk. Studies with combined gemcitabine and radiotherapy in head and neck cancers also showed a high rate of complete response with a high rate of normal tissue toxicity even

Table 8. Phase II studies of new agents + XRT in stage IIIB NSCLC

Study Group	Dosage Schedule	No. of Patients	Response Rate (%)	Median Survival (mos)	1 Yr Survival Rate (%)
Langer et al. [110]	C (AUC 7.5) + T (175-225 mg/m² over 3 h) q 3 wks x 2 cycles followed by C (AUC 7.5) + T (67.5-175 mg/m²) q 3 wks + XRT (60 Gy/30 Gy/5days/wk	29 (16 evaluable)	59	NR	62
Isokongas et al. [111]	C (200 mg/m² D1) + T (135 mg/m² over 1 h) q 3 wk x 3 followed by CDDP (30 mg/m² D1,2,3) +T (30 mg/m² D1,2,3) + XRT 56 Gy 2Gy/fx	27 (21 evaluable)	78	12n	36(2yr)
Greco et al. [112]	CDDP (60 mg/m² q 3 wk) + T (135 mg/m² q 3 wk) + VP16 (weekly) + XRT	33	82	14+	65
Choy et al. [113]	T (60 mg/m²/wk x 6) + XRT (2 Gy 5 days/wk x 6)	33 (29 evaluable)	86	20	61
Choy et al. [114]	C (AUC 2) weekly x 7 + T (50 mg/m²/wk x 7 wks + XRT 60 Gy 2 Gy/fx followed by C (AUC 6) + T (200 mg/m²) x 2 cycles	39 (37 evaluable)	75.7	20.5	NR
Belani et al. [115]	C (100 mg/m²/wk) + T (45 mg/m²/wk) x 6 wks + XRT (1.8 Gy fx 5d/wk total 60-65 Gy)	38	NR	36+	63
Choy et al. [116]	C (AUC 2) weekly + T (50 mg/m²/wk x 6) + HRT 1.2 Gy BID - total 69.6 Gy followed by C (AUC 6) + T (200 mg/m²) x 2 cycles	32 (22 evaluable)	77.2	NR	NR
Comella et al. [117]	CDDP (30 mg/m²/wk x 6) + T (45 mg/m²/wk) + HRT (1.2 Gy BID x 5 d/wk x 5 - 60 Gy total	25	60	16	66

Table 8. (continued)

		25	80	14+	60
Lau et al. [118]	T (25 mg/m²/d q 4 days x 12 doses) + XRT				
Pisch et al. [119]	T (30 mg/m²/d x 4 days) + CDDP (100 mg/m² D5) + XRT (1.5 Gy 2x/d - total 60)	7	100	NR	NR
Rigas et al. [120]	C (AUC 6) + T (200 mg/m²) q 3 wks x 2 cycles followed by T (2.5 mg/fx escalating to 10 mg/fx daily) + XRT 68.6 Gy in 34 fx	17 (12 evaluable)	75	NR	NR
Koukourakis et al. [121]	D (20 mg/m² escalating weekly) + XRT (64 Gy in 5 wks, concomitant boost technique)	30	73	NR	NR
Masters et al. [125]	V (20-25 mg/m²/wk) + CDDP (100 mg/m² q 3 wks) + XRT (2 Gy/d x 30 days)	37 (37 evaluable)	47	10	28%
Zatloukal et al. [126]	V 25 mg/m² D1,8,15 + CDDP 80 mg/m² D1 every 4 wks x 2 cycles followed by V 12,5 mg/m² D1,8,15 + CDDP 80 mg/m² D1 every 4 wks x 2 cycles with XRT (2 Gy/d for 30 fx – total 60 Gy)	20 (16 evaluable)	62.5	NR	NR
Viallet et al. [127]	V (30 mg/m²/wk 1,3,4,5 and 15 mg/m² wk 2) + CDDP (100 mg/m² wk 1,5) + XRT (2 Gy/d in wk 7,8 and 2 Gy BID in wk 9,10)	42 (33 evaluable)	42	NR	NR
Nakagawa et al.[128]	I (30 mg/m² escalating) + C (20 mg/m²/d x 5) every 4 wks + XRT 60 Gy 2 Gy/d	23	69.6	NR	NR

Abbreviations: C, Carboplatin; AUC, Area under Curve; T, Paclitaxel; CDDP, Cisplatin; VP16, Etoposide; D, Docetaxel; V, Vinorelbine; I, Irinotecan with a gemcitabine dose of 300 mg/m^2/wk [123]. A phase II study of gemcitabine (1000 mg/mm^2/wk x 6 weeks) with XRT (2 Gy/fx 5 days/wk total 60 Gy) in 8 patients resulted in 3 treatment-related deaths (2 pulmonary toxicity and 1 hemorrhage secondary to the radiation), pneumonitis and esophagitis in 3 patients and other side effects related to XRT in the remaining 2 patients [124].

Two phase I/II studies evaluating the combination of weekly vinorelbine and cisplatin (100 mg/m^2 q 3 wks) with radiotherapy showed an objective response of 42% in 32 evaluable patients in the first study and 73% in 33 evaluable patients in the second study [125,126]. The first study showed a median survival of 10 months with 1, 2 and 3 year survival rates of 28%, 15.6% and 6% respectively. Another study combined vinorelbine (25 mg/m^2 D1, 8, 15 – reduced to 12.5 mg/m^2 during cycles 2 and 3) with cisplatin (80 mg/m^2 D1) every 4 weeks for 4 cycles. Radiation therapy (60 Gy/ 30 fx/6 wks) was initiated on D4 of cycle 2. An overall response rate of 62.5% with 18.7% CR was seen in 16 evaluable patients [127]. A Japanese phase I/II study combining weekly irinotecan (escalating from 30 mg/m^2/wk) and carboplatin (20 mg/m^2/d for 5 days) every 4 weeks with concurrent TRT (2 Gy/day to 60 Gy total) in 23 assessable patients, showed an overall objective response of 69.6% (2 CR/13PR) [128]. Median survival time was not reached in all eligible patients.

The combination of a new agent with radiotherapy in locally advanced, unresectable stage III patients appears to be effective with some studies showing response and 1 year survival rates greater than 60%. More studies combining paclitaxel with a platinum agent have been initiated. The dosing schedule of paclitaxel remains undefined, though it appears that weekly paclitaxel achieves the highest response rates. Randomized trials need to be undertaken to determine the optimum approach. Studies using the other new agents have only been recently initiated and too early to be evaluated. The CALGB is currently doing a randomized phase II study of gemcitabine or paclitaxel or vinorelbine with cisplatin as induction chemotherapy followed by concomitant chemoradiotherapy in stage IIIB NSCLC patients [129]. Randomized trials are necessary to see if new agents are better than old ones and to determine the best way to combine these new agents.

Therapy in advanced but potentially operable stage IIIA

The five year survival rates for patients with clinical stage IIIA N2 NSCLC treated with surgery alone is poor (10-20%). Postoperative radiotherapy improves local control but fails to improve survival [130]. The poor survival and high rate of distant relapse made studies of preoperative chemotherapy logical. Phase II studies of such an approach provided encouraging results (see Table 9). The Memorial Sloan-Kettering Cancer Center, administering 2 or 3 cycles of neoadjuvant mitomycin, vinblastine and cisplatin chemotherapy, reported an objective response rate of 77% to chemotherapy, a complete resection rate of 78%, with a pathologic CR of 14% and a 5 year survival rate of 17% for all the patients. Nearly all the 5 year survivors were in the subgroup of patients undergoing complete resection, showing a 5 year survival of 26% [131] (see Table 9). The group in Toronto using the same chemotherapy regimen reported a 71% response rate and a 51% complete resection rate [132]. The median survival and 5 year survival rate were 21.3 months and 20%, respectively (Table 9). The CALGB administered two cycles of vinblastine/cisplatin prior to complete resection, followed by chest irradiation in patients who had incomplete resection or no response to chemotherapy in 74 patients with stage IIIA disease [133] (Table 9). The objective response plus stable disease rate was 88%. Eighty-six percent of patients were treated by surgery, with 36% achieving a complete resection. The 3 year overall survival rate was 23%, with median survivals of 20.9 months in patients undergoing complete resection and 17.8 months in those with incomplete resection compared with 8.5 months in patients who were not resected.

The benefit of chemotherapy prior to surgery in stage IIIA patients was confirmed in two prospective phase III randomized trials comparing neoadjuvant cisplatin-based chemotherapy followed by surgery to surgery alone. Both studies showed a highly statistically significant improvement in survival for the chemotherapy groups [132,133]. The Spanish trial compared cisplatin + ifosfamide + mitomycin C for 3 cycles followed by surgery to surgery alone [134]. The median (26 months vs. 8 months) and the 3 year survival (25% vs. 0%) favored the chemotherapy. In the study from the MD Anderson Cancer Center, the preoperative chemotherapy consisted of cisplatin + cyclophosphamide + etoposide for 3 cycles before surgery or surgery alone [135]. Postoperative chemotherapy was also administered and postoperative radiotherapy allowed at the physician's discretion. Survival results again favored the chemotherapy with improved median (64 months vs. 11 months) and 3 year survival (56 vs. 15%). Both of these studies had a very small number of patients (60 in each study) because the statisticians closed the studies at an early stopping rule due to the highly statistically significant improvement in survival. This indicates that the cisplatin-based chemotherapy used in these studies (which is inferior to paclitaxel, vinorelbine or gemcitabine-based therapy in stage IV disease) decreased the recurrence rate by 33% to more than 50%. This reduction in hazard rate is greater than the magnitude of the reduction observed in breast cancer patients receiving adjuvant therapy.

Since the combination of chemotherapy and radiotherapy is effective in locally advanced, inoperable stage IIIB patients, it seemed logical to try all three modalities in operable stage III patients. A Southwest Oncology Group (SWOG) phase II study combining cisplatin and etoposide with concurrent radiotherapy reported an 85% resectability for the stage IIIA (N2) group and an 80% resectability for the IIIB group. Two and three year survival rates were 37% and 27%, respectively [136]. A recent

Table 9. Selected phase II neoadjuvant studies in stage IIIA NSCLC

Study Group (ref)	Treatment	No. of Patients	Response Rate (%)	Median Survival (mos)	Percent Survival (yr) +
MKSCC [131]	MVP	136	77	19	17(5)
Toronto [132]	MVP	55	71	21	20(5)
CALGB [133]	VP	74	88*	20.9	33(3)
SWOG [136]	EP + RT	75	88*	13	27(3)
Germany [137]	EP + EP+RT	52	67	20	31(4)

* includes stable disease and responders
Abbreviations: MSKCC, Memorial Sloan Kettering Cancer Center ; CALGB, Cancer and Leukemia Group B ; SWOG, Southwest Oncology Group
Chemotherapy: MVP, mitomycin, vinblastine, cisplatin ; EP, etoposide, cisplatin ; RT, radiation therapy ; VP, vinblastine, cisplatin
+, percent of patients alive at year indicated in parenthesis

phase II study in Germany evaluated patients with unresectable stage IIIA and IIIB disease treated with 3 cycles of cisplatin (60 mg/m^2 d1, 7) and etoposide (150 mg/m^2 d3, 4, 5) every 3 weeks initially followed by 1 cycle of cisplatin (50 mg/m^2 d2, 9) and etoposide (100 mg/m^2 d4, 5, 6) along with concurrent twice-daily hyperfractionated accelerated radiotherapy (1.5 Gy BID 5d/wk x 3 wks) then definitive surgery [137] (see Table 9). Of the 94 patients evaluable, 53% achieved complete resection with 26% attaining a pathologic CR. The median survival was 20 months for stage IIIA, 18 months for stage IIIB and 42 months for those who underwent complete resection. Calculated 4 year survival rates were 31%, 26% and 46%, respectively. This study showed a survival benefit with the addition of hyperfractionation compared to standard radiotherapy.

The optimal combined therapy approach for stage IIIA patients remains undefined. Excellent results have been achieved with chemotherapy plus surgery, with chemotherapy plus radiotherapy and with all three modalities. Future randomized trials will be necessary to clarify the optimal approach. An intergroup study is currently in progress to determine whether all 3 modalities are better than combined modality with chemotherapy plus radiotherapy. Future trials should also address whether chemotherapy + radiotherapy or chemotherapy + surgery is preferred for stage IIIA N2 NSCLC patients.

Since new agents are more efficacious than older agents in stage IV patients, they will need to be evaluated in combination therapy for stage IIIA patients. Preliminary results of such studies are now ongoing.

A German study used the combination of carboplatin (AUC 6) and paclitaxel (200 mg/m^2) every 21 days for 3 cycles in locally advanced stage IIIA (T3N2) and IIIB (T4, N0-2) [138]. Three of 7 patients with IIIA and 5 of 16 patients with IIIB achieved PR. Five (71%) with IIIA and 8 (50%) with IIIB underwent thoracotomy with complete tumor resection. A study at the University of Pennsylvania Cancer Center evaluated the use of preoperative paclitaxel with G-CSF in stage IIIA-N2 NSCLC patients [139]. Two cycles of paclitaxel (250 mg/m^2 over 24 h) were given preoperatively and 4 cycles post operatively. Of the seventeen patients eligible, 88% responded to preoperative chemotherapy with 41% undergoing complete resection. Patients who were incompletely or unresected received either radiation alone, radiation + chemotherapy, or chemotherapy alone. With maximum follow-up of 37 months, estimated median survival was 18 months (23 months resected, 13 months not resected). O'Rourke et al. [140] administered vinorelbine (35 mg/m^2 every other week and 17.5 mg/m^2 on days 8 and 22) with cisplatin

(100 mg/m^2 on days 1, 29, 71, and 113) therapy preoperatively in patients with inoperable stage IIIA or IIIB NSCLC. Thirty-three patients were entered and 27 evaluable. An objective response of 44% (3 CR) was achieved with 10 patients undergoing surgery.

A French study evaluated induction chemotherapy with cisplatin and vinorelbine followed by concurrent chemoradiotherapy with daily carboplatin and radiotherapy in stage IIIB NSCLC patients [141]. Patients received cisplatin (120 mg/m^2 q 4 wks) with vinorelbine (30 mg/m^2/wk wks 1-9, except wks 3 and 7 where dose was decreased to 15 mg/m^2) followed by daily carboplatin (15 mg/m^2) with concurrent radiotherapy (2 Gy/fx-total 66 Gy). An overall response rate of 58% (4 CR, 52 PR) was achieved after induction chemotherapy. Response rate to the overall schedule was 52% of evaluable cases. Median survival was 10 months with 1 and 2 year survival rates of 44% and 23%, respectively.

The use of these new agents alone or in combination with radiotherapy preoperatively in locally advanced stage IIIB and IIIA appears effective in increasing complete responses and survival rates. The results of the intergroup study determining which combined approach is most effective will be eagerly awaited. Randomized trials using these agents should be undertaken in future trials. An Intergroup study combined induction chemotherapy with combination chemotherapy containing either cisplatin > 100 mg/m^2 or carboplatin > 400 mg/m^2 followed by either surgery or XRT in patients who achieved a response. Of the 200 patients entered, 107 patients were randomized (55.5%) [142]. An overall response rate of 57% (9CR/97 PR) was achieved.

Chemotherapy for stage IB, IIA and IIB NSCLC

Surgery is the primary therapy for patients with stage I and II NSCLC, providing cure rates exceeding 70% only for pathologic stage IA (T1, N0, M0) disease. The majority of patients with stage IB to IIIA NSCLC will recur after surgical therapy and the majority of these recurrences are in distant sites [130]. Less than 25% of first recurrences are in regional sites alone, irrespective of the histology of the primary tumor. Thus, effective systemic therapy must be part of any adjuvant or neoadjuvant therapy to have a major impact on survival.

Chest radiotherapy has been used as both preoperative and postoperative therapy. Neither approach has led to improved survival nor overall cure rates, as proven by multiple randomized trials and meta-analysis of these trials [3]. Preoperative radiotherapy with doses greater than 45 Gy increases the operative morbidity and mortality and should not be used alone or with chemotherapy [143]. Postoperative radiotherapy in stage IB-IIIA NSCLC has been found to reduce the rate of local recurrence but has no benefit in overall survival. A randomized trial by the LCSG, investigating the efficacy of postoperative mediastinal irradiation in completely resected squamous cell carcinoma of the lung demonstrated a reduction in local recurrence (1% vs. 21%) but this improvement did not translate into a survival benefit since most of the failures were distant [144]. Because local recurrences may cause symptoms and morbidity, some investigators believe its routine use is justified, especially in patients with N2 disease where the local failure rate is higher. Others prefer careful observations with periodic chest X-rays and radiotherapy reserved for those with regional failure. A recent meta-analysis of 9 randomized clinical trials comparing surgery versus surgery followed by radiotherapy assessed the role of postoperative radiotherapy in the treatment of NSCLC [145]. This meta-analysis showed a 21% relative increase in the risk of death, equivalent to an absolute detriment of 7% at 2 years reducing overall survival from 55% to 48%. Thus, it would seem inappropriate to offer patients postoperative radiotherapy.

The earliest studies of postoperative adjuvant chemotherapy used alkylating agents alone or in combination [3]. These studies showed no benefit for the postoperative chemotherapy and in several studies, including the one above, survival was actually shortened. A meta-analysis of all postoperative adjuvant studies with alkylating agent based therapy confirmed an increased hazard ratio for death and a shortened survival [3]. These therapies were also relatively toxic and these facts led to considerable pessimism for the role of adjuvant chemotherapy.

After cisplatin-based chemotherapy was shown to have activity in advanced NSCLC, it was evaluated as postoperative therapy in resected patients. Many trials used the CAP regimen consisting of cyclophosphamide, adriamycin and low dose cisplatin (40 mg/m^2). Some of these trials showed survival advantages for the chemotherapy but others did not. A meta-analysis of these trials showed that the cisplatin therapy reduced the hazard rate of death by 13%, translating into an absolute improvement in the 5 year survival rate of 5% [3]. Given the small number of patients in these studies, this survival increase was of borderline statistical significance (p = 0.08). Physicians in the UK were surveyed after being shown these data and less than 5% indicated that they would recommend this chemotherapy for their patients [146]. In contrast, when such data were explained to patients, 95% would elect to receive adjuvant chemotherapy which would offer a 5% improvement in survival [147]. This was similar to a prior study where patients with cancer were more likely to opt for cytotoxic chemotherapy with minimal chance of benefit than people without cancer, including medical and nursing professionals [148].

A number of additional and larger adjuvant trials with postoperative cisplatin based therapy are in progress or were recently completed. Some of these trials employed chemotherapy alone and some employed both chemotherapy and chest radiotherapy. There are no published results of trials using chemotherapy regimens based on the newer agents such as paclitaxel, docetaxel, vinorelbine or gemcitabine. Combinations with these agents are more effective than older cisplatin-based regimens in advanced disease [7]. Thus, results of trials with these new combinations are eagerly awaited. In the US and Canada, an intergroup randomized trial compares surgery alone to surgery followed by chemotherapy with vinorelbine and cisplatin.

Clinical stage T2N0, T1N1, T2N1, and T3N0-1 have a poor 5 year survival when treated with surgery alone (36%, 34%, 23% and 8%, respectively) [2]. Since the combination of carboplatin and paclitaxel is active in advanced NSCLC, this combination was tried in earlier stage disease. A multicenter Bi-modality Lung Oncology (BLOT) phase II trial of induction paclitaxel and carboplatin in early stage (T2N0, T1-2N1, and selected T3N0-1) NSCLC was conducted in several institutions in the United States [149]. Paclitaxel (225 mg/m^2 over 3 hours D1) and carboplatin (AUC 6 D1) were given every 21 days for 2 cycles prior to surgery followed by 3 cycles of the same combination chemotherapy in completely resected patients who did not progress on preoperative chemotherapy. Sixty-four patients have been entered and a 55% response was noted after induction chemotherapy (1 CR/33Pr) and 82% [49] underwent complete resection. Final results should be available within a few years. A randomized intergroup study is planned.

Conclusions

New drug combinations are superior to older chemotherapy regimens in advanced NSCLC, increasing survival and improving quality of life compared to best supportive care. New agent based chemotherapy improves survival from four months to about 10 months, one year survival from 10% to 40-50%, and 2 year survival to about 20%. Since several new combinations produce similar results, the optimal two drug combination will be defined when ongoing randomized trials are completed. Three drug combinations which include two new agents have produced encouraging results. Future randomized trials will need to compare these three drug combinations to the best two drug combinations and compare alternating approaches to standard two drug combinations.

In stage III patients, the addition of combination chemotherapy to radiotherapy prolongs survival in stage IIIB patients with median survivals of about 14-16 months and 5 year survival rates of about 15-20% compared to 5% with radiotherapy alone. Newer agents in combination with radiotherapy have shown higher median and one year survival rates compared to prior cisplatin-based regimens, with median survivals of about 18 months and one year survival rates of about 62%. Some studies have shown an increased resectability rate in patients with locally advanced disease. In stage IIIA patients, chemotherapy alone or in combination with radiotherapy prior to surgery has been shown to improve survival. Future studies will determine whether all three modalities are superior to chemotherapy + surgery or chemotherapy + radiotherapy. Results of studies using the new agents will be eagerly anticipated.

In patients with resectable IB, IIA, IIB NSCLC, postoperative cisplatin-based chemotherapy produced a modest survival advantage. Preliminary trials with newer chemotherapy-based regimens are ongoing and results are pending. Neoadjuvant chemotherapy using in combination these new agents in such groups of patients are also ongoing with preliminary results showing promise.

Lung cancer diagnosis should not be viewed with pessimism. The role of chemotherapy in lung cancer patients should be viewed with optimism and thus be offered to lung cancer patients.

References

1. Parker SL, Tong T, Bolden S, Wingo PA (1997) Cancer Statistics. Cancer J Clin 47: 5-27
2. Mountain CF (1997) Revisions in the international system for staging lung cancer. Chest 111:1710-1717
3. Non-small Cell Collaborative Group (1995) Chemotherapy in non-small cell lung cancer. Meta-analysis using updated data in individual patients from 52 randomized clinical trials. Brit Med J 311:899-909
4. Bunn PA Jr (1989) The expanding role of cisplatin in the treatment of non-small cell lung cancer. Semin Oncol 16(Suppl 6):10-21
5. Billingham LJ, Cullen MH, Woods J et al (1997) Mitomycin, ifosfamide and cisplatin in non-small cell lung cancer. Results of a randomized trial evaluating palliation and quality of life. Lung Cancer 18(Suppl 1):A9
6. Ellis PA, Smith IE, Hardy JR et al (1995) Symptom relief with MVP (mitomycin C, vinblastine and cisplatin) chemotherapy in advanced non-small cell lung cancer. Brit J Cancer 71:366-370

7. Bunn PA Jr, Kelly K (1998) New chemotherapeutic agents prolong survival and improve quality of life in non-small cell lung cancer. Review of the literature and future directions. Clin Cancer Res 5:1087-1100

8. Vokes EE (1995) Integration of Vinorelbine into Chemotherapy Strategies for Non-Small Cell Lung Cancer. Oncology 9:565-575

9. LeChevalier T, Pujol JL, Douillard JY et al (1994) A three arm trial of vinorelbine (Navelbine) plus cisplatin, vindesine plus cisplatin, and single agent vinorelbine in the treatment of non-small cell lung cancer: An expanded analysis. Semin Oncol 21:28-33

10. Crawford J, O'Rourke M, Schiller J et al (1996) Randomized trial of vinorelbine compared with fluorouracil plus leucovorin in patients with stage IV non-small cell lung cancer. J Clin Oncol 14:2777-2784

11. Pronzato P, Landucci M, Vaira F et al (1994) Failure of vinorelbine to produce responses in pretreated non-small cell lung cancer patients. Anticancer Res 14:1413-1416

12. Rinaldi M, Della Giulia M, Venturo I et al (1994) Vinorelbine as single agent in the treatment of advanced non-small cell lung cancer. Proc Am Soc Clin Oncol 13:A360

13. Santoro A, Maiorino L, Santoro M (1994) Second line with vinorelbine in the weekly monotherapy for the treatment of advanced non-small cell lung cancer. Lung Cancer 11(Suppl 1):A130

14. Tononi A, Panzini I, Oliverio G et al (1997) Vinorelbine chemotherapy in non-small cell lung cancer: experience in elderly patients. J Chemother 9(4):304-308

15. Gridelli C, Perrone F, Gallo C et al: Vinorelbine is well tolerated and active in the treatment of elderly patients with advanced non-small cell lung cancer. A two-stage phase II study. E J Cancer 33: 392-397, 1997

16. Veronesi A, Crivellari D, Magri MD et al (1996) Vinorelbine treatment of advanced non small cell lung cancer with special emphasis on elderly patients. Eur J Cancer 32A:1809-1811

17. Furuse K, Fukuoka M, Hara N et al (1998) Vinorelbine in the Treatment of Elderly patients with advanced non-small cell lung cancer. Proc Am Soc Clin Oncol 17:A1862

18. Perrone F, Rossi A, Ianniello GP et al (1998) Vinorelbine plus best supportive care (BSC) vs BSC in the treatment of advanced non-small cell lung cancer elderly patients. Results of a phase III randomized trial. Proc Am Soc Clin Oncol 17:A1752

19. Chang AY, Kubota K, Kawahara M et al (1993) A phase II study of Taxol, merbarone and piroxantrone in stage IV non-small cell lung cancer: the Eastern Cooperative Oncology Group results. J Natl Cancer Inst 85:388-394

20. Murphy WK, Fosella F, Winn et al (1993) Phase II study of Taxol in patients with untreated advanced non-small cell lung cancer. J Natl Cancer Inst 85:384-387

21. Gatzemeier U, Heckmayr M, Neuhauss R et al (1995) Phase II study of paclitaxel for the treatment of advanced inoperable non-small cell lung cancer. Lung Cancer 12(Suppl 2):101-106

22. Hainsworth JD, Hopkins L, Thomas M et al (1994) Taxol administered by one hour infusion: Preliminary results of a phase I/II study comparing two dose schedules. Lung Cancer 11(Suppl 11):A96

23. Akerley W, Choy H, Safran H et al (1997) Weekly paclitaxel in patients with advanced lung cancer: preliminary data from a phase II trial. Semin Oncol 24(Suppl 12):10-13

24. Chang A, Boros L, Asbury R et al (1998) Weekly moderate-dose paclitaxel in stage IV non-small cell lung cancer. Proc Am Soc Clin Oncol 17:A1806

25. Murphy WK, Fosella FV, Winn RJ et al (1994) Phase II study of Taxol in patients with non-small cell lung cancer who have failed platinum containing chemotherapy. Proc Am Soc Clin Oncol 13:A363
26. Ruckdeschel J, Wagner H, Williams C et al (1994) Second line chemotherapy for resistant metastatic non-small cell lung cancer: The role of Taxol. Proc Am Soc Clin Oncol 13:A357
27. Hainsworth JD, Thompson DS, Greco FA (1995) Paclitaxel by 1 hr infusion: An active drug in metastatic non-small cell lung cancer. J Clin Oncol 13:1609-1614
28. LeChevalier T, Mattson K, Bosquee L et al (1997) Phase II study of docetaxel (Taxotere) in locally advanced or metastatic non-small cell lung cancer (NSCLC); Interim report on 204 patients. Lung Cancer 18(Suppl 1):A83
29. Fossella FV, Lee JS, Hong WK (1997) Management strategies for recurrent non-small cell lung cancer. Semin Oncol 24:455-462
30. Gandara DR, Vokes E, Green M et al (1997) Docetaxel (Taxotere) in platinum-treated non-small cell lung cancer (NSCLC): confirmation of prolonged survival in a multicenter trial. Proc Am Soc Clin Oncol, 16:A1632
31. Fossella F, Devore R, Kerr R et al (1998) Randomised phase III study of Taxotere (100 mg/m^2 and 75 mg/m^2) versus Vinorelbine or Ifosfamide in non-small cell lung cancer patients, previously treated with platinum-based chemotherapy. Proc Am Soc Clin Oncol 17:A1859
32. Manegold C: Single agent gemcitabine versus cistaplin/etoposide with inoperable, locally advanced, or metastatic non-small cell lung cancer. Semin Oncol 25 (suppl 9): 1=-22, 1998
33. Perng RP, Chen YM, Ming-Liu J et al (1997) Gemcitabine versus the combination of cisplatin and etoposide in patients with inoperable non-small cell lung cancer in a phase II randomized study. J Clin Oncol 15:2097-2102
34. Crino L, Mosconi AM, Scagliotti GV et al: Gemcitabine as second-line treatment for relapsing or refractory advanced non-small cell lung cancer: a phase II trial. Semin Oncol 25 (suppl 9): 23-26, 1998
35. Rosvold R, Langer CJ, Schilder R et al (1998) Salvage therapy with gemcitabine in advanced non-small cell lung cancer progressing after prior carboplatin-paclitaxel. Proc Am Soc Clin Oncol 17:A1797
36. Martin C, Artizzoni A and Rosso R: Gemcitabine: safety profile and efficacy in non-small cell lung cancer unaffected by age. Aging 9: 297-303, 1997
37. CPT-11 Cooperative Group Study (1991) A phase II study of CPT-11, a camptothecin derivative, in patients with primary lung cancer. Jpn J Cancer Chemother 18:1013-1019
38. Nakai H, Fukuoka M, Furuse K et al (1991) An early phase II study of CPT-11 for primary lung cancer. Jpn J Cancer Chemother 18:607-612
39. Niitani H, Fukuoka M, Nagao K (1994) Clinical development of irinotecan (CPT-11) in lung cancers. Lung Cancer 11(Suppl 2):30-31
40. Wozniak AJ, Crowley JJ, Balcerzak SP et al: Randomized trial comparing cisplatin with cisplatin plus vinorelbine in the treatment of advanced non-small cell lung cancer: A Southwest Oncology Group Study. J Clin Oncol 16: 2459-2465, 1998
41. Bonomi P, Kim K, Kugler K et al (1997) Results of a Phase III Trial comparing taxol-cisplatin (TC) regimens to etoposide-cisplatin (EC) in non-small cell lung cancer (NSCLC) Lung Cancer 18(Suppl 1):A28
42. Bunn PA (1989) Review of therapeutic trials of carboplatin in lung cancer. Semin Oncol 16:27-33

43. Garst, J, Crawford J, O'Rourke M et al (1996) Vinorelbine (NVB) and carboplatin for the treatment of patients with advanced non-small cell lung cancer (NSCLC): a phase II response, toxicity and survival study. Proc Am Soc Clin Oncol 15:A1233
44. Masotti A, Borzellino G, Zannini G et al (1995) Efficacy and toxicity of vinorelbine-carboplatin combinations in the treatment of advanced adenocarcinoma or large cell carcinoma of the lung. Tumori 81:112-116
45. Pronzato P, Ghio E, Losardo PL et al (1996) Carboplatin and vinorelbine in advanced non-small cell lung cancer. Cancer Chemother Pharmacol 37:610-612
46. Pennucci MC, Baldini E, Portalone L et al (1996) Cisplatin, vindesine, mitomycin vs. cisplatin, ifosfamide, navelbine vs. carboplatin, navelbine for stage IIIB/IV non-small cell lung cancer patients: a randomized phase II FONICAP trial. Proc Am Soc Clin Oncol 14:A1107
47. Giaccone P, Splinter TA, Debruyne C et al (1998) Randomized study of palitaxel-cisplatin versus cisplatin-teniposide in patients with advanced non-small cell lung cancer. J Clin Oncol 16(6):2133-2141
48. Gatzemeier U, von Pawel J, Gottfried M et al (1998) Phase II comparative study of high-dose cisplatin versus a combination of paclitaxel and cisplatin in patients with advanced non-small cell lung cancer. Proc Am Soc Clin Oncol 17:A1748
49. Langer CJ, Millenson M, Rosvold E et al (1997) Paclitaxel (1 hour) and carboplatin (AUC 7.5) in advanced non-small cell lung cancer: A phase II study of the Fox Chase Cancer Center and Its Network. Semin Oncol 24(Suppl 12):81-88
50. Greco FA, Hainsworth JD (1998) One hour paclitaxel plus carboplatin in advanced non-small cell lung cancer : Preliminary results of a Multicenter study. Oncology 12(Suppl 2):71-73
51. Belani CP, Natale RB, Lee JS et al (1998) Randomized phase III trial comparing cisplatin/etoposide versus carboplatin/paclitaxel in advanced and metastatic non-small cell lung cancer. Proc Am Soc Clin Oncol 17:A1751
52. Ukena D, Leutz M, Schroder R et al (1997) Intensified treatment of stage IV non-small cell lung cancer (NSCLC): Weekly chemotherapy with paclitaxel and carboplatin. Lung Cancer 18(Suppl 1):A122
53. Georgoulias V, Androulakis N, Dimopoulos C et. al: First-line treatment of advanced non-small cell lung cancer with docetaxel and cisplatin: a multicenter phase II study. Ann Oncol 9: 331-334, 1998
54. Mattson K, Vansteenkiste J, Saarinen A et al (1997) A phase II study of docetaxel (taxotere) alternating with cisplatin with full doses of both drugs for advanced NSCLC. Lung Cancer 18(Suppl 1):A64
55. Orcel B, Antoine EC, Benhammouda A et al (1997) Interim results of a sequential administration of docetaxel (taxotere) followed by Cisplatin-vindesine in chemotherapy naïve patients with locally advanced or metastatic non-small cell lung cancer (NSCLC). Lung Cancer 18 (Suppl 1):A197
56. Belani CP, Einzig A, Bonomi P et al (1997) Multi-institutional phase II trial of docetaxel and carboplatin combination in patients with stage IIIB and IV non-small cell lung cancer (NSCLC). Lung Cancer 18(Suppl 1):A52
57. Capozzoli MJ, Belani CP, Einzig A et al (1998) Multi-institutional phase II trial of docetaxel and carboplatin combination in patients with stage IIIB and IV non-small cell lung cancer. Proc Am Soc Clin Oncol 17:A1845
58. Peters GJ, Bergman AM, Ruiz van Haoeren VWT et al (1995) Interaction between cisplatin and gemcitabine in vitro and in vivo. Semin Oncol 22(Suppl 11):72-79

59. Lopez Cabrerizo MP, Cardenal F, Artal A et al (1997) Gemcitabine plus cisplatin versus etoposide plus cisplatin in advanced non-small cell lung cancer: A randomized trial by the Spanish Lung Cancer Group. Lung Cancer 18(Suppl 1):A27

60. Sandler A, Nemunaitis J, Dehnam C et al (1998) Phase III study of cisplatin with or without gemcitabine in patients with advanced non-small cell lung cancer. Proc Am Soc Clin Oncol 17:A1747

61. Crino L, Conte P, De Marinis F et al (1998) A randomized trial of gemcitabine cisplatin versus mitomycin, ifosfamide and cisplatin in advanced non-small cell lung cancer. Proc Am Soc Clin Oncol 17:A1750

62. Carmichael J, Allerheiligen S, Walling J (1996) A phase I study of gemcitabine and carboplatin in non-small cell lung cancer. Semin Oncol 23(Suppl 10):55-59

63. Ng EW, Sandler AB, Einhorn LH (1998) A phase II study of carboplatin plus gemcitabine in non-small cell lung cancer. Proc Am Soc Clin Oncol 17:A1801

64. Rapp E, Pater JL, Willan A et al (1988) Chemotherapy can prolong survival in patients with advanced non-small cell lung cancer-Report of a Canadian multicenter randomized trial. J Clin Oncol 6:633-641

65. Georgoulias V, Kourousis C, Kakolyris S et al (1997) Second-line treatment of advanced non-small cell lung cancer with paclitaxel and gemcitabine: a preliminary report on an active regimen. Semin Oncol 24(4 Suppl 12):61-66

66. Breton JL, Jacoulet P, Pellae-Cosset et al (1997) Phase I study of paclitaxel (P) over 1 hr infusion in combination with vinorelbine (V) in advanced non small cell lung cancer (NSCLC). Lung Cancer 18 (Suppl 1):A202

67. Chang AY, DeVore R, Gu C et al (1997) Paclitaxel and vinorelbine in non-small cell lung cancer. In vitro and clinical studies. Oncology 11(Suppl 12):31-34

68. Georgoulias V, Kourousis C, Androulakis N et al (1998) Frontline treatment of advanced non-small cell lung cancer with docetaxel and gemcitabine: A multicenter phase II trial. Proc Am Soc Clin Oncol 17:A1819

69. Miller VA, Grant SC, Ng K et al (1998) Phase I trial of docetaxel and vinorelbine with filgrastim in patients with advanced non-small cell lung cancer. Proc Am Soc Clin Oncol 17:A1813

70. Trillet-Lenoir V, Monnier A, Douillard JY et al (1996) Interim results of a phase II study of docetaxel (Taxotere) and vinorelbine in chemotherapy naïve patients with advanced non-small cell lung carcinoma (NSCLC)(abstr 450P). Ann Oncol 7(Suppl 5):95

71. Kourousis C, Androulakis N, Kakolyris S et al (1996) First line treatment of non-small cell lung carcinoma (NSCLC) with docetaxel and vinorelbine: A phase II study (abstr 1441P). Ann Oncol 7(Suppl 5):93

72. Lorusso V, Mancarella S, Carpagnano F et al (1998) Gemcitabine plus vinorelbine in patients with stage IIIB-IV non small cell lung cancer. A phase II study. Proc Am Soc Clin Oncol 17:A1808

73. Esteban E, Llano JLG, Vieitex JM et al (1998) Phase I/II study of gemcitabine plus vinorelbine in non-small cell lung cancer. Proc Am Soc Clin Oncol 17:A1855

74. Isokangas OP, Mattson K, Joensuu H et al (1998) A phase II study of vinorelbine and gemcitabine in inoperable stage IIIB-IV NSCLC. Proc Am Soc Clin Oncol 17:A1882

75. Lilenbaum RC, Schwartz MA, Cano R et al (1998) Gemcitabine and navelbine in advanced non-small cell lung cancer. Proc Am Soc Clin Oncol 17:A1901

76. Kudoh S, Negoro S, Masuda N et al (1997) Phase I/II study of docetaxel and irinotecan (CPT-11) for previously untreated advanced non-small cell lung cancer (NSCLC). Lung Cancer 18(Suppl 1):A144

77. Kelly K (1998) The Fox Chase Cancer Center and Free University Investigator's Workshop and Consensus Conference. St. Thomas, US Virgin Islands, March 26-27

78. Hainsworth JD, Erland JB, Hon JK et al (1998) Phase I/II trial of paclitaxel (1 hour infusion), carboplatin and gemcitabine in the treatment of advanced non-small cell lung cancer. Proc Am Soc Clin Oncol 17:A1811

79. Frasci G, Comella P, Panza N et al (1998) Cisplatin-gemcitabine-paclitaxel in advanced non-small cell lung cancer. A dose finding study. Proc Am Soc Clin Oncol 17:A1850

80. Sorensen JB, Stenbyggard LE, Hansen HH et al (1998) Biweekly paclitaxel, gemcitabine and cisplatin in non-resectable non-small cell lung cancer. Proc Am Soc Clin Oncol 17:A1930

81. Greco FA (1998) The Fox Chase Cancer Center and Free University Investigator's Workshop and Consensus Conference. St. Thomas, US Virgin Islands, March 26-27

82. Comella P, Panza N, Frasci G et al (1997) Gemcitabine (GEM)-cisplatin (CDDP)-vinorelbine (VNR) combination in advanced non-small cell lung cancer (NSCLC). A phase II randomized study. Lung Cancer 18:A231

83. Gonzalez-Baron M, Garcia MJ, Chacon JI et al (1998) A phase II study of gemcitabine, cisplatin and vinorelbine in patients with advanced non-small cell lung cancer. Proc Am Soc Clin Oncol 17:A1802

84. Dorta J, Martin G, Constenla M et al (1998) A phase II study of gemcitabine, cisplatin and vinorelbine in patients with advanced non-small cell lung cancer. Proc Am Soc Clin Oncol 17:A1853

85. Viallet J, Laberge F, Martins H et al (1996) A phase II trial of docetaxel alternating with cisplatin and vinorelbine in non small cell lung cancer. Ann Oncol 7(Suppl 5):A440P

86. Georgoulias V, Kourousis C, Androulakis N et al (1997) Docetaxel(Taxotere) and vinorelbine in the treatment of non-small cell lung cancer. Semin Oncol 24 (Suppl 14):9-14

87. Masters G, Mauer AM, Hoffman PC et al: A phase I-II study of paclitaxel, ifosfamide, and vinorelbine with filgrastim (rhG-CSF) support in advanced non-small cell lung cancer. Ann Oncol 9: 677-680, 1998

88. Castellano D, Lianes P, Calzas J et al (1998) Non-cisplatin based chemotherapy for advanced non small cell lung cancer: A phase II study with gemcitabine, ifosfamide and vinorelbine. Proc Am Soc Clin Oncol 17:A1847

89. Comella P, Frasci G, DeCataldis G et al: Cistaplin/carboplatin + etoposide + vnorelbine in advanced NSCLC. A randomised phase II. Gruppo Oncologico Compano. Br J Cancer 74: 1805-1811, 1998

90. Zarogoulidis K, Papagiannis A, Constantinidis TC et al (1997) Paclitaxel, carboplatin and mitomycin as first line treatment in patients with advanced non-small cell lung cancer (NSCLC). Lung Cancer 18(Suppl 1):A227

91. Zaniboni A, Meriggi F, Rizzi A et al (1997) Paclitaxel, ifosfamide and carboplatin for the treatment of stages IIIB and IV non-small cell lung cancer: Preliminary results. Semin Oncol 24(Suppl 12):70-72

92. Donnellan P, Duffy K, Murray R et al (1997) Combination of docetaxel (Taxotere), ifosfamide and cisplatin in non-small cell lung cancer (NSCLC). Lung Cancer 18 (Suppl 1): A228

93. Perol M, Guerin JC, Thomas P et al (1996) Multicenter randomized trial comparing cisplatin-mitomycin-vinorelbine versus cisplatin-mitomycin-vindesine in advanced non-small cell lung cancer. 'Groupe Francais de Pneumo-cancerologie' Lung Cancer 14:119-134

94. Mohedano N, Sanchez-Rovira P, Medina B et al (1997) Phase II trial of gemcitabine in combination with cisplatin and ifosfamide in advanced non-small cell lung cancer (NSCLC). Lung Cancer 18(Suppl 1):A159

95. Barneto IC, De la Haba J, Gosalbez B et al (1997) Phase II activity of cisplatin (CDDP) plus ifosfamide (IFO) and gemcitabine (GEM) in non small cell lung cancer (NSCLC). Preliminary results. Lung Cancer 18 (Suppl 1):A204

96. Jaakkimainen L, Goodwin PJ, Pater J et al (1990) Counting the costs of chemotherapy in a National Cancer Institute of Canada randomized trial in nonsmall-cell lung cancer. J Clin Oncol 8:1301-1309

97. Evans WK (1997) Treatment of NSCLC with chemotherapy is controversial because of low response and high cost. Lung Cancer 18(Suppl2):117-118

98. Pritchard RS, Anthony SP (1996) Chemotherapy plus Radiotherapy Compared with Radiotherapy Alone in the Treatment of Locally Advanced, Unresectable, NSCLC. A meta-analysis. Ann Int Med 125:723-729

99. Dillman RO, Seagren SL, Herndon J et al (1990) A randomized trial of induction chemotherapy plus high-dose radiation versus radiation alone in stage III non-small cell lung cancer. N Engl J Med 323:940-945

100. Dillman RO, Herndin J, Seagren SL et al (1996) Improved survival in stage III non-small cell lung cancer: seven year follow-up of cancer and leukemia group B (CALGB) 8433 trial. J Natl Cancer Inst 88:1210-1215

101. Sause WT, Kolesar P, Taylor S et al (1998) Five-year results; Phase III trial of regionally advanced unresectable non-small cell lung cancer, RTOG 8808, ECOG 4588, SWOG 8992. Proc Am Soc Clin Oncol 17:A1743

102. Le Chevalier T, Arriagada R, Quiox E et al (1991) Radiotherapy alone versus combined chemotherapy and radiotherapy in unresectable non-small cell lung cancer: First analysis of a randomized trial in 353 patients. J Natl Cancer Inst 83:417-423

103. Schaake-Koning C, Van Den Bogert W, Dalesio O et al (1992) Effects of concomitant cisplatin and radiotherapy in inoperable non-small cell lung cancer. N Engl J Med 326:524-530

104. Jeremic B, Shibamoto Y, Acinovic L et al (1995) Randomized trial of hyperfractionated radiation therapy with or without concurrent chemotherapy for stage III non-small cell lung cancer. J Clin Oncol 13:452-458

105. Jeremic B, Shibamoto Y, Acinovic L et al (1996) Hyperfractionated radiation therapy with or without concurrent low dose daily carboplatin/etoposide for stage III non-small cell lung cancer: A randomized study. J Clin Oncol 14:1065-1070

106. Takada Y, Furuse K, Fukuoka YH et al (1997) A randomized phase III study of concurrent versus sequential thoracic radiotherapy (TRT) in combination with mitomycin, vindesine, and cisplatin in unresectable stage III non-small cell lung cancer (NSCLC). Lung Cancer 18(Suppl 1):A294

107. Leonard C, Chan DC, Chou PC et al (1996) Paclitaxel enhances in vitro radiosensitivity of squamous carcinoma cell lines of the head and neck. Cancer Res 56:5198-5204

108. McGinn CJ, Shewach DS, Lawrence TS (1996) Radiosensitizing nucleosides. J Natl Cancer Inst 88:1193-1203

109. Okishio K, Kudoh S, Kurihara N et al (1996) Irinotecan (CPT-11) enhances the radiosensitivity of lung cancer cells in vitro. Cellular Pharmacol 3:247-252

110. Langer CJ, Movsas B, Hudes R et al (1997) Induction Paclitaxel and carboplatin followed by concurrent chemoradiotherapy in patients with unresectable, locally advanced non-small cell lung carcinoma: Report of Fox Chase Cancer Center Study 94-001. Semin Oncol 24(Suppl 12):89-95

111. Isokangas OP, Joensuu H, Halme M et al: Paclitaxel (Taxol) and carboplatin followed by concomitant paclitaxel, cisplatin and radiotherapy for inoperable stage III NSCLC. Lung Cancer 20: 127-123, 1998

112. Greco FA, Stroup SL, Gray JR et al (1996) Paclitaxel in combination with radiotherapy in patients with unresectable stage III non-small cell lung cancer. J Clin Oncol 14:1642-1648

113. Choy H, Safran H, Akerley W et al: Phase II trial of weekly paclitaxel and concurrent radiation therapy for locally advanced non-small cell lung cancer. Clin Cancer Res 4: 1931-1936, 1998

114. Choy H, Ackerley W, Safran H et al: Multiinstitutional phase II trial of paclitaxel, carboplatin, and concurrent radiation therapy for locally advanced non-small cell lung cancer. J Clin Oncol 16: 3316-3322, 1998

115. Belani CP, Aisner J, Day R et al (1997) Promising long term outcome of weekly paclitaxel and carboplatin with simultaneous thoracic radiotherapy (TRT) for locally advanced non-small cell lung cancer (NSCLC). Lung Cancer 18(Suppl 1):A242

116. Choy H, DeVore RF, Hande KR et al: Preliminary analysis of a phase II study of paclitaxel, carboplatin, and hyperfractionated radiation therapy for locally advanced inoperable non-small cell lung cancer. Semin Oncol 24 (suppl 12): 21-26, 1997

117. Comella G, Frasci G, Scoppa G et al (1997) Weekly paclitaxel/cisplatin with concurrent radiotherapy in patients with locally advanced non-small cell lung cancer: A phase I study. Semin Oncol 24(Suppl 12):113-116

118. Lau D, Ryu J, Gandara D et al (1997) Twice-weekly paclitaxel and radiation for stage III non-small cell lung cancer. Semin Oncol 24(Suppl 12):102-109

119. Pisch J, Pagluica T, Malamud S et al (1997) Uninterrupted twice a day irradiation with concomitant chemotherapy and G-CSF for advanced lung cancer. Phase I-II study. Lung Cancer 18(Suppl 1):A262

120. Rigas J, Leopold K, Maurer LH et al (1997) Daily paclitaxel and thoracic radiation for the treatment of stage II-IIIB NSCLC. Lung Cancer 18(Suppl 1):A268

121. Koukourakis MI, Kourousis C, Kamilaki M et al: Weekly docetaxel and concomitant boost radiotherapy for non-small cell lung cancer. A phase I/II dose escalation trial. Eur J Cancer 34(6): 838-844, 1998

122. Gregor A (1997) Gemcitabine plus radiotherapy for non-small cell lung cancer. Semin Oncol 24(8)39-41

123. Lawrence T, Eisbruch A and Shewach DS: Gemcitabine-mediated radiosensitization. Semin Oncol 24 (2 suppl 7): 24-28, 1997

124. Scalliet P, Goor C, Galdermans D et al (1998) Gemzar (gemcitabine) with thoracic radiotherapy. A phase II pilot study in chemonaive patients with advanced non-small cell lung cancer. Proc Am Soc Clin Oncol 17:A1923

125. Masters G, Haraf DJ, Hoffman PC et al: Phase I study of vinorelbine, cisplatin, and concomitant thoracic radiation in the treatment of advanced chest malignancies. J Clin Oncol 16(6): 2157-2163, 1998

126. Viallet J, Rousseau P, Souhami L et al (1995) A phase I/II trial of neoadjuvant chemotherapy with cisplatin and vinorelbine (Navelbine) followed by accelerated thoracic irradiation in inoperable non-small cell lung cancer. Proc Am Soc Clin Oncol 14:A1169

127. Zatloukal P, Petruzelka L, Zemanova M et al (1998) Vinorelbine plus cisplatin and concurrent radiotherapy in advanced non-small cell lung cancer. Proc Am Soc Clin Oncol 17:A1947

128. Nakagawa K, Yamamoto, Kudoh S et al (1998) Irinotecan (CPT-11) and carboplatin with concurrent thoracic radiotherapy for unresectable stage III non-small cell lung cancer. Preliminary results. Proc Am Soc Clin Oncol 17:A1909

129. Vokes EE, Leopold KA, Herndon JE et al (1997) A CALGB randomized phase II study of gemcitabine or paclitaxel or vinorelbine with cisplatin as induction chemotherapy (Inc CT) and concomitant chemoradiotherapy (XRT) in stage IIIB non-small cell lung cancer (NSCLC): feasibility data (CALGB #9431). Proc Am Soc Clin Oncol 16:A1636

130. Bunn PA Jr (1994) The Treatment of Non-Small Cell Lung Cancer: Current Perspectives and Controversies, Future Directions. Semin Oncol 21(Suppl 6):49-59

131. Martini N, Kris M, Flehinger B et al (1993) Preoperative chemotherapy for stage IIIA (N2) lung cancer: The Sloan Kettering experience with 136 patients. Ann Thorac Surg 55:1365-1374

132. Burkes R, Ginsberg, Shepherd F et al (1992) Induction chemotherapy with mitomycin C, vindesine and cisplatin for stage III unresectable non-small cell lung cancer: results of the Toronto phase II trial. J Clin Oncol 10:580-586

133. Sugarbaker DJ, Herndon J, Kohman LJ et al (1995) Results of Cancer and Leukemia Group B Protocol 8935: multiinstitutional phase II trimodality trial for stage IIIA (N2) NSCLC. J Thorac Cardiovasc Surg 109:473-485

134. Rosell R, Gomez-Codina J, Camps C et al (1994) A randomized trial comparing preoperative chemotherapy plus surgery with surgery alone in patients with non-small cell lung cancer. N Engl J Med 330:153-158

135. Roth JAB, Fossella F, Komaki R et al (1992) A randomized trial comparing perioperative chemotherapy and surgery with surgery alone in resectable stage IIIA non-small cell lung cancer. J Natl Cancer Inst 86:673-680

136. Albain KS, Rusch V, Crowley J et al (1995) Concurrent cisplatin/etoposide plus chest radiotherapy followed by surgery for stages IIIA and IIIB non-small cell lung cancer: Mature results of Southwest Oncology Group phase II study 8805. J Clin Oncol 13:1880-1892

137. Eberhardt W, Wilke H, Stamatis G et al (1998) Preoperative chemotherapy followed by concurrent chemoradiation therapy based on hyperfractionated accelerated radiotherapy and definitive surgery in locally advanced non-small cell lung cancer: Mature results of a phase II trial. J Clin Oncol 16:622-634

138. Ukena D, Leutz M, Huwer H et al (1997) Induction chemotherapy with paclitaxel and carboplatin in locally advanced stage IIIA/IIIB non-small cell lung cancer (NSCLC). Lung Cancer 18(Suppl 1):A230

139. Friedland D, Greenberg R, Miller W et al (1997) Phase II trial of perioperative paclitaxel plus granulocyte-colony stimulating factor in mediastinoscopy staged IIIA-N2 non-small cell lung cancer. Lung Cancer 18(Suppl 1):A283

140. O'Rourke MA, Klassy JA, Denham CA et al (1997) An evaluation of a two drug combination of navelbine and cisplatin as neoadjuvant therapy for patients presenting with inoperable stage IIIA or IIIB non-small cell lung cancer. Proc Am Soc Clin Oncol 16:A1717

141. Bardet E, Douillard JY, Riviere A et al (1997) Induction chemotherapy (ICT cisplatin and vinorelbine) followed by a combination of daily irradiation and carboplatine (CBDCA) in stage IIIB non-small cell lung cancer (NSCLC): Final analysis of a phase II trial. Lung Cancer 18(Suppl 1):A352

142. Splinter TAW, Kirkpatrick A, van Meerbeeck J et al (1998) Randomized trial of surgery versus radiotherapy in patients with stage IIIA non-small cell lung cancer after

a response to induction chemotherapy. Intergroup study 08941. Proc Am Soc Clin Oncol 17:A1742

143. Wagner H Jr, Lad T, Piantadosi S (1991) Randomized phase II evaluation of preoperative radiation therapy and preoperative chemotherapy with mitomycin C, vinblastine and cisplatin in patients with technically unresectable IIIA and IIIB non-small cell lung Cancer. Lung cancer 7:157

144. Weisenburger JH, Lung Cancer Study Group (1986) Effects of postoperative mediastinal radiation on completely resected stage II and stage III epidermoid carcinoma of the lung. N Engl J Med 315:1377

145. Stewart LA, Burdett S, Souhami RL (1998) Post operative radiotherapy (PORT) in non-small cell lung cancer: A meta-analysis using individual patient data from randomised clinical trials. Proc Am Soc Clin Oncol 17:A1760

146. Crook A, Duffy A, Girling DJ et al (1997) Survey on the treatment of non-small cell lung cancer in England and Wales. Lung Cancer 18(Suppl 1):9

147. Yellan SB, Cella DF (1995) Someone to live for: Social well being, parenthood states, and decision making in oncology. J Clin Oncol 13:1255-1264

148. Slevin ML, Stubbs L, Plant HJ et al (1990) Attitudes to chemotherapy: comparing views of patients with cancer with those of doctors, nurses and general public. BMJ 2/300(6737):1458-1460

149. Pisters KMW, Ginsberg RJ (1998) Phase II trial of induction paclitaxel & carboplatin in early stage (T2N0, T1-2N1, & selected T3N0-1) non-small cell lung cancer. Proc Am Soc Clin Oncol 17:A1738

Part IV
Urological Tumors

Update in testicular cancer

L. H. Einhorn

Introduction

Germ cell tumors are relatively uncommon, accounting for only 1% of male malignancies in the United States. The highest worldwide incidence is in Scandinavian countries; by contrast, testicular cancer is rare in African Americans. The primary age group is 15-35 for nonseminomatous tumors and a decade older for seminoma. Thus, the potential for loss of productive years of life has always made testis cancer important both medically and economically.

In 1998, there will be approximately 8,000 newly diagnosed cases in the United States. This contrasts sharply with the 317,000 cases of prostate cancer in 1996. Most important clinical questions have been addressed and answered in testis cancer by randomized phase III studies, whereas many relevant issues remain unresolved in cancer of the prostate.

Despite the paucity of cases, this tumor has become an extremely important oncological disease. Firstly, it is the most common carcinoma in young men ages 15 to 35 and thus, has the potential to greatly shorten productive years of life compared to most other more common carcinomas. Secondly, available serum markers (alphafetoprotein and human chorionic gonadotropin) allow the clinician to make important and accurate treatment-related decisions. Thirdly, it has been demonstrated that surgical resection of radiographically persistent disease can improve the cure rate. Fourthly, germ cell tumors have become an excellent testing ground for active experimental drugs (e.g. cisplatin, VP-16, and ifosfamide, all of which were approved by the FDA primarily upon data in testicular cancer). This is an important disease because it has become a model for a curable neoplasm. The goal of chemotherapy in germ cell tumors is never merely palliation or prolongation of survival, but cure.

Testis cancer has long been a model for a curable neoplasm [1, 2]. Germ cell tumors are uniquely chemosensitive and chemocurable. Surgery also plays a major role, both as primary treatment and for postchemotherapy resection. Orchiectomy plus retroperitoneal lymph node dissection has a higher cure rate than any other type of cancer surgery with nodal metastases.

There are many published updates and reviews concerning the management of germ cell tumors in textbooks and journals, including a recent review article from Memorial Sloan Kettering Cancer Center [3]. This paper will review past and present accomplishments, current chemotherapy strategies, and emphasize complicated and controversial surgical issues.

Early Chemotherapy Studies

Prior to the usage of cisplatin combination chemotherapy, standard chemotherapy for disseminated testicular cancer consisted of dactinomycin, alone or in combination with methotrexate and chlorambucil. Thirty years ago Dr. Li and colleagues at Memorial Sloan Kettering recognized that testis cancer was chemosensitive, with a 50% objective response rate including 10% to 20% complete remissions (C.R.) and a 5% to 10% cure rate [4]. Samuels and colleagues at M.D. Anderson later evaluated vinblastine + bleomycin, a synergistic regimen in preclinical studies, and achieved a 25% long-term disease-free survival [5]. However, the most important event in chemotherapy of germ cell tumors was the discovery of cisplatin by Dr. Rosenberg [6]. In early clinical trials, this drug was very toxic with only modest activity in various solid tumors when used in chemorefractory and heavily pre-treated patients. Investigators at Roswell Park evaluated cisplatin in previously treated patients with germ cell tumors and obtained 3 complete and 3 partial remissions in 11 patients [7].

With this background, in August 1974, we began our initial cisplatin + vinblastine + bleomycin (PVB) study at Indiana University, utilizing the established two-drug synergistic regimen of vinblastine + bleomycin, and simply adding the then experimental promising drug cisplatin [8]. The PVB regimen fulfilled the requirements for a successful combination chemotherapy regimen: single agent activity for each component of the PVB regimen, different and unique mechanism of action for the three agents, separate and non-overlapping toxicity, allowing administration of each drug in full dosage, and evidence of preclinical synergism (vinblastine + bleomycin).

PVB Studies

From 1974 to 1976, we initiated and completed our first PVB study [8]. As was traditional in the mid-70's, induction therapy was followed by maintenance chemotherapy (vinblastine 0.3 mg/kg monthly for a total of 2 years of chemotherapy). Four courses of PVB induction chemotherapy were utilized.

Thirty-three of 47 (70%) patients attained a C.R. and an additional 5 patients (11%) were rendered disease-free by post-PVB surgical resection of radiographically persistent disease.

A subsequent phase III study addressed whether we could reduce the significant neuromuscular and myelosuppressive toxicity of vinblastine by decreasing the dosage from 0.4 to 0.3 mg/kg and still maintain therapeutic efficacy. As expected, the lower dose of vinblastine was associated with a significant reduction in toxicity, and the C.R. and cure rates were similar with the two arms.

Our subsequent PVB study challenged one of the basic tenets of oncology, the utilization of maintenance therapy. Patients achieving a disease-free status were randomized to a standard arm of 21 months of maintenance vinblastine versus an experimental arm of just 12 weeks of PVB with no further therapy. One hundred thirteen patients entered this study at Indiana University or participating institutions in the Southeastern Cancer Study Group. The relapse rate was only 5%, with or without maintenance vinblastine [9].

PVB versus Cisplatin plus VP-16 plus Bleomycin (BEP)

Etoposide (VP-16) is an epipodophyllotoxin derivative with definite single agent activity in refractory testicular cancer [10]. In 1978, we began our initial salvage chemotherapy studies with cisplatin plus VP-16 in patients who were not cured with PVB or similar induction therapy. VP-16, unlike vinblastine, is essentially devoid of neuromuscular toxicity. Schabel and colleagues demonstrated remarkable synergism with cisplatin plus etoposide in preclinical models [11].

From 1981 through 1984, the Southeastern Cancer Study Group conducted a randomized prospective study comparing PVB and BEP as initial induction chemotherapy [12]. No maintenance therapy was given in either arm, and if the markers were normal postchemotherapy but there were persistent radiographic abnormalities, appropriate surgery was done. If carcinoma was found, 2 more courses of the original induction regimen were given, deleting bleomycin.

A total of 244 patients from 24 institutions entered this trial. Of 121 patients treated with PVB, 74 (61%) had a C.R., and another 15 (13%) became disease-free after resection of teratoma (10 patients) or carcinoma (5 patients). Among the 123 patients given BEP, 74 (60%) had a C.R., and 28 (23%) became free of disease after resection of teratoma (22 patients) or carcinoma (6 patients). Thus, 74% became disease-free after treatment with PVB and 83% after BEP. Nine patients on PVB and 6 receiving BEP subsequently had recurrences. In the subgroup of advanced disseminated disease, there was a survival advantage for BEP (p = 0.02).

Granulocytopenic toxicity, including granulocytopenic fever, was similar in the two arms. There was a major reduction in neuromuscular toxicity, as manifested by paresthesia, abdominal cramps, ileus, and myalgias. This was significant not only statistically, but also clinically. On the basis of this study, which demonstrated a reduction in morbidity and superior survival, we have utilized BEP since 1984 as first-line therapy for disseminated testicular cancer and have abandoned PVB.

Subsequent Studies

Good-Risk (Minimal-Moderate Disease)

Several groups have designed staging systems that attempt to discriminate good-risk from poor-risk disease [13,14]. We began a phase III study in 1984 evaluating the standard 4 courses of BEP versus 3 courses (9 weeks) of BEP in good-risk (minimal or moderate extent) disease. One hundred eighty-four patients entered this study, and 97% achieved an NED status confirming the accuracy of minimal and moderate extent disease as "good-risk". An identical 92% of patients on each arm are continuously NED [15]. We have recently updated this study for the 118 patients entered at Indiana University (median follow-up 9 years). There remain no differences between the two arms, with only 4 deaths in each arm. Furthermore, for patients with serum HCG less than 1,000 mIU/ml, there were only 2 deaths out of 104 patients [16].

The Eastern Co-operative Oncology Group (ECOG) completed a phase III study in good-risk disease randomizing patients to a standard arm consisting of BEP for 3 courses versus the identical therapy, but with the deletion of bleomycin. One hundred seventy-one patients were evaluable, and 94% attained an NED status with the three drug regimen compared to 88% for cisplatin + VP-16 (p = 0.20). The failure-free survival favored the bleomycin arm, 86% versus 69% (p = 0.004). Overall survival was also superior for the three drug regimen, 95% versus 86% (p = 0.011) [17].

A large European study randomized 419 good prognosis nonseminomatous patients to four cycles of cisplatin + etoposide with or without 30 units of bleomycin weekly for 12 weeks. The European version of BEP (and EP) in this study utilized a dosage of 120 mg/M^2 days 1, 3, and 5 (360 mg/M^2) compared to an etoposide dosage of 100 mg/M^2 for 5 days (500 mg/M^2) in the United States. Eighty-seven percent on EP achieved a disease-free status, compared to 95% with BEP (p = 0.0075). Due to the low number of unfavorable events, there was no statistically significant difference in overall survival (p = 0.262) [18].

Investigators at Memorial Sloan Kettering Cancer Center (MSKCC) randomized 164 patients with good prognosis germ cell tumors to 4 courses of cisplatin + etoposide (100 mg/M^2 x 5) versus the five drug VAB-6 regimen. Therapeutic results were equivalent, but there was a statistically and clinically significant reduction in toxicity favoring EP [19]. Based upon this phase III study, 4 courses of EP became the standard therapy for good prognosis disease at MSKCC. Subsequent updates have confirmed the high cure rate with this regimen [20, 21].

Another approach to reduce toxicity in good prognosis disease was to substitute the less toxic carboplatin for cisplatin. A large European study randomized 598 patients with good prognosis nonseminomatous disease to 4 cycles of BEP with the etoposide dosage 120 mg/M^2 days 1-3 versus CEB with substitution of carboplatin using AUC (area under curve) of 5. There were 10 deaths on the BEP arm versus 27 with CEB (p = 0.003) [22].

Investigators at MSKCC and Southwest Oncology Group (SWOG) evaluated 4 courses of etoposide + either cisplatin or carboplatin (500 mg/ M^2 every 4 weeks). The VP-16 dosage was 100 mg/M^2 for 5 consecutive days on both arms. Two hundred sixty-five evaluable patients were analyzed. Although the initial NED rate was similar for both arms (90% vs. 88%), the relapse rate was 3% versus 12% and the continuous NED rate was 87% versus 76% favoring the cisplatin arm (p = 0.005) [23].

There are two appropriate and standard approaches for good-risk disease, namely BEP x 3 or EP x 4. Our personal preference is for the abbreviated 3 courses of cisplatin combination chemotherapy. Nine weeks (270 units) of bleomycin in good-risk disease is essentially devoid of any clinically significant pulmonary toxicity [15-17]. Neither 3 courses of EP nor substitution of carboplatin for cisplatin is appropriate. Since 98% of patients with minimal or moderate extent disease and serum HCG less than 1,000 mIU/ml are alive and disease-free following 3 courses of BEP, 4 courses of BEP represent overtreatment in this patient population [16].

Definition of Poor-Risk (Advanced) Disease

Several investigators have proposed classifications to stratify patients with disseminated germ cell tumors into good and poor risk categories. The strategy for good risk disease was to maintain the approximately 90% cure rate and reduce cost and toxicity. As mentioned previously, 3 courses of BEP or 4 courses of EP constitutes standard therapy. It would be very difficult to document that an alternative regimen could improve these results.

Poor risk disease is a more heterogeneous patient population, and has been defined based upon tumor markers, volume of metastatic disease, and multiplicity of anatomic sites [13,14]. These patients will have a 40-60% cure rate with standard therapy. In this group, the impetus has been to evaluate more aggressive chemotherapy in phase II and phase III studies to try to improve the therapeutic outcome. Unfortunately, thus far, no chemotherapy regimen has been documented to be superior to the standard 4 courses of BEP.

Recently, an international group was convened to develop a consensus classification for poor risk (and good risk) germ cell tumors. Data were available on 5,862 patients, with median follow-up time 5 years. Only 14% of these patients comprised the poor risk category, with a 41% 5 year disease-free survival and overall 48% 5 year survival [24]. The cure rate with standard BEP is probably 10% higher, since the intergroup consensus included older regimens (e.g. PVB and VAB regimens) that did not include etoposide. This new definition (Table 1) is now incorporated in the current American intergroup trial for poor risk disease.

Table 1. Poor risk disease (all nonseminomatous patients)

1. LDH > 10 times upper limit of normal, HCG > 50,000 IU/ml, or AFP > 10,000 Ng ml
2. Any primary mediastinal nonseminomatous germ cell tumor
3. Non-pulmonary visceral metastases (bone, liver, brain, etc.)

Advanced Disease

In poor risk (advanced) disease, utilizing the Indiana classification [13], an intergroup study addressed the therapeutic question to test whether double dose (40 mg/M^2 x 5) cisplatin could improve the cure rate. One hundred fifty-three patients were evaluable. As expected, patients receiving double dose cisplatin experienced considerably more toxicity than standard BEP. Unfortunately, there was no evidence of therapeutic superiority for the high dose cisplatin arm, with 62.2% continuously NED with high dose and 63.6% with standard BEP [25].

A successor intergroup study in advanced disease was completed in 1992. The standard arm of BEP was compared to an experimental arm of VP-16 + ifosfamide + cisplatin (VIP). The VIP regimen was chosen because of its success as salvage therapy after PVB and/or BEP. This represented a similar philosophy for ifosfamide compared to VP-16; namely single agent activity, incorporation as a curative salvage regimen, and then evaluation as first-line therapy. Three hundred four patients entered this intergroup study. With a minimal follow-up of 2 years, there was no difference, as 56% are continuously NED with VIP and 57% with BEP [26].

The current intergroup study for poor risk disease utilizes the new international staging system [24]. The control arm consists of 4 courses of standard BEP versus the experimental arm of BEP x 2 followed by 2 courses of very high dose carboplatin, etoposide and cyclophosphamide with peripheral stem cell rescue. Since only 14% of patients fulfill the category of poor risk, it is very important that as many eligible patients as possible enter this important study. Participants include Indiana University, MSKCC, and the American Co-operative groups.

Salvage Therapy

Our concept for salvage therapy has always been to use cisplatin plus other active agents not previously utilized, as long as there was not progression during cisplatin combination chemotherapy. Cisplatin + etoposide was initiated in 1978 as salvage therapy after PVB. Our initial salvage therapy after BEP had been vinblastine 0.11 mg/kg day 1 and 2 + ifosfamide 1.2 grams/M^2 x 5 + cisplatin 20 mg/M^2 x 5 (VeIP) every 3 weeks for 4 courses. Between 1984 and 1989, 135 patients received this regimen as second-line therapy. Sixty-seven patients (49.6%) achieved NED status (no evidence of disease), including 15 (11%) who were NED after postchemotherapy resection of teratoma and 10 (7.4%) NED after postchemotherapy resection of carcinoma. Thirty-two (23.7%) are continuously NED with minimal follow-up of 5 years. Thirty of 100 testicular primaries are continuously NED, compared to 2 of 3 extragonadal seminoma and 0 of 32 nonseminomatous extragonadal patients [27].

High dose therapy with carboplatin and VP-16 and autologous bone marrow transplant (ABMT) was first started at Indiana University in 1986. Initially, this was used as a last attempt at curative therapy (third-line or later or following progression during cisplatin therapy). Six of these first 40 patients are 5+ years continuously NED [28]. We now utilize peripheral stem cells and G-CSF, and we are able to safely administer carboplatin 700 mg/M² x 3 + etoposide 750 mg/M² x 3. We currently utilize this therapy as initial salvage chemotherapy. Twenty-five of 49 patients (51%) are continuously disease-free for 1+ years with this approach [29]. However, we continue to use VeIP as initial salvage for seminoma, as 19 of 23 (83%) achieved an NED status and 13 of 23 (56%) are continuously NED with this regimen as second-line chemotherapy [30].

Complicated Testicular Cancer Issues

I.   Management of NSGCT clinical stage I, but with elevated HCG and/or AFP, is a rare clinical situation; namely, normal radiographic studies, but elevated HCG or AFP (after accounting for proper time to normalize postorchiectomy). In the past, standard therapy was RPLND. However, investigators from both Indiana University [31] and MSKCC [32] have concluded that chemotherapy (alone) is optimal treatment (4 courses of EP or 3 courses of BEP). In reality, these patients have a high probability of having disease outside, rather than inside the RPLND field as the cause of their elevated marker, thus making chemotherapy a logical choice.

II.   Management of residual mass postchemotherapy in a patient with seminoma: at MSKCC, if the persistent mass is 3 cm. or larger, RPLND is recommended [33]. At Indiana University, we would simply follow such patients with repeat abdominal C.T. every 3 months the first year, every 4 months the second year, and once or twice a year for the next 3 years [34].

A recent series from Royal Marsden also supported the policy of observation in these patients, and documented that postchemotherapy irradiation was not beneficial [35].

III. Should patients presenting with large (> 3 cm) retroperitoneal masses undergo a postchemotherapy RPLND if they achieve a C.R. with chemotherapy? At MSKCC, 22 patients in this category underwent postchemotherapy RPLND and 2 had persistent carcinoma and 3 teratoma [36]. It is unknown how many received a non-etoposide containing regimen. At Indiana, we have retrospectively reviewed 36 such patients treated with chemotherapy alone. Thirty-four of 36 (94%) are continuously NED with median follow-up 5 years. There was only one relapse, as the other patient not continuously NED developed a second primary [37]. Thus, we do not feel that surgery should ever be performed postchemotherapy if a C.R. is achieved, regardless of the size of the initial mass.

IV. Should the presence or absence of teratoma in the orchiectomy specimen influence the decision about postchemotherapy RPLND for residual mass? Obviously, the presence of teratoma in the orchiectomy specimen, especially if the dominant cell type, strongly suggests a postchemotherapy residual mass will also contain teratoma. We retrospectively evaluated this issue at Indiana University. Seventy-nine patients with teratoma in the orchiectomy and a residual postchemotherapy mass underwent RPLND. As expected, most had teratoma (65 of 79; 82%); 10 (13%) had necrosis and 4 (5%) had carcinoma. Forty-four patients had no teratoma in the orchiectomy specimen and less than a 90% volumetric regression with chemotherapy, and underwent subsequent RPLND. In this category, despite no teratoma in the orchiectomy specimen, 18 of 44 (41%) had teratoma in the RPLND specimen, 4 had residual cancer, and the remaining 50% necrosis [37].

V. Do patients with testis cancer experience late relapse? Testicular cancer is a rapidly proliferating and uniquely chemo-sensitive tumor. We now recognize the fact that approximately 2-3% of patients who are disease-free at 2 years will experience a late relapse and about half of those relapses will be beyond 5 years. This is often manifested by a rising alphafetoprotein on a routine evaluation. Unfortunately, with very rare exceptions, these patients are not curable with chemotherapy. Proper management for these patients is to find where their disease is radiographically and attempt to surgically resect their disease [38]. It is important to recognize that testicular cancer patients require lifelong follow-up. Our current policy postchemotherapy is routine history and physical exam including palpation of contralateral testis, serum HCG and AFP, and posteroanterior and lateral chest X-ray every 2 months the first year, every 4 months the second year, every 6 months years 3-5, and then annually. If a postchemotherapy resection contained bulky (> 5 cm) teratoma, abdominal C.T.'s are done at least every 3 months the first year, every 6 months the second year, and annually years 3-5.

Summary

Testicular cancer has become a model for a curable neoplasm. Our studies with cisplatin combination chemotherapy allow us to conclude that: (1) short duration intensive induction therapy with the most active agents in optimal dosage is more important than maintenance therapy; (2) modest dose escalation increases toxicity without improving therapeutic efficacy; (3) it is possible to develop curative salvage therapy for refractory germ cell tumors, and (4) preclinical models predicting synergism, such as vinblastine + bleomycin or cisplatin + VP-16 have clinical relevance. Finally, testicular cancer has also become a model for new drug development. Cisplatin was approved by the FDA for testis and ovarian cancer, and etoposide and ifosfamide for refractory germ cell tumors. The success of these studies confirms the importance of the continued search for new investigational drugs in all solid tumors.

References

1. Einhorn LH (1981) Testicular cancer: A model for a curable neoplasm. Cancer Research 41:3275-3280
2. Einhorn LH (1990) Treatment of testicular cancer: A new and improved model. J Clin Oncol 8:1777-1781
3. Bosl GJ, Motzer RJ (1997) Testicular germ cell cancer. NEJM 337:242-253
4. Li MC, Whitmore WF, Golbey R et al (1960) Effects of combined drug therapy on metastatic cancer of the testis. JAMA 174:145-153
5. Samuels ML, Lanzotti VJ, Holoye PY et al (1976) Combination chemotherapy in germinal cell tumors. Cancer Treat Rev 3:185-204
6. Rosenberg B, VanCamp L, Krigas T (1965) Inhibition of cell division in e. coli by electrolysis products from a platinum electrode. Nature 205:678-699
7. Higby DJ, Wallace HJ, Albert DJ et al (1974) Diamminedichloroplatinum: A phase I study showing responses in testicular and other tumors. Cancer 33:1219-1225
8. Einhorn LH, Donohue JP (1977) Combination chemotherapy with cis-diamminedichloroplatinum, vinblastine, and bleomycin in disseminated testicular cancer. Ann Int Med 87:293-298
9. Einhorn LH, Williams SD, Troner M, Greco FA, Birch R (1981) The rise of maintenance therapy in disseminated testicular cancer: A Southeastern Cancer Study Group Protocol. NEJM 305:717-731
10. Fitzharris BM, Kaye SB, Saverymuttu S et al (1980) VP-16 as single agent in advanced testicular tumors. Eur J Cancer 16:1193-1197

11. Schabel FM Jr, Trader MW, Laster WR Jr et al (1979) Cisplatin: combination chemotherapy and cross-resistance studies with tumors of mice. Cancer Treat Rep 63:1459-1473

12. Williams SD, Birch R, Irwin L, Greco A, Loehrer PJ, Einhorn LH (1987) Disseminated germ cell tumors: chemotherapy with cisplatin plus bleomycin plus either vinblastine or etoposide. NEJM 316:1435-1440

13. Birch R, Williams SD, Cone A, Einhorn LH et al (1986) Prognostic factors for favorable outcome in disseminated germ cell tumors. J Clin Oncol 4:400-407

14. Bosl GJ, Geller NL, Cirrincione C et al (1983) Multivariate analysis of prognostic variables in patients with metastatic testicular cancer. Cancer Res 43:3403-3407

15. Einhorn LH, Williams, SD, Loehrer PJ et al (1989) Evaluation of optimal duration of chemotherapy in favorable prognosis disseminated germ cell tumors: An SECSG Protocol. J Clin Oncol 7:387-391

16. Saxman S, Finch D, Gonin R, Einhorn LH (1998) Long-term follow-up of a phase III study of 3 versus 4 cycles of bleomycin, etoposide, and cisplatin in favorable prognosis germ cell tumors: The Indiana University experience. J Clin Oncol 16:702-706

17. Loehrer PJ, Einhorn LH, Elson P et al (1995) The importance of bleomycin in favorable prognosis disseminated germ cell tumors: An Eastern Cooperative Oncology Group Trial. J Clin Oncol 13:470-476

18. de Wit R, Stoter G, Kaye SB et al (1997) Importance of bleomycin in combination chemotherapy for good-prognosis testicular nonseminoma: A randomized study of the European Organization for Research and Treatment of Cancer Genitourinary Tract Cancer Cooperative Group. J Clin Oncol 15:1837-1843

19. Bosl GJ, Geller NL, Bajorin D, Leitner SP, Yagoda A et al (1988) A randomized trial of etoposide + cisplatin versus vinblastine + bleomycin + cisplatin + cyclophosphamide + dactinomycin in patients with good-prognosis germ cell tumors. J Clin Oncol 6:1231-1238

20. Bajorin DF, Geller NL, Weisen SF, Bosl GJ (1991) Two-drug therapy in patients with metastatic germ cell tumors. Cancer 67:28-32

21. Xiao H, Mazumdar M, Bajorin DF et al (1997) Long-term follow-up of patients with good-risk germ cell tumors treated with etoposide and cisplatin. Proc Amer Soc Clin Oncol 16:321

22. Horwich A, Sleijfer DT, Fossa SD, Kay SB, Oliver RTD et al (1997) Randomized trial of bleomycin, etoposide, and cisplatin compared with bleomycin, etoposide, and carboplatin in good-prognosis metastatic nonseminomatous germ cell cancer: A Multi-institutional Medical Research Council/European Organization for Research and Treatment of Cancer Trial. J Clin Oncol 15:1844-1852

23. Bajorin D, Sarosdy MF, Pfister DG et al (1993) Randomized trial of etoposide and cisplatin versus etoposide and carboplatin in patients with good-risk germ cell tumors. J Clin Oncol 11:598-608

24. International Germ Cell Collaborative Group (1997) International germ cell consensus classification: A prognostic factor-based staging system for metastatic germ cell cancers. J Clin Oncol 15:594-603

25. Nichols CR, Williams SD, Einhorn LH et al (1991) Randomized study of cisplatin dose intensity in advanced germ cell tumors: An SECSG and SWOG protocol. J Clin Oncol 9:1163-1172

26. Nichols CR, Loehrer PJ, Einhorn LH et al (1997) Phase III study of BEP versus VIP in advanced stage germ cell tumors: An intergroup trial. J Clin Oncol 16:1287-1293

27. Loehrer PJ, Gonin R, Nichols CR, Weathers T, Einhorn LH (1992) Vinblastine plus ifosfamide plus cisplatin as initial salvage therapy in recurrent germ cell tumor. J Clin Oncol 16:2500-2504

28. Broun ER, Nichols CR, Einhorn LH et al (1992) Long-term follow-up of salvage chemotherapy in relapsed and refractory germ cell tumors using high dose carboplatin and etoposide with autologous bone marrow support. Annals Intern Med 117:124-128

29. Bhatia S, Cornetta K, Broun R, Nichols C, Abnour R, Einhorn LH (1998) High dose chemotherapy with peripheral stem cell or autologous transplant as initial salvage chemotherapy for testicular cancer. Proc Amer Soc Clin Oncol 17:321 (abstr)

30. Miller KD, Loehrer PJ, Gonin R, Einhorn LH (1997) Salvage chemotherapy with vinblastine, ifosfamide, and cisplatin in recurrent seminoma. J Clin Oncol 15:1427-1431

31. Saxman SB, Nichols CR, Einhorn LH et al (1996) The management of patients with clinical stage I nonseminomatous testicular tumors and persistently elevated serologic markers. J Urol 155:587-589

32. Davis BE, Herr HW, Fair WR, Bosl GJ (1994) The management of patients with nonseminomatous germ cell tumors of the testis with serologic disease only after orchiectomy. J Urol 152:111-114

33. Sheinfield J, Puc HS et al (1997) Surgery for a post-chemotherapy residual mass in seminoma. J Urol 157:860-862

34. Schultz SM, Einhorn, LH, Conces D et al (1989) Management of post-chemotherapy residual mass in patients with advanced seminoma: Indiana University Experience. J Clin Oncol 7:1497-1503

35. Horwich A, Paluchowska B, Norman A et al (1997) Residual mass following chemotherapy of seminoma. Ann Oncol 8:37-40

36. Toner GC, Panciek DM, Heelan RT et al (1990) Adjunctive surgery after chemotherapy for nonseminomatous germ cell tumors: recommendations for patient selection. J Clin Oncol 8:1683-1694

37. Debono DJ, Heilman DK, Einhorn LH, Donohue JP (1997) Decision analysis for avoiding post-chemotherapy surgery in patients with disseminated nonseminomatous germ cell tumors. J Clin Oncol 15:1455-1464

38. Baniel J, Foster RS, Gonin R, Messemer JE, Donohue JP, Einhorn LH (1995) Late relapse of testicular cancer. J Clin Oncol 13: 1170-1176

Screening for Prostate Cancer: the good, the bad and the ugly

L. Denis

Abstract

Background

Mortality from prostate cancer is a large, worldwide burden and the value of population screening for prostate cancer is unknown. A consensus meeting on screening and global strategy for prostate carcinoma, held in Antwerp in 1994, resulted in a collaboration among European centres to pursue the formation of a multinational randomized screening trial. This trial is known as the "European Randomized Study of Screening for Prostate Cancer (ERSPC)".

Methods

Based on a number of feasibility trials conducted in Antwerp, Rotterdam and Finland, a number of pitfalls and problems of a randomized screening study were confronted. Today six centres in six European countries coordinate their work and analysis of the results and others are lining up to join this massive effort. A recent step forward joined ERSPC with the screening activities of the US National Cancer Institute (NCI) to result in the International Prostate Screening Trials Evaluation Group (IPSTEG).

Results

A sustained policy to achieve a common work strategy and data analysis has been reached and the first study results of the trial aiming to screen 180.000 men showed the potential to finish the trial by the year 2004 based on the evaluation of over 200.000 men.

Conclusions

Data collected from six collaborating centres lead to a consensus on the methodology of a population screening supported by a number of committees to focus on the quality of the study and on the quality of life of the participants in the study.

General Aspects of the Screening Controversy

Screening for prostate cancer is highly controversial in contrast to screening for breast and cervical cancer in women. This observation is somewhat surprising if one realizes that after more than 30 years of trials on breast cancer screening important questions remain on the age limitations, the treatment of early stage disease and cost-efficacy as well as quality control of diagnosis and treatment of both types of tumors [1, 2].

Even more surprising, in view of the fact that for the estimated new cancer cases in the US SEER program for 1998, after the 1997 downward revision for incidence of prostate cancer, respectively breast cancer in females matches prostate cancer in men in incidence (30% vs. 29%) in absolute numbers (178.700 vs. 184.500) in estimated cancer deaths in both sexes (16% vs. 13%) and in cancer death numbers (43.500 vs. 39.200) [3, 4].

These figures are not exclusive to the US since mortality rates in both the US and Europe range between 20 and 30 deaths/100.000 men per year (roughly between 35.000 and 40.000 deaths per year) with an expected increase in incidence and mortality in the underdeveloped world by increasing longevity of the male population, increased efficacy of diagnostic tests and unfortunately a real increase in prostate cancer risk [5, 6].

Of course, one cannot miss the huge discrepancy between incidence/mortality rate in the US and Europe. The explanation is almost certainly the greater use of cancer detection techniques in the US resulting in a considerable shift of cancer stages at the time of diagnosis to non-metastatic disease [7, 8].

Despite these impressive numbers the cited controversy continues as we have no reliable results from randomized prospective screening programs showing a prostate cancer mortality reduction, survival benefit and increased levels of quality of life for the aging male population after screening. We tried to settle the issue in 1994 by the organization of a Consensus Workshop on Screening and Global Strategy for Prostate Cancer in Antwerp, Belgium [9].

The major goal of the workshop was to provide answers to the following questions.

1. Is there an acceptable method for early detection of prostate cancer available on a population basis?

2. Do the current results provide encouragement for proceeding to develop widespread, randomized trials?
3. What is the proper way to conduct such efforts and what other important issues should be considered?
4. What are the bases for the treatment of patients with prostate cancer when discovered?

The answers from the different working parties confirmed Prostate Specific Antigen (PSA) determination as the most appropriate tumor marker for prostate cancer, the shift in detected cancers to earlier stages as a platform to increase the cure rate, the complexity of quality control on planned randomized trials and that 85 to 90% of the cancers are clinically important cancers admitting, however, that watchful waiting is an accepted form of treatment in well defined patients.

There are three viewpoints actively pursued by their protagonists which we label as good, bad and ugly not exactly in the moral meaning of the words, since we could classify them also as optimist, pessimist and indifferent. It is evident that the viewpoint of the optimist is frequently shared by the urologist who by this specialty is responsible for the diagnosis and treatment of the patients with prostate cancer, that submit themselves to his expertise in complete trust.

There is no discussion that prostate cancer in the localized stage of the disease is curable by local therapy and incurable in advanced stages. Ten year survival rates of patients with localized diseases after radical prostatectomy range from 95% for pT1 and 70% for pT2 disease, decreasing immediately to 60% for the next stage of extension through the capsule [10].

These encouraging results have been confirmed in several large US demonstration trials correctly termed "early detection trials" [11,12].

Based on the analysis of 208.234 cases diagnosed between 1973 and 1993 in population based Surveillance, Epidemiology and End Results Program (SEER), Smart concluded that indirect evidence suggested that screening in men over 50 years of age decreases the incidence of distant disease which may influence the mortality rate [13].

Based on the same figures showing increased five year prostate cancer survival rates, the American Cancer Society Prostate Task Force proposed to keep the ACS 1992 guidelines to offer PSA and digital rectal examination (DRE) annually to each male at age 50 and to younger men at high risk with the 1997 added restriction that these males would have a ten year life expectancy [14].

At the same time the Task Force however acknowledged the need to answer a number of critical research questions opening the constructive dialogue with the pessimistic, some prefer the realistic view, that only the completion of a well designed prospective randomized screening trial with decreasing mortality as an endpoint will allow for a definite recommendation on screening for prostate cancer as a general health screening policy [15,16].

Here both views find consensus on the need to answer the clinical research questions on the enhancement of PSA testing, differentiating the clinical aggressive tumors, eliminating length and lead time bias and selecting the appropriate treatment which may be watchful waiting in selected patients. One of the most efficient ways to move forward seems to be the international consultations patronized by the World Health Organizations, the International Union against Cancer, and the International Consultation on Urological Diseases. The proceedings and specifically the executive summaries of the 18 expert committees including health economic aspects and quality of life prepare adequate data to extract guidelines or information for evidence based cancer care or clinical research [17].

A social reality is the misunderstanding of the term "screening", which involves examining and classifying asymptomatic men as likely or unlikely to have the disease. The organized examination of large groups form the basis for a population screening. It is another realistic point of view to resist population screening by awaiting the final results of the ongoing randomized studies, but in the meantime advocate "case finding" in a clinical population consisting of men who consult for lower urinary tract problems (LUTS), mainly caused by benign prostate hyperplasia (BPH) prevalent in males over 50 years of age. The American College of Physicians recommends description of the possible advantages and/or harms of screening, diagnosis and treatment of prostate cancer and encouragement to enroll eligible men in ongoing trials [18].

One element overlooked in these recommendations is the impact of the US demonstration trials on the general population including the medical profession.

In the follow-up of a nationwide prospective cohort study of 51.529 males enrolled in the Health Professionals Study, the detection of organ confined tumor rose abruptly by 86% in 1991 after the publication of a study advocating screening with PSA in prostate cancer [19].

It is far more difficult to find a common ground for consultation with professionals who want to ignore the public health problem of prostate cancer. One recent example prefers watchful waiting over screening based on the presumption that in screening a majority of latent cases will be detected leading to overdiagnosis and subsequent overtreatment, that localized prostate cancer has no impact on survival and last that there is no evidence of an effect of treatment of even that increased mortality is caused by treatment mortality [20].

Unfortunately these statements echoed in other contributions ignore the vast wealth of data from radical prostatectomy specimen that only a small proportion of screen detected cancers can be labelled as incidental or serendipitous (latent used by the author) compatible with autopsy or surgical incidental cancers with a usual colume of less than 0.02 cm³ [21-23].

Analysis of evidence based data has established that we are able to cure poorly differentiated aggressive cancers in a subclinical stage that deserve aggressive treatment with curative intent [24, 25].

The reverse is also true that we do include part of the detected cancers in the watchful waiting treatment but based on diagnostic information rather than on panicky thinking. Worst, however, is the indifference to the fact that prostate cancer mortality can be solved by the established randomized trials in prostate cancer screening as the European Randomized Study of Screening for Prostate Cancer (ERSPC) and the Prostate, Lung, Colorectal and Ovarian Screening Study (PLCO), with all the quality control added only topped by statements that indeed mortality is high but the waiting time until prostate cancer death is not unfavourable [20].

These reports are not unique and we do face clinical research questions in a randomized prospective fashion, but there is a difference in stating that screening is ethically unacceptable if the purpose is to provide evidence of no harm [26] or advising to halt funding of screening for prostate cancer [27].

Among the many side studies emanating from the ERSPC we were able to establish the satisfaction and lack of anxiety of the participants in both the Antwerp and Rotterdam sites of the study [28, 29], a factor that next to the cost-efficacy aspects of a screening study will complement the information needed to define screening policy for health authorities in the future. The projections are that prostate cancer is likely to be the most common cause of male cancer death in the developed world by the year 2010. It is astonishing that the health policy makers of Sweden with one of the highest death rates by prostate cancer, or the United Kingdom with the closest death rate to the incidence rate do not intend to take preventive action. The most cynical is probably the region of Flanders where screening is accepted as a valuable scientific study, popular with the population but unfortunately cut in funding since all resources had to go into immediate clinical application grants, even realizing that prostate cancer is the number two male cancer in incidence and death. This death rate is still increasing but in men over 70 years of age so why care is the motto.

Where do we stand on screening for prostate cancer?

The principles for launching a population screening laid down in 1968 still stand [30], and the main advantages and disadvantages [31] are presented in Tables 1 and 2.

There is general agreement that sensitivity and specificity of any given test cannot be improved together and that high specificity is desirable in a screening setting. It is also important to acknowledge that the predictive value of any test is dependant on the prevalence of the disease screened for [32].

Lead time bias means early diagnosis with identical outcome and length time bias means more chances to detect slow growing tumors, make the interpretation of screening benefits difficult and support a randomized trial with an appropriate control group [13].

Screening is a delicate medical activity involving a population rather than an individual and one has to understand that sensitivity/specificity is usually chosen to detect the maximal numbers of clinical relevant but also curable cancers with a minimal number of diagnostic tests aiming to decrease the number of biopsies. In other words, the indication for a pros-

Table 1. The principles of screening

I.	The condition sought should be an important health problem
II.	There should be an accepted treatment for the patients with the recognized disease
III.	Facilities for diagnosis and treatment should be available
IV.	There should be a recognisable latent or early symptomatic stage
V.	There should be a suitable test or examination available
VI.	The test should be acceptable to the population
VII.	The natural history of the disease from pre- to clinical disease should be adequately understood
VIII.	There should be an agreed policy on whom to treat as patients
IX.	The cost of case-finding (including diagnosis and treatment of patients diagnosed) should be economically balanced in relation to possible expenditure on medical care as a whole
X.	Case-finding should be a continuing process and not a once-for-all-activity

Table 2. Advantages and disadvantages of screening

A.	*Advantages*
I.	Possible cure for cases detected by screening
II.	Less radical treatment with identical cure rate
III.	Reassurance for those with negative test results
IV.	Cost saving by treating upfront
B.	*Disadvantages*
I.	Longer morbidity for cases whose prognosis is unaltered (length and lead bias)
II.	Overtreatment of clinically unimportant cancers
III.	False reassurance for those with false-negative results
IV.	Diversion of scarce resources to screening programme
V.	Hazards of screening test (biopsy, anxiety)

tate biopsy based on a particular value of serum PSA is established on the entry criteria for the trial rather than on an individual assessment of patient and tumor characteristics. Still completing such a trial is important in order to decide on a policy pattern for general use of diagnosis and treatment of patients with prostate cancer.

A well executed trial will also provide data on cost effectiveness which are lacking in studies that diagnose and treat select cohorts of patients. The effect measure is based on the number of relevant, curable cancers and the increased survival benefit. Due to competing causes of death at the median age of prostate cancer patients, this overall effect measure is preferentially expressed in specific mortality reduction instead of survival benefit [33].

Population screening decisions depend on demonstration studies and randomized screening trials [9]. A number of demonstration studies followed by radical prostatectomy provided the needed scientific platform to correlate the diagnostic tests with the inclusion of the biopsy with the final tumor pathology leading to the uncontested acceptance of PSA as an effective diagnostic and prognostic factor in assessing the risk in the presence and progression of prostate cancer. They can show an impact on mortality rates through monitoring existing cancer registries but fail to indicate the specific amount due to a lack of a control in screened populations.

These studies bring additional information on the prediction value of the used tests as ultrasound (TRUS), DRE and various gimmicks of PSA to increase specificity of screening, including the free PSA (fPSA), and they continue to provide a constant source of reliable information in evaluation of data in diagnosis and treatment.

High 10 to 15 year survival rates after treatment by surgery or radiotherapy have been reported [34].

Newer technologies as brachytherapy and cryotherapy are under evaluation hoping to reduce the complications associated with invasive treatment. Observations on watchful waiting reported inferior results, but series involving selected cohorts of males over 70 years of age with well differentiated tumors were interesting enough to launch several randomized trials on treatment or watchful waiting providing some extra understanding in this complex problem.

Two large randomized screening trials have been established and joined in IPSTEG in 1997 to share quality control in monitoring, epidemiology, markers, pathology and causes of death committees.

The PLCO study was launched in 1994 and is based on volunteers who after randomization receive annual PSA and DRE screening for a total of four years and half to the usual community care. The trial has a planned sample size of 74.000 men aged 55-74 to show a 20% reduction in prostate cancer mortality at 10 years. The cut off for biopsy for PSA is 4 mg/ml. The compliance so far is good and PSA contamination in the community hovers around 12% which is identical to most European centres [35].

The ERSPC was initiated in 1994 after a number of feasibility studies in Antwerp and Rotterdam. Six European centres from Belgium, the Netherlands, Finland, Portugal, Spain and Sweden are involved and others are awaiting clearance to join. Men between 55 and 69 are invited from population registries to join and randomized to a screen and control group. The cut off PSA has been set at 3 mg/ml as the sole biopsy indication. Eliminating DRE and TRUS from the screening will result in a substantial decrease of biopsies and a relative loss of a few cancers leading to increased screen performance. A sample of 180.000 men is anticipated to be increased if PSA contamination would rise in the control groups. The current follow-up is ten years, hopefully to be reduced, and rescreens are planned between 2 and 4 years [36].

The Canada Quebec trial was supported to join this multinational effort but their premature presentation at the 1998 ASCO meeting might hamper their successful development.

It is clear that the strength of advance planning and continuous coordinated quality control based on a minimal data set forms a guarantee for a final overview analysis. Still it is a herculean task, and different regulations on human experimentation, differences in baseline mortality and policies over treatment have to be evaluated to obtain an optimal objective result. It is therefore of substantial support that the European Cancer Leagues in their 17th ECL Annual Conference in Madrid adopted the following resolution on their 'European Well Man's Programme' on prostate cancer. No positive advice should be given for any type of random screening for the prostate but patience and especially support (with attention and money) is recommended for the ERSPC. This public support from the Leagues representing the interest of the cancer patient is a big boost to continue this complex journey to the truth.

Part V
Melanoma

The Development of Cancer Vaccines for the Treatment of Metastatic Melanoma

F. M. Marincola, S. A. Ronseberg

Introduction

Immunization against pathogens induces humoral as well as cellular immune responses. While the former is directed toward extra-cellular invaders, the latter is directed toward proteins produced by pathogens following their infection of permissive cells. Like other intracellular proteins, viral products are enzymatically degraded into short peptides (9-11 amino acids in length) and presented on the surface of infected cells in association with Major Histocompatibility Complex (MHC) class I molecules: a requirement for T cell recognition. Vaccines aimed at prevention of disease might be particularly effective because they can arm the host with powerful neutralizing antibodies against subsequent infections which results in a dramatic reduction in the load of pathogen reaching the target cell. After the pathogen is hidden in the host's cells, the immune system relies predominantly on T cell function. Clearing of the infection will at this point depend on the balance between the efficiency of the T cell response and the protective strategies adopted by the pathogen [1].

Contrary to viral responses, tumor antigens come from within the cell and it is, therefore, likely that the cellular response is the prevalent immunological defense of the organism against tumors [2]. Recently, serological analysis of recombinant cDNA expression libraries has shown that the host can develop antibodies against cancer specific proteins expressed by autologous tumor cells [3]. The anti-tumor role of these antibodies that recognize intra-cellular proteins, however, is not clear. Most experimental models suggest that the cellular rather than the humoral arm of the immune response plays a major role in the elimination of cancer [4]. For instance, adoptive transfer of T lymphocytes from immune animals can induce resistance to tumor challenge and, in some cases, actual elimination of established cancer. With the identification of the human T cell growth factor, Interleukin-2 (IL-2), stable human T cell lines were expanded that could specifically recognize autologous tumor cells [5].

Empirically, cultures of tumor infiltrating lymphocytes (TIL) expanded *in vitro* from metastatic melanoma lesions and adoptively transferred into patients in combination with IL-2 could mediate tumor regression [6]. Because of the ease with which tumor specific TIL could be obtained from melanoma patients and their potential therapeutic relevance, melanoma has served as the prototype model for human tumor immunology. Thus, in the last decade strategies for the immunization of patients against cancer were focused at the enhancement of T cell reactivity against melanoma.

The focus on cellular immune responses, combined with the astonishing pace of bio-technological advances, resulted in unprecedented progress in the understanding of the immunologic aspects of tumor-host interactions in patients with melanoma. An important achievement was the demonstration of the existence of tumor specific antigens that could be recognized by the autologous host. This demonstration settled the most controversial question that had previously dominated tumor immunology. Furthermore, it unveiled a surprising biological characteristic of tumor immunity. Unexpectedly, the mechanisms regulating tumor/host interactions are profoundly intertwined with the complex biology of autoimmune phenomena. Host immune surveillance against neoplastic growth was suggested long ago on the assumption that tumor cells are seen as foreign by the host [7]. The modern understanding of the immunology of melanoma suggests that self/non-self discrimination is not adequate to explain observed phenomena as most melanoma associated antigens (MAA) that have been identified are non-mutated self-molecules expressed by normal cells [8].

The major advances of the last few years can be summarized as follows. Several MAA and their peptide epitopes recognized by HLA class I-restricted CTL have been identified [9, 10]. Many MAA were noted to be non mutated molecules naturally expressed by normal cells of melanocytic lineage [8]. These epitopes could be utilized to demonstrate, by *in vitro* sensitization experiments a high frequency of MAA reactive T cells in PBL of patients with melanoma [11, 12]. (MAA specific CTL could also be elicited from normal, non-tumor bearing individuals though with lower frequency than from patients with melanoma [12]). The same epitopes could be utilized to enhance MAA specific T cell reactivity *in vivo* when administered in combination with Incomplete Freund's Adjuvant (IFA) [13, 14]. Epitope-based vaccinations showed clinical effectiveness when combined with the administration of IL-2 [15].

Treatment of Patients with Metastatic Melanoma with Non-Specific Biologic Response Modifiers

The five-year survival of patients with metastatic melanoma is less than 2% with a median survival of about 6 months. Although combination chemotherapy can induce objective regressions of melanoma in approximately 20% of patients, this treatment is rarely, if ever, curative [16]. Alternative approaches include the administration of biological response modifiers such as IFN-α and IL-2 [17]; however, their success rate is limited. The adoptive transfer of TIL in combination with systemic IL-2 administration can mediate regression in 35 to 40% of patients with advanced melanoma [6]. Results with cancer vaccines aimed at active immunization have been, until recently, disappointing. Most attempts at active immunization against cancer have involved whole tumor cells or tumor cell fragments though it would be desirable to immunize specifically against unique tumor antigens that distinguish malignant from normal cells. Most importantly, the therapeutic effect of these approaches has been, at best, anecdotal and the immunologic effect difficult to document due to the lack of a known target antigen for monitoring. Administration of high-dose IL-2 has resulted in complete responses in patients with metastatic renal cell cancer and metastatic melanoma. Treatment of 283 consecutive patients in the Surgery Branch, National Cancer Institute (NCI) with high-dose IL-2 (720,000 IU/kg every 8 hours) resulted in 7% complete responses and 10% partial responses in patients with metastatic melanoma. Complete responses were most often durable with several patients remaining disease free more than five years [18]. Administration of IL-2 was associated with high systemic toxicity. Lethal complications were mostly of cardiac or septic origin. Since cardiac screening and use of prophylactic antibiotics were instituted, no treatment-related mortality occurred in over 700 consecutive patients [19]. Like IFN, IL-2 administration has anti-tumor effects. However, while the activity of IFN is partly due to a direct anti-proliferative effect on tumor cells, IL-2 does not have direct activity on cancer cells but works through stimulation of the immune system [20]. In 1992, 10 years after the first administration of IL-2, the US Food and Drug Administration licensed IL-2 for the treatment of patients with metastatic renal cancer, and in 1998 for treatment of patients with metastatic melanoma [19].

Tumor Infiltrating Lymphocytes and the Identification of MAA

The *in vitro* expansion of lymphocytes with IL-2 identified 2 categories of tumor-reactive T cells: Lymphokine-Activated Killer (LAK) cells and tumor specific CTL. LAK cells could be easily generated by culturing peripheral blood monocytes (PBMC) in IL-2 (6,000 IU/ml) [21]. Tumor specific CTL were obtained from TIL expanded from single cell suspensions of tumor grown in IL-2 [22]. LAK cells are not antigen specific and killing of "abnormal" cells is not MHC-restricted. Although able to kill tumor targets *in vitro*, LAK cells did not prove useful for the treatment of patients with metastatic melanoma and renal cancer. A randomized trial, in which IL-2 was administered alone or with LAK cells [21] failed to show differences in response rates or survival.

The identification of TIL responsible for partial or complete responses in patients treated with IL-2 has played an important role in the identification of many tumor antigens [5, 22, 23]. Treatment of 86 patients with metastatic melanoma using TIL plus IL-2 resulted in 34% objective response rates including patients who had previously failed treatment with high-dose IL-2 alone [18]. The identification of MAA was a direct consequence of efforts aimed at the characterization of TIL. Kawakami et al. [24] showed that the majority of TIL recognized "shared" antigens because they could kill melanoma cell lines from other patients expressing the relevant MHC (HLA in humans) molecule. The region encoding for the HLA class I molecules is located in chromosome 6 in humans and includes three loci termed HLA-A, -B and -C. HLA class I molecules are expressed by most normal cells while the expression on tumor cells is heterogeneous [25]. Each of the HLA genes is extremely polymorphic, with multiple alleles at each locus [26]. The most direct consequence of HLA polymorphism is that most individuals are heterozygous for each HLA locus and since there are three loci, most individuals express six functionally different HLA alleles on the cell surface. Most of the HLA polymorphism is clustered within the peptide binding and T cell receptor (TCR)-interacting domain [27]. In this functional region, the $\alpha1$ and $\alpha2$ chains form a platform composed of a flat β-pleated sheet representing the floor of a groove between two parallel α-helical sides. This groove is the binding site for antigenic epitopes consisting of peptide fragments 8-10 amino acids in length [27]. HLA alleles are very stringent with respect to ligand specificity and the stringency of the requirements for TCR/HLA interaction is referred to as "HLA restriction". HLA restricted recognition of MAA was formally proved by transduction of the appropriate

HLA allele (restriction element) for a particular TIL into melanoma cells which did not express such alleles. Recognition of the transfected tumor cell (but not the wild type) by the TIL constituted a formal proof of the HLA restricted recognition of shared MAA [24].

The observation that MAA recognized by TIL were shared in most melanomas and that normal melanocytes could be recognized by the same TIL suggested that MAA were non-mutated, lineage specific molecules. These findings encouraged efforts to identify these MAA with the assumption that they could be broadly used for anti-melanoma immunization. Two techniques were used for the identification of MAA. In the first approach, a cDNA library from a melanoma was established. Genes from this library were then stably transfected into non-melanoma cells (not expressing the MAA). The transfected target was then tested for recognition by TIL specific for the melanoma from which the cDNA library was generated. The cDNA clones that caused recognition upon transfection were then isolated and sequenced for identification of the antigen. An alternative technique involved the screening of cDNA libraries with a monkey cell (COS-7) previously transfected with the appropriate HLA restriction element. Transient transfection of pools of cDNA clones into the highly transfectable COS-7 allowed rapid screening of a large number of pooled genes [28]. The identified reactive pool was sub-cloned into single genes also transfected in COS-7. Sequencing then identified the gene responsible for TIL. This method was subsequently adopted for the identification of most MAA recognized by T cells [18]. A difference between the first MAA (MAGE-1) identified by Boon and colleagues and the MAA identified at the Surgery Branch, NCI, was the type of T cell used for the identification. While TIL were routinely used at the NCI, Boon and colleagues utilized T cells expanded *in vitro* from PBMC stimulated with autologous tumor. Interestingly, these two methods yielded two major categories of MAA. The first category includes Tumor Differentiation Antigens (TDA) which were predominantly identified using TIL. TDA include antigens such MART-1/MelanA, gp100/Pmel17, tyrosinase and TRP-1 and TRP-2 expressed by melanoma and melanocytes [29-32] but not other malignancies and normal tissues [33]. The predominant recognition of TDA over other MAA by TIL suggests an immunodominant role. Furthermore, the association of *vitiligo* (localized depigmentation of the skin due to destruction of melanocytes) with response to immunotherapy [34] suggests that clinically relevant immune responses are directed against TDA. Tumor specific antigens (TSA) are other common MAA. TSA are not expressed by normal melanocytes but are found in testes (cancer-testis antigens) and in a subset of patients with melanoma or other malignancies. TSA include the MAGE, BAGE and GAGE families and the newly identified NY-ESO-1 [35].

Clinical Applications of MAA

Several MAA identified to date [9, 10] are summarized in Table 1. Although the identification of the first MAA occurred in association with HLA-A*0101 [28] due to the prevalence of HLA-A*0201 in the melanoma population [36, 37], a significant number of MAA were subsequently identified in association with this allele. These include MART-1/Melan A [38, 39], gp100/Pmel 17 [40], tyrosinase [41], MAGE-3 [42], N-Acetylglucosaminyltransferase V [43], and NY-ESO-1 [44]. Among them, MART-1 has received particular attention because of its "immunodominance" in the context of HLA-A*0201 [38]. Approximately 90% of TIL originated from HLA-A*0201 patients recognize the MART-1 27-35 (AAGIGILTV) [45]. gp100 is the second most commonly recognized MAA by TIL. Analysis of 217 fresh metastatic melanoma specimens showed heterogeneous expression of MART-1 and gp100 *in vivo* [31]. However, the majority of lesions expressed these MAA in at least 50-75% of their cells. Because of the frequency of their expression in tissues and their immunodominance in HLA-A*0201 patients, these two MAA have been the focus of vaccination efforts at our institution.

To analyze the immune response to MART-1, ten MART-1-derived 9-mer peptides containing the HLA-A*0201 binding motif were screened for ability to induce specific CTL *in vitro* [11]. Tumor-lytic CTL could be generated from PBCM of melanoma patients using minimal epitopic determinants. Among the ten peptides, only MART-1 27-35 could consistently induce CTL reactivity against melanoma cells demonstrating stringent epitope/HLA allele requirements for MART-1 immunodominance. Further analysis of MAA reactive CTL that originated from PBMC of melanoma patients or healthy donors provided the first evidence of an enhanced level of sensitization against MAA in tumor-bearing hosts compared with normal individuals [12]. MART-127-35 specific reactivity could be generated *in vitro* in 13 of 13 melanoma patients but only in 5 of 9 healthy donors (p < 0.001). FluM158-66 specific T cells could be generated with similar efficiency in patients with melanoma. Furthermore, specific activity against MART-1 27-35 could be detected with fewer *in vitro* sensitizations of PBMC from in melanoma patients compared with PBMC from healthy, non-tumor bearing, donors.

Table. 1. Differentiation Antigens of the Melanocytic Lineage
(expressed by > 80% of melanoma lesions)

Site		Restriction Element	Epitope	Reference
MART-1	27-35	**HLA-A*0201**	**AAGIGILTV**	*Kawakami et al. [39, 45]
(118 aa)	32-40	HLA-A*0201	ILTVILGVL	Castelli et al. [76]
gp100	154-162	**HLA-A*0201**	**KTWGQYWQV***	Kawakami et al. [60]
(661 aa)	209-217	**HLA-A*0201**	**ITDQVPFSV***	Kawakami et al. [60]
	280-288	**HLA-A*0201**	**YLEPGPVTA***	Cox et al. [77]
	457-466	HLA-A*0201	LLDGTATLRL*	Kawakami et al. [60]
	476-485	HLA-A*0201	VLYRYGSFSV*	Kawakami et al. [60]
		HLA-A*03**	ALLAVGATK*	Skipper et al. [56]
Tyrosinase	1-9	HLA-A*0201	MLLAVLYLL*	Wolfel et al. [41]
(530 aa)	192-200	HLA-B*4403	YEIWRDIDF*	Brichard et al. [58]
	206-214	HLA-A*24**	AFLPWHRLF*	Kang et al. [57]
	369-377	HLA-A*0201	YMNGTMSQV*	Visseren et al. [78]
M14	??	HLA-A2?/A11	QDLTMKYQIF	Morioka et al. [79]

Tumor Specific (expressed by 30-70% of melanoma lesions)

MAGE-1		HLA-A*01**	EADPTGHSY*	Van d. Bruggen et al. [28]
(30%)		HLA-C*1601	SAYGEPRKL*	Van d. Bruggen et al. [80]
MAGE-3		HLA-A*01**	EVDPIGHLY*	Gaugler et al. [59]
(70%)		HLA-A*02**	FLWGPRALV*	Van d. Bruggen et al. [42]
BAGE		HLA-C*1601	AARAVFLAL*	Boel et al. [81]
(20%)				
GAGE-1		HLA-Cw6	YRPRPRRY*	Van d. Eynde [82]
(24%)				
NY-ESO		HLA-A*0201	(Q)SLLM-	Jager et al. [44]
(30%)			WITQC(FL)	

Epitopes from mutated gene products (uncommon)

gp75		HLA-A*31**	MSLQRQFLR*[1]	Wang et al. [83]
(TRP1)				
β-Catenin		HLA-A*2402	SYLDSGIHF*	Robbins et al. [85]
NA17-A		HLA-A*0201	VLPDVFIRCV	Guillox et al. [43]

Epitopes expressed differentially by melanoma cells

p15		HLA-A24	AYGLDFYIL*	Robbins et al. [85]

* Recognized on tumor cells by TIL and/or *in vitro* sensitized CTL. Underlined: peptide eluted from tumor cells; in brackets: size of molecule; bold: "immunodominant".
1. This epitope results from an alternative open reading frame of a non-mutated gene

These findings suggested that MAA had immunostimulatory properties not only at tumor site (as suggested by the TIL phenomenon) but also systemically.

At least five HLA-A*0201 restricted peptide sequences could be identified for the larger gp100 molecule that could be used *in vitro* to generate melanoma specific CTL [46]. gp100 epitopes were not as efficient as MART-1 27-35 for *in vitro* induction of anti-gp100 CTL reactivity [46]. Therefore, to enhance *in vitro* immunogenicity single amino acid substitutions were made to identify peptides with higher affinity for HLA-A*0201. Modified peptides were compared with the parental for increased immunogenicity based on their ability to induce anti-tumor lymphocytes *in vitro*. Based on these studies a candidate peptide was identified (G9-209-2M: IMDQVPFSV, natural sequence: ITDQVPFSV) which had increased immunogenic reactivity *in vitro* and *in vivo*. Because of the immunologic properties described above most vaccination studies performed at our institution have utilized MART-1 27-35 or G9-209-2M.

HLA-A*0201 is the predominant allele in the Northern American Caucasian [36, 37] and peptide-based vaccinations restricted to HLA-A*0201 expressing patients were initiated by administering the MART-1 27-35. MART-1 27-35 was administered sub-cutaneously (4 times at 3-week intervals in an emulsification with incomplete Freund's adjuvant). Although retinal expression of MART-1 has been documented by PCR, immunohistochemical techniques have failed to demonstrate protein expression in normal retina [47]. Furthermore, eye evaluation of patients undergoing effective vaccination with TDA has failed to identify any retinal damage that could be related to the vaccination [48]. The immunologic effectiveness of MART-1 27-35 vaccination was analyzed by comparing *in vitro* reactivity of PBMC obtained before and after vaccination. PBMC were analyzed in 18 patients by weekly *in vitro* sensitization with irradiated autologous PBMC pulsed with MART-1 27-35. In 15 post-vaccination CTL cultures, a more than threefold increase in specific release of IFN-γ was noted, compared with pre-vaccination. Nine HLA-A*0201 melanoma patients were then treated with the native g209 peptide and 11 patients were treated with g209-2M. Thirty-one additional patients were finally treated with g209-2M in combination with high dose intravenous IL-2. A lower percentage of patients that received the native g209 exhibited successful immunization compared to patients immunized with g209-2M. Recognition of peptide correlated with recognition of tumor cells and was far greater in patients receiving the modified peptide. Paradoxically, in spite of the strong CTL responses observed, no clinical responses were noted in patients vaccinated with MART-127-35, 1 of 9 patients immunized with the 209 peptide achieved a transient response and no patients immunized with g209-2M achieved tumor regression. When high dose IL-2 was combined with the administration of g209-2M, 13 of 31 patients (42%) had objective responses [15].

In summary, vaccination of melanoma patients with synthetic peptide modified to increase binding to MHC molecules such as g209-2M was able to mediate the generation of anti-tumor lymphocytes and when administered with IL-2 resulted in tumor regression [15]. Present studies address the expansion of such treatments to other cohorts of patients expressing other HLA types (A1, A3, A24, A31) by utilizing epitopes identified in association with such alleles and derived from various MAA including gp 100 (A2, A3), tyrosinase (A1,A2 and A24) and TRP-1 (A31).

Vaccination across the HLA Polymorphism

One disadvantage of epitope-based vaccination is the exclusiveness of the relationship between peptide and HLA alleles. HLA are among the most polymorphic of the human genes and because this polymorphism is clustered in the functional peptide-binding region, the binding of antigenic peptides is necessarily restricted to specific HLA alleles. This limits the interactions between CTL and antigen to specific sequences for each HLA allele. Because of the intrinsic limitations posed by HLA polymorphism [49-52], a vaccination strategy based on endogenous processing and presentation of whole T cell antigen (containing the maximum epitopic potential) could broaden the application of MAA vaccines. An ideal vaccine might be engineered that could be offered regardless of the patient's HLA phenotype and without identification of immunogenic epitopes. Therefore, the concept of whole antigen vaccination is an attractive alternative to peptide-based vaccination. To be successful, this strategy requires that individual molecules function as immunogen with comparable efficiency in association with various HLA alleles. Few lines of evidence, however, suggest that MAA can comparably induce T cell reactivity in association with different HLA alleles. For example, there is no evidence that MART-1 can be recognized in association with HLA alleles other than A*0201. We compared the ability of MART-1 to elicit non HLA-A*0201 restricted T cell responses using an autologous antigen presentation system consisting of dendritic cells (DC) infected with recombinant vectors encoding for MART-1 [53]. When stimulated in conditions in which A*0201 restricted anti-melanoma reactivity could be frequently observed, no reactivity could be elicited in association with other HLA-A class I alleles no matter how structurally similar to A*0201. Clonal analysis of HLA-A*0201 restricted, MART-1 specific CTL confirmed that its immunodominance is strongly restricted to the AAGIGILTV / HLA-A*0201 combination. Thus, whole protein vaccination for small molecular weight antigens may provide no further advantage over a peptide-based approach [54, 55]. For larger MAA recognized by HLA-A*0201 restricted CTL, epitopic determinants associated with other HLA-A class I alleles have been identified such as HLA-A3 for gp100/pMel 17 [56], HLA-A24 and -B44 for Tyrosinase [57, 58] and HLA-A1 for MAGE-3 [59]. However, responses to these epitopes are generally observed less frequently. For example, tyrosinase, which is predominantly recognized by HLA-A24 restricted TIL [57], is probably not a dominant immunogen in association with HLA-A*0201 as none of 10 HLA-A*0201 restricted TIL cultures analyzed recognized this MAA [60]. It is possible, however, that whole protein vaccination may have a role for larger molecules whose immunologic potential has been demonstrated for particular HLA class I phenotypes. Thus, adenoviruses expressing whole MAA have been constructed and used to immunize patients with metastatic melanoma. A phase I clinical trial was started in 1996 in which 54 patients received escalating doses of adenovirus encoding either MART-1 or gp100. This recombinant vector was administered either alone or in combination with high dose intravenous IL-2. The immune response was compared in PBMC and serum obtained before and after immunization. One of 16 patients with metastatic melanoma receiving adeno-MART-1 experienced a complete response. Other objective responses (two complete and two partial responses) occurred in patients receiving IL-2 simultaneously. No consistent evidence of immunization to MART-1 or gp-100 could be demonstrated in contrast with the results previously described for peptide vaccines. It is possible that the high titer of neutralizing antibodies generated by the exposure to the virus eliminated the vector before it could generate antigen for immunization. Similar results were seen with Poxvirus vectors.

Enhancing T Cell Response with the use of Dendritic Cells (DC)

As previously discussed, the *in vivo* administration of synthetic peptides emulsified in IFA could specifically enhance systemic CTL responses but, administered alone, was not sufficient to induce clinical responses. Pre-clinical models have shown that the administration of peptide alone is not very efficient [61] and the choice of an appropriate adjuvant capable of enhancing the immunogenic stimulus may play an important role. Among possible adjuvants, DC play a critical role in antigen presentation *in vivo* [62]. Several groups have shown that DC can function as an efficient adjuvant for MHC class I restricted anti-tumor sensitization *in vivo* [63-67]. Bone marrow derived murine dendritic cells pulsed with MHC class I restricted soluble β-galactosidase [66] or ovalbumin peptides [65], or with acid-eluted tumor peptides [64] could induce long-lasting immunity against tumors. These studies have suggested that peptide pulsed DC are more efficient in inducing anti-tumor protection in mice than immunization with peptide alone [65, 66] or emulsified in IFA [67]. Sallusto and Lanzavecchia [68] have shown that monocytes derived from the peripheral circulation can be readily activated into DC by culture with granulocyte/ macrophage colony-stimulating factor and interleukin-4. This method allows for easy preparation of large numbers of autologous DC from the peripheral blood of patients. By using DC we could easily sensitize *in vitro* PBMC from melanoma patients against several HLA-A*0201 restricted epitopes [69]. We are now conducting a phase I immunization protocol in which DC pulsed with 10 μM MART-127-35 or 10 μM G209-2M. Patients receive four successive immunizations at intervals of three weeks with the same number of DC. Three patients have so far completed treatment with the administration of 3 x 107 DC pulsed with MART-127-35 and 3 x 107 DC pulsed with G9-209-2M, and four patients with 1 x 108 DC pulsed with MART-127-35 and 1 x 108 DC pulsed with G9-209-2M. A cohort receiving the high dose of DC in combination with high dose IL-2 is presently being enrolled. Of the seven evaluable patients one achieved a temporary partial response. However, in contrast to direct peptide vaccination, evidence of *in vitro* sensitization could only be demonstrated in one patient (who did not respond to treatment).

Future Challenges

Many possible mechanisms could be responsible for the inability of the MAA specific CTL generated by peptide vaccination to eliminate tumors *in vivo*. It is possible that the characteristics of antigen presentation exercised by tumors are not optimal to maintain T cells in a status of activation at the tumor site [70]. Alteration in TCR and signal transduction *in vivo* may lead to immunosuppression of cancer patients [71]. It is possible that the characteristics of most MAA, which are non-mutated self-molecules, may induce central tolerance [8]. Lack of CTL localization at tumor site has been shown to correlate with lack of response to adoptive therapy with melanoma specific CTL [72]. Expression of apoptotic signals [73] or immunosuppressive cytokines [74, 75] or loss of expression of HLA [25] or target antigens [31] may also lead to ineffectiveness of CTL elicited by vaccination.

During the last decade a major achievement of tumor immunology has been the identification of molecules immunologically responsible for cancer regression. The identification of MAA has lead to their exploitation as vaccines with the purpose of enhancing T cell reactivity against cancer. In comparison, relatively little has been done to identify the reasons for the ineffectiveness of tumor specific T cells *in vivo* and significant effort is needed to study this problem.

References

1. Zinkernagel RM (1996) Immunology taught by viruses. Science 271:173
2. Yewdell JW, Bennink JR (1990) The binary logic of antigen processing and presentation to T cells. Cell 62:203
3. Old LJ, Chen YT (1998) New Paths in Human Cancer Serology. J Exp Med 187:1163
4. Restifo NP, Wunderlich JR (1996) Principles of tumor immunity: biology of cellular immune responses. In: De Vita VT, Hellmans, Rosenberg SA (eds) Biologic therapy of cancer. JB Lippincott Co, Philadelphia, p 3
5. Knuth A, Danowski B, Oettgen HF, Old LJ (1984) T-cell-mediated cytotoxicity against autologous malignant melanoma: analysis with interleukin 2-dependent T-cell cultures. Proc Natl Acad Sci USA 81:3511
6. Rosenberg SA, Yannelli JR, Yang JC, Topalian SL, Schwartzentruber DJ, Weber JS, D.R. Parkinson, C.A. Seipp, J.H. Einhorn, D.E. White (1994). Treatment of patients with metastatic melanoma with autologous tumor-infiltrating lymphocytes and interleukin 2. J Natl Cancer Inst 86:1159
7. Burnet FM (1970). The concept of immunological surveillance. Prog Exp Tumor Res 13:1
8. Kawakami Y, Rosenberg SA (1996). T-cell recognition of self peptides as tumor rejection antigens. Immunol Res 15:179

9. Rosenberg SA (1997) Cancer vaccines based on the identification of genes encoding cancer regression antigens. Immunol Today 18:175

10. Boon T, Coulie PG, Van den Eynde B (1997) Tumor antigens recognized by T cells. Immunol.Today 18:267

11. Rivoltini L, Kawakami Y, Sakaguchi K, Southwood S, Sette A, Robbins PF, Marincola FM, Salgaller M, Yannelli JR, Appella E, Rosenberg SA (1995) Induction of tumor reactive CTL from peripheral blood and tumor infiltrating lymphocytes of melanoma patients by in vitro stimulation with an immunodominant peptide of the human melanoma antigen MART-1. J Immunol 154:2257

12. Marincola FM, Rivoltini L, Salgaller ML, Player M, Rosenberg SA (1996). Differential anti-MART-1/MelanA CTL activity in peripheral blood of HLA-A2 melanoma patients in comparison to healthy donors: evidence for in vivo priming by tumor cells. J Immunother 19:266

13. Cormier JN, Salgaller ML, Prevette T, Barracchini KC, Rivoltini L, Restifo NP, Rosenberg SA, and Marincola FM (1997) Enhancement of cellular immunity in melanoma patients immunized with a peptide from MART-1/Melan A. Cancer J Sci Am 3:37

14. Salgaller ML, Marincola FM, Cormier JN, Rosenber SA (1996) Immunization against epitopes in the human melanoma antigen gp100 following patient immunization with synthetic peptides. Cancer Res 56:4749

15. Rosenberg SA, Yang JC, Schwartzentruber D, Hwu P, Marincola FC, Topalian SL, Restifo NP, Dufour E, Schwartzberg L, Spiess P, Wunderlich J, Parkhurst MR, Kawakami Y, Seipp C, Einhorn JH, White D (1998) Immunologic and therapeutic evaluation of a synthetic tumor associated peptide vaccine for the treatment of patients with metastatic melanoma. Nat Med 4:321

16. Mc CE C.M. Mc (1996) Systemic chemotherapy for the treatment of metastatic melanoma. Semin.Oncol 23:744

17. Marincola FM, Rosenberg SA (1995) Biologic Therapy with Interleukin-2. Clinical Applications-Melanoma. In: De Vita VT, Hellmans, Rosenberg SA (eds) Biologic Therapy of Cancer. JB Lippincott Company, Philadelphia, PA, p 250

18. Rosenberg SA (1997) Keynote address: perspective on the use of Interleukin-2 in cancer treatment. Cancer J Sci Am 3:S2

19. Marincola FM (1994) Interleukin-2. Biol Ther Cancer Updates 4 (3):1

20. Lotze MT (1991) Interleukin-2: Basic principles. In: De Vita VT, Hellmans, Rosenberg SA (eds) Biologic Therapy of Cancer. JB Lippincott Co, Philadelphia, p 123

21. Rosenberg SA, Lotze MT, Yang JC, Topalian SL, Chang AE, Schwartzentruber DJ, Aebersold P, Leitman S, Linehan WM, Seipp CA, White D (1993) Prospective randomized trial of high-dose interleukin-2 alone or in conjunction with lymphokine-activated killer cells for the treatment of patients with advanced cancer. J Natl Cancer Inst 85:622

22. Rosenberg SA, Spiess P, Lafreniere R (1986) A new approach to the adoptive immunotherapy of cancer with tumor-infiltrating lymphocytes. Science 233:1318.

23. Itoh K, Tilden AB, Balch CM (1986) Interleukin-2 activation of cytotoxic T-lymphocytes infiltrating into human metastatic melanomas. Cancer Res 46:3011

24. Kawakami Y, Zakut R, Topalian SL, Stotter H, Rosenberg SA (1992) Shared human melanoma antigens. Recognition by tumor-infiltrating lymphocytes in HLA-A2.1-transfected melanomas. J Immunol 148:638

25. Ferrone S, Marincola FM (1995) Loss of HLA class I antigens by melanoma cells: molecular mechanisms, functional significance and clinical relevance. Immunol Today 16:487

26. Zemmour J, Parham P (1993) HLA Class I nucleotide sequences, 1992. Immunobiology 187:70
27. Bjorkman PJ, Parham P (1990) Structure, function, and diversity of class I major histocompatibility complex molecules. Annu Rev Biochem 59:253
28. Van der Bruggen P, Traversari C, Chomez P, Lurquin C, De Plaen E, Van den Eynde B, Knuth A, Boon T (1991) A gene encoding an antigen recognized by cytolytic T lymphocytes on a human melanoma. Science 254:1643
29. Chen Y-T, Stockert E, Tsang S, Coplan KE, Old LJ (1995) Immunophenotyping of melanomas for tyrosinase: implications for vaccine development. Proc Natl Acad Sci USA 92:8125
30. Marincola FM, Hijazi YM, Fetsch P, Salgaller ML, Rivoltini L, Cormier J, Simonis TB, Duray PH, Herlyn M, Kawakami Y, Rosenberg SA (1996) Analysis of expression of the melanoma associated antigens MART-1 and gp100 in metastatic melanoma cell lines and in in situ lesions. J Immunother 19:192
31. Cormier JN, Hijazi YM, Abati A, Fetsch P, Bettinotti M, Steinberg SM, Rosenberg SA, Marincola FM (1998) Heterogeneous expression of melanoma-associated antigens (MAA) and HLA-A2 in metastatic melanoma in vivo. Int J Cancer 75:517)
32. Cormier JN, Abati A, Fetsch P, Hijazi YM, Rosenberg SA, Marincola FM, Topalian SL (1998) Comparative analysis of the in vivo expression of tyrosinase, MART-1/Melan-A, and gp100 in metastatic melanoma lesions: implications for immunotherapy. J Immunother. 21:27
33. Fetsch PA, Kleiner D, Marincola FM, Abati A (1997) Analysis of melanoma associated antigen MART-1 in normal tissues and in selected non-melanomatous neoplasms. Modern Path 10:43
34. Barnaba V, Franco A, Paroli M, Benvenuto R, De Petrillo G, Burgio VL, Santilio I, Balsano C, Bonavita MS, Cappelli G (1994) Selective expansion of cytotoxic T lymphocytes with a CD4+CD56+ surface phenotype and a T helper type 1 profile of cytokine secretion in the liver of patients chronically infected with Hepatitis B virus. J.Immunol. 152:3074
35. Chen YT, Scanlan MJ, Sahin U, Tureci O, Gure AO, Tsang S, Williamson B, Stockert E, Pfreundschuh M, Old LJ (1997) A testicular antigen aberrantly expressed in human cancers detected by autologous antibody screening. Proc Natl Acad Sci USA 94:1914
36. Marincola FM, Shamamian P, Rivoltini L, Salgaller ML, Reid J, Restifo NP, Simonis TB, Venzon D, White DE, Parkinson DR (1996) HLA associations in the anti-tumor response against malignant melanoma. J Immunother 18:242
37. Player MA, Barracchini KC, Simonis TB, Rivoltini L, Arienti F, Castelli C, Mazzocchi A, Belli F, Marincola FM (1996) Differences in frequency distribution of HLA-A2 sub-types between American and Italian Caucasian melanoma patients: relevance for epitope specific vaccination. J Immunother 19:357
38. Kawakami Y, Eliyahu S, Delgado CH, Robbins PF, Rivoltini L, Topalian SL, Miki T, Rosenberg SA (1994) Cloning of the gene coding for a shared human melanoma antigen recognized by autologous T cells infiltrating into tumor. Proc Natl Acad Sci USA 91:3515
39. Coulie PG, Brichard V, Van Pel A, Wolfel T, Schneider J, Traversari C, Mattei S, De Plaen E, Lurquin C, Szikora JP et al (1994) A new gene coding for a differentiation antigen recognized by autologous cytolytic T lymphocytes on HLA-A2 melanomas [see comments]. J Exp Med 180:35

40. Kawakami Y, Eliyahu S, Delgado CH, Robbins PF, Sakaguchi K, Appella E, Yannelli JR, Adema GJ, Miki T, Rosenberg SA (1994) Identification of a human melanoma antigen recognized by tumor-infiltrating lymphocytes associated with in vivo tumor rejection. Proc Natl Acad Sci USA 91:6458

41. Wolfel T, Van Pel A, Brichard V, Schneider J, Seliger B, Meyer KH zum Buschenfelde, and Boon T (1994) Two tyrosinase nonapeptides recognized on HLA-A2 melanomas by autologous cytolytic T lymphocytes. Eur J Immunol 24:759

42. Van der Bruggen P, Bastin J, Gajewski T, Coulie PG, Boel P, De Smet C, Traversari C, Townsend A, Boon T (1994) A peptide encoded by human gene MAGE-3 and presented by HLA-A2 induces cytolytic T lymphocytes that recognize tumor cells expressing MAGE-3. Eur J Immunol 24:3038

43. Guilloux Y, Lucas S, Brichard VG, Van Pel A, Viret C, De Plaen E, Brasseur F, Lethe B, Jotereau F, Boon T (1996) A peptide recognized by human cytolytic T lymphocytes on HLA-A2 melanomas is encoded by an intron sequence of the N-acetylglucosaminyltransferase V gene. J Exp Med 183:1173

44. Jager E, Chen YT, Drijfhout JW, Karbach J, Ringhoffer M, Jager D, Arand M, Wada H, Naguchi Y, Stockert E, Old LJ, Knuth A (1998) Simultaneous humoral and cellular immune response against Cancer-Testis antigen NY-ESO-1: definition of human histocompatibility leukocyte antigen (HLA)-A2-binding peptide epitopes. J Exp Med 187:265

45. Kawakami Y, Eliyahu S, Sakaguchi K, Robbins PF, Rivoltini L, Yannelli JR, Appella E, Rosenberg SA (1994) Identification of the immunodominant peptides of the MART-1 human melanoma antigen recognized by the majority of HLA-A2-restricted tumor infiltrating lymphocytes. J Exp Med 180:347

46. Salgaller ML, Afshar A, Marincola FM, Rivoltini L, Kawakami Y, Rosenberg SA (1995) Recognition of multiple epitopes in the human melanoma antigen gp 100 by peripheral blood lymphocytes stimulated in vitro with synthetic peptides. Cancer Res 55:4972

47. Nicotra MR, Nistico P, Mangoni A, Di Filippo F, Marincola FM, Natali PG (1997) Melan-A/MART-1 antigen expression in cutaneous and ocular melanomas. J Immunother. 20:466

48. Kim CJ, Chan CH, Rosenberg SA (1998) Ophtalmologic evaluation in patients undergoing immunization with melanoma associated antigens. J.Immunother (in press)

49. del Guercio MF, Sidney J, Hermanson G, Perez C, Grey HM, Kubo RT, Sette A (1995) Binding of a peptide antigen to multiple HLA alleles allows definition of an A2-like supertype. J Immunol 154:685

50. Rivoltini L, Loftus DJ, Barracchini K, Arienti F, Mazzocchi A, Biddison WE, Salgaller ML, Appella E, Parmiani G, Marincola FM (1996) Binding and presentation of peptides derived from melanoma antigens MART-1 and gp100 by HLA-A2 subtypes: implications for peptide-based immunotherapy. J Immunol 156:3882

51. Sidney J, Grey HM, Southwood S, Celis E, Wentworth PA, del Guercio MF, Kubo RT, Chesnut RW, Sette A (1996) Definition of an HLA-A3-like supermotif demonstrates the overlapping peptide-binding repertoires of common HLA molecules. Hum Immunol 45:79

52. Rotzschke O, Falk K, Stevanovic S, Jung G, Rammensee HG (1992) Peptide motifs of closely related HLA class I molecules encompass substantial differences. Eur J Immunol 22:2453

53. Kim CJ, Prevette T, Cormier J, Overwijk W, Roden M, Restifo NP, Rosenberg SA, Marincola FM (1997) Dendritic cells infected with poxviruses encoding MART-1/ MelanA sensitize T lymphocytes in vitro. J Immunother 20:276

54. Kim CJ, Parkinson DR, Marincola FM (1998) Immunodominance across the HLA polymorphism: implications for cancer immunotherapy. J Immunother 21(1): 1-16

55. Bettinotti M, Kim CJ, Lee K-H, Roden M, Cormier JN, Panelli MC, Parker KC, Marincola FM (1998) Stringent allele/epitope requirements for MART-1/Melan A immunodominance: implications for peptide-based immunotherapy. J Immunol 161: 877-889

56. Skipper JC, Kittlesen DJ, Hendrickson RC, Deacon DD, Harthun NL, Wagner SN, Hunt DF, Engelhard VH, Slingluff CL, Jr (1996) Shared epitopes for HLA-A3-restricted melanoma-reactive human CTL include a naturally processed epitope from Pmel-17/gp100. J Immunol 157:5027

57. Kang X, Kawakami Y, el-Gamil M, Wang R, Sakaguchi K, Yannelli JR, Appella E, Rosenberg SA, Robbins PF (1995) Identification of a tyrosinase epitope recognized by HLA-A24- restricted, tumor-infiltrating lymphocytes. J Immunol 155:1343

58. Brichard VG,Herman J , Van Pel A, Wildmann C, Gaugler B, Wolfel T, Boon T, Lethe B (1996) A tyrosinase nonapeptide presented by HLA-B44 is recognized on a human melanoma by autologous cytolytic T lymphocytes. Eur J Immunol 26:224

59. Gaugler B, Van den Eynde B, van der Bruggen P, Romero P, Gaforio JJ, De Plaen E, Lethe B, Brasseur F, Boon T (1994) Human gene MAGE-3 codes for an antigen recognized on a melanoma by autologous cytolytic T lymphocytes. J Exp Med 179:921

60. Kawakami Y, Eliyahu S, Jennings C, Sakaguchi K, Kang X, Southwood S, Robbins PF, Sette A, Appella E, Rosenberg SA (1995) Recognition of multiple epitopes in the human melanoma antigen gp100 by tumor-infiltrating T lymphocytes associated with in vivo tumor regression. J Immunol 154:3961

61. Vitiello A, Ishioka G, Grey HM, Rose R, Farness P, LaFond R, Yuan L, Chisari FV, Furze J, Bartholomeuz R et al (1995) Development of a lipopeptide-based therapeutic vaccine to treat chronic HBV infection. I. Induction of a primary cytotoxic T lymphocyte response in humans. J Clin Invest 95:341

62. Steinman RM (1991) The dendritic cell system and its role in immunogenicity. Annu Rev Immunol 9:271

63. Young JW, Inaba K (1996) Dendritic cells as adjuvants for class I major histocompatibility complex-restricted antitumor immunity. J Exp Med 183:7

64. Zitvogel L, Mayordomo JI, Tjandrawan T, Deleo AB, Clarke MR, Lotze MT, and Storkus WJ (1996) Therapy of murine tumors with tumor peptide-pulsed dendritic cells: dependence on T cells, B7 costimulation, and T helper cell 1-associated cytokines [see comments]. J Exp Med 183:87

65. Celluzzi CM, Mayordomo JI, Storkus WJ, Lotze MT, Falo LD, Jr (1996) Peptide-pulsed dendritic cells induce antigen-specific CTL- mediated protective tumor immunity. J Exp Med 183:283

66. Paglia P, Chiodoni C, Rodolfo M, Colombo MP (1996) Murine dendritic cells loaded in vitro with soluble protein prime cytotoxic T lymphocytes against tumor antigen in vivo. J Exp Med 183:317

67. Mayordomo JI, Zorina T, Storkus WJ, Zitvogel L, Celluzzi C, Falo LD, Melief CJ, Ildstad ST, Kast WM, Deleo AB et al (1995) Bone marrow-derived dendritic cells pulsed with synthetic tumour peptides elicit protective and therapeutic antitumour immunity. Nat Med 1:1297

68. Sallusto F, Lanzavecchia A (1994) Efficient presentation of soluble antigen by cultured human dendritic cells is maintained by granulocyte/macrophage colony- stim-

ulating factor plus interleukin 4 and downregulated by tumor necrosis factor alpha. J Exp Med 179:1109

69. Scher RL, Koch WM, W.J. Richtsmeier (1993) Induction of the intercellular adhesion molecule (ICAM-1) on squamous cell carcinoma by interferon gamma. Arch Otolaryngol Head Neck Surg 119:432

70. Fuchs EJ, Matzinger P (1996) Is cancer dangerous to the immune system? Semin.Immunol. 8:271

71. Zea AH, Curti BD, Longo DL, Alvord WG, Strobl SL, Mizoguchi H, Creekmore SP, O'Shea JJ, Powers GC, Urba WJ, Ochoa AC (1995) Alterations in T cell receptor and signal transduction molecules in melanoma patients. Clin Cancer Res 1:1327

72. Pockaj BA, Sherry RM, Wei JP, Yannelli JR, Carter CS, Leitman SF, Carasquillo JA, Steinberg SM, Rosenberg SA, Yang JC (1994) Localization of 111indium-labeled tumor infiltrating lymphocytes to tumor in patients receiving adoptive immunotherapy. Augmentation with cyclophosphamide and correlation with response. Cancer 73:1731

73. Hahne M, Rimoldi D, Schroter M, Romero P, Schreier M, French LE, Schneider P, Bornand T, Fontana A, Lienard D, Cerottini J-C, Tschopp J (1996) Melanoma cell expression of Fas (Apo-1/CD95) ligand: Implications for tumor immune escape. Science 274:1363

74. Wojtowicz-Praga S (1997) Reversal of tumor-induced immunosuppression: a new approach to cancer therapy. J Immunother 20:165

75. Wang RF, Robbins PF, Kawakami Y, Kang XQ, Rosenberg SA (1995) Identification of a gene encoding a melanoma tumor antigen recognized by HLA-A31-restricted tumor-infiltrating lymphocytes. J Exp Med 181:799

76. Castelli C, WJ Storkus, Maeurer MJ, Martin DM, Huang EC, Pramanik BN, Nagabhushan TL, Parmiani G, Lotze MT (1995) Mass spectrometric identification of a naturally processed melanoma peptide recognized by CD8+ cytotoxic T lymphocytes. J Exp Med 181:363

77. Cox AL, Skipper J, Chen Y, Henderson RA, Darrow TL, Shabanowitz J, Engelhard VH, Hunt DF, Slingluff CL Jr (1994) Identification of a peptide recognized by five melanoma-specific human cytotoxic T cell lines. Science 264:716

78. Visseren MJW, van Elsas A, van der Voort EIH, Ressing MA, Kast WM, Schrier PI, and MeliefJM (1995) CTL specific for the tyrosinase autoantigen can be induced from healthy donor blood to lyse melanoma cells. J Immunol 154:3991

79. Morioka N, Kikumoto Y, Hoon DS, Morton DL, Irie RF (1994) A decapeptide from human melanoma is recognized by CTL in melanoma patients. J Immunol 153:5650

80. Van der Bruggen P, Szikora JP, Boel P, Wildmann C, Somville M, Sensi M, Boon T (1994) Autologous cytolytic T lymphocytes recognize a MAGE-1 nonapeptide on melanomas expressing HLA-Cw*1601. Eur J Immunol 24:2134

81. Boel P, Wildmann C, Sensi ML, Brasseur R, Renauld JC, Coulie P, Boon T, and van der Bruggen P (1995) BAGE: a new gene encoding an antigen recognized on human melanomas by cytolytic T lymphocytes. Immunity. 2:167

82. Van den Eynde B, Peeters O, De Backer O, Gaugler B, Lucas S, Boon T (1995) A new family of genes coding for an antigen recognized by autologous cytolytic T lymphocytes on a human melanoma. J Exp Med 182:689

83. Wang RF, Parkhurst MR, Kawakami Y, Robbins PF, Rosenberg SA (1996) Utilization of an alternative open reading frame of a normal gene in generating a novel human cancer antigen. J Exp Med 183:1131

84. Rubinfeld B, Robbins P, el-Gamil M, Albert I, Porfiri E, Polakis P (1997) Stabilization of beta-catenin by genetic defects in melanoma cell lines. Science 275:1790

85. Robbins PF, el-Gamil M, Li YF, Topalian SL, Rivoltini L, Sakaguchi K, Appella E, Kawakami Y, Rosenberg SA (1995) Cloning of a new gene encoding an antigen recognized by melanoma- specific HLA-A24-restricted tumor-infiltrating lymphocytes. J Immunol 154:5944

The Role of Interferon in the Adjuvant Treatment of Cutaneous Melanoma

N. Cascinelli, F. Belli

Cutaneous melanoma presents antigens capable of eliciting a host-immune response, and regression of primary melanoma seems to reflect these interactions of the tumor with the immune system. Due to those specific features, melanoma is well suited to immunological intervention with interferons (IFNs). The exact mechanism of activity of IFN and expecially IFN-α in melanoma is not known, but it may act by enhancing the expression of tumor antigens and antitumour activity against melanoma cells, as well as having both direct antiproliferative and immunomodulatory effects [1]. The antiproliferative effects of IFN-α arise from its capacity of inhibition in the expression of cellular oncogenes and of DNA synthesis, while the immunomodulating effects of IFNs include enhancement of macrophage, cytotoxic T cell, and natural killer cell activity. Many studies suggest that IFN may manifest all these various types of anti-neoplastic function.

Furthermore, from a clinical point of view, IFN administered alone to patients with metastatic and advanced melanoma has already achieved meaningful results in some series of patients [2-5].

On this basis, in the recent past many trials were designed and performed in the USA and Europe in which IFNs were administered to individuals with melanoma at high risk of relapse, who may be most sensitive to the antiproliferative and immunomodulatory effects of this agent, and able to tolerate it for protracted periods of time.

Mainly stage II and III patients (AJCC classification) (Table 1) were considered to be included into these large cooperative multicentric studies.

Main characteristics and results of the most important trials are reported in Table 2.

Table 1. Criteria for the American Joint Committee on Cancer (AJCC) four-stage classification system

IA	Localised melanoma ≤ 0.75 mm or Clark's level II* (T1N0M0)
IB	Localised melanoma 0.76-1.5 mm or Clark's level III* (T2N0M0)
IIA	Localised melanoma 1.51-4 mm or Clark's level IV* (T3N0M0)
IIB	Localised melanoma > 4 mm or Clark's level V* (T4N0M0)
III	Limited nodal metastases involving only one regional lymph node basin, or fewer than five in-transit metastases without nodal metastases (any T, N1M0)
IV	Advanced regional metastases (any T, N2M0) or any patient with distant metastases (any T any N, M1 or M2)

*When the thickness and level of invasion criteria do not coincide within a T classification, thickness should take precedence

Adjuvant Interferon in Stage II Disease

Up to now two studies reported a significant disease-free survival benefit for low-dose IFN-α2a maintenance therapy in patients with stage II disease. The largest of these prospectively randomized studies, comparing low-dose IFN-α2a with no maintenance therapy (Table 2), is that performed by the French Cooperative Group on Melanoma including 499 patients [6-8], while similar results were reported by Pehamberger [9, 10] in a study involving 311 patients.

In both of these studies, patients were randomized to receive either low-dose IFN-α2a or no maintenance therapy. In the French study, IFN-α2a was given at a dose of 3 MU s.c. three injections a week (t.i.w.) for 18 months, while in the Austrian study, a higher cumulative dose was given during the first 3 weeks (IFN-α2a, 3 MU s.c. daily), followed by IFN-α2a, 3 MU t.i.w. for 1 year.

Recently, Grob presented the disease-free survival and overall survival results of the study based on a relatively long follow-up. Grob reported the continued impact of IFN-α2a on disease free interval (p = 0.03), with a relative reduction in the risk of relapse of 16% at 5 years. A relative reduction in the risk of death at 5 years was also reported.

The results of the Austrian study confirm the disease-free interval benefit reported for IFN-α2a in the French study. A statistically significant disease-free survival benefit was reported for an intention-to-treat analysis at a mean follow-up of 41 months (p = 0.02). Overall survival data for this study were not indicated.

Table 2. Main adjuvant IFN clinical studies

Group / Author	IFN Schedule	Pts	Results
WHO no. 16/Cascinelli [21]	IFNα 3 MU s.c. t.i.w. for 3 years	444	DFS (-); OS (-)
NCCTG no. 83-7052/Cregan et al. [20]	IFNα 20 MU/m² i.m. t.i.w. for 12 weeks	262	DFS (-); OS (-)
ECOG no. 1684/Kirkwood et al. [17]	IFNα 20 MU/m² per day i.v. for 1 month followed by 10 MU/m² s.c. t.i.w. for 48 weeks	287	DFS (+); P = 0.0002; OS (+); P = 0.023
ECOG no. 1690/INT no. 2055/Kirkwood	IFNα as in ECOG no. 1684 versus IFNα 3 MU s.c. t.i.w. for 2 years	642	Closed Jan 1995
ECOG no. 1694/Kirkwood	IFNα as in ECOG no. 1684 versus ganglioside vaccine		Ongoing
France, Grob et al., [7]	IFNα 3 MU s.c. t.i.w. for 18 months	493	DFS (+); P = 0.03; OS (-)
EORTC no. 18871/Kleeberg []	IFNα 1 MU/day s.c. for 1 year versus IFNγ 0.2 mgday s.c. for 1 year versus Iscador	830	Closed 1996
EORTC no. 18952/Eggermont []	IFNα 10 MU/day s.c. for 5 days/week for 4 weeks, followed by 10 MU s.c. t.i.w. for 1 year versus IFN(5 MU s.c. t.i.w. for 2 years		Ongoing
Austria/Pehamberger et al. [10]	IFNα 3 MU s.c. daily for 3 weeks, then t.i.w. for 12 months	311	DFS (+); P = 0.02; OS = (?)

Abbreviations: WHO = World Health Organization; NCCTG = North Central Clinical Trials Group; ECOG = Eastern Cooperative Oncology Group; INT = Intergroup; EORTC = European Organization for Research and Treatment of Cancer; t.i.w. = three times a week; s.c. = subcutaneous; i.m. = intramuscularly; i.v. = intravenously; DFS = disease free survival; OS = overall survival

Adjuvant Interferon in Stage III Disease

Evidence of regional lymphnode metastases is certainly the factor that most worsens the prognosis of patients with melanoma submitted to radical surgery: the risk for these patients to be affected by microscopical localisations at different sites is high and evaluable in about 80-85% of cases [11]. That is why in the last 20 years a great number of studies were set up in order to evaluate the beneficial effects of an adjuvant treatment in patients submitted to radical surgery for regional metastases from cutaneous melanoma.

Unfortunately until now, with few exceptions, all the clinical studies adopting chemo, immunological or chemo-immunological schedules of adjuvant therapy did not achieve convincing results [12-16].

As mentioned before the various and complex biologic activities that IFN can express against cancer cells and especially against melanoma cells justify the great interest dedicated to such a biologic agent in these recent years in many clinical studies performed in Europe and the USA.

At least six large phase III studies have been undertaken or are currently underway that compare IFN-α adjuvant therapy with no treatment in patients with stage III disease (Table 2). These different trials have investigated different regimens of IFN-α, ranging from high-dose regimens, associated with significant toxicity and requiring dose reductions in many patients, to very well-tolerated low-dose regimens.

In the following paragraphs the main trials performed in this field will be considered.

ECOG EST 1684

In this study, high-dose IFNα, was administered for 1 year, following excision of the primary tumour. The planned dose was an induction regimen consisting of 20 MU/m^2 i.v. five times a week given for 4 weeks, followed by a maintenance regimen of 10 MU/m^2 s.c. t.i.w. given for 11 months.

After a median follow-up period of 6.9 years there was a significant increase in relapse free survival from 1 to 1.7 years (P = 0.002) as well as in overall survival from 2.8 to 3.8 years (P = 0.023) (Fig. 1).

Estimated 5-year relapse-free survival rates on IFNα were 37% versus 26% on observation, and the 5-year survival rates were 46% and 37%, respectively [17].

The intensity of this regimen required dose reductions (37% of patients in induction phase, 36% of patients in maintenance phase), and 26% of

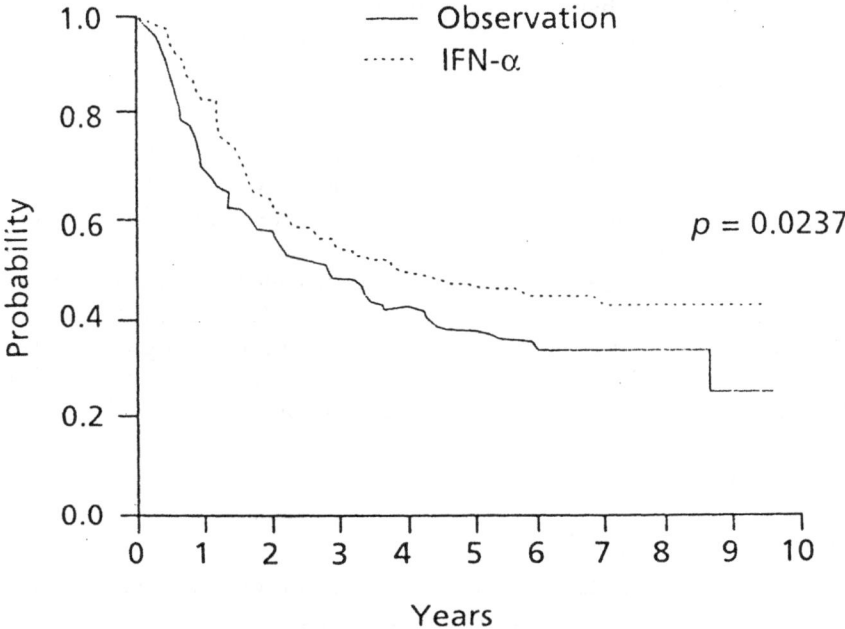

Fig. 1. Overall survival curves in ECOG EST 1684 study

patients withdrew from treatment. The median and mean doses for the initial month were 18 MU/m², and the median and mean doses for the maintenance period were 9 MU/m².

When reasons other than toxicity were included, dose delay or reduction occurred in 50% and 48%, respectively. The most common toxicities were of constitutional, haematological and neurological origin. Toxic deaths due to hepatotoxicity occurred in two patients in whom follow-up was not performed according to the protocol. The benefits in terms of relapse-free and overall survival have to be balanced against these substantial toxicities and the costs of treatment. In an elegant study using a survival analysis adjusted for quality of life (quality-adjusted time without symptoms and toxicity; Q-TWIST) it was suggested that the clinical benefit of IFNα treatment at this dose and schedule outweigh the toxic effects [18].

The cost-efficiency of therapy is another important consideration. This has been analysed for the ECOG EST 1684 study [19]. Kirkwood reported that the cost per quality-adjusted year of survival for this therapy is comparable with that of adjuvant therapy in breast cancer and colon cancer, and therefore is likely to be acceptable in most countries.

NCCTG n° 83-7052

Creagan et al. [20] investigated the value of a short course of IFNα therapy at 20 MU/m^2 intramuscularly three times a week for 12 weeks in patients with ≥ 1.7 mm melanoma or completely resected regional nodes. Although this study showed no difference in disease-free and overall survival, the disease-free survival was significantly increased in node-positive patients from 11 months to 17 months. This result has to be interpreted with caution since it concerns a retrospective subgroup analysis. Compared with the low regimens, toxicity was more pronounced in this trial, with severe flu-like symptoms, loss of ≥ 10% baseline body weight and worsening of baseline performance status in 44%, 10% and 45% of patients, respectively.

WHO Melanoma Programme Trial 16

This is a randomized study aimed at evaluating the efficacy and tolerability of low dose IFN in stage III melanoma patients.

The patients included in the treatment arm were given: IFNα-2A, 3 millions IU subcutaneously t.i.w. starting 30-35 days after surgery till the appearance of clinical or radiological detectable, local or distant, recurrences (Fig. 2).

The discontinuation of treatment was considered for the patients without evidence of recurrent disease if major toxicity occurred, otherwise the treatment was carried out for 3 years.

Lymphonode dissection was performed on the basis of clinical diagnosis of axillary, inguinal or cervical lymphnode involvement following current worldwide criteria of radical surgical oncology.

Site, number and pattern of diffusion of involved nodes were accurately registered. The series was stratified by center, number of positive nodes (one, two or three, more than three), and pattern of pathological diffusion (intra or extracapsular).

Each patient was closely checked to detect the appearance of new local or distant recurrences or the onset of toxic effects due to therapy with scheduled follow-up controls.

The aim of this study was to evaluate the toxicity and tolerance of chronic three times a week therapy with IFNα2A and to evaluate the effi-

RADICAL SURGERY

HISTOLOGY N+

STRATIFICATION

1= Center
2= Clinic met. lymphnodes
3= Number of positive nodes
4= Extent of nodal involvement

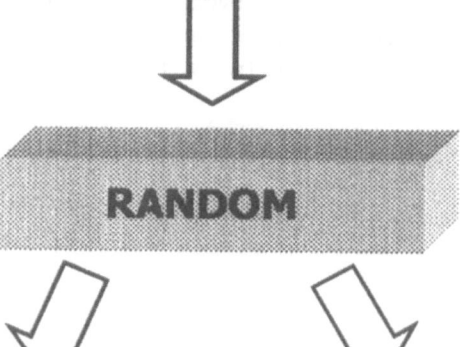

No further treatment   rIFNα - 2A, 3 MIU 3 times a week
                            until relapse or onset of major toxic
                            effects, or otherwise for 3 years

Fig. 2. Study Design of WHO Melanoma Programme Clinical Trial 16

cacy of adjuvant therapy with IFNα-2A in patients at high risk of relapse after radical surgery.

The statistical evaluation of this open study was done at Istituto Nazionale Tumori of Milan and to evaluate a difference of 15% at 5 years at a statistically significant level with an α error of 5% and a power (1-β) of 90%, more than 200 patients per arm were forecasted.

From June 1990 to January 1994 474 patients, 443 of them fully eligible and evaluable, were accrued with the participation of 23 centers of the WHO Melanoma Programme.

Disease-free survival of patients receiving IFN treatment was not affected by the treatment, moreover product limit 5-year cumulative survival observed in patients submitted to node dissection was only 39.3% compared with the 33.7% of patients receiving interferon after surgery. The difference was not statistically significant (P = 0,46 Wilcoxon test: $\chi^2 = 0.54$) (Figs. 3 and 4). No differences in the two study arms were observed in any subsets of patients identified by age, sex, number of involved nodes or type of diffusion. Multivariate analysis of survival showed that administration of low dose of interferon for three years had no impact on survival of these patients, even if corrected for age, sex, number of positive nodes or type of diffusion.

The toxicity due to treatment was extremely slim. The most frequent symptoms claimed by patients consisted of fever, asthenia and malaise. Usually they were of mild or moderate intensity and no patient requested discontinuation of dosing because of toxicity. It should be underlined

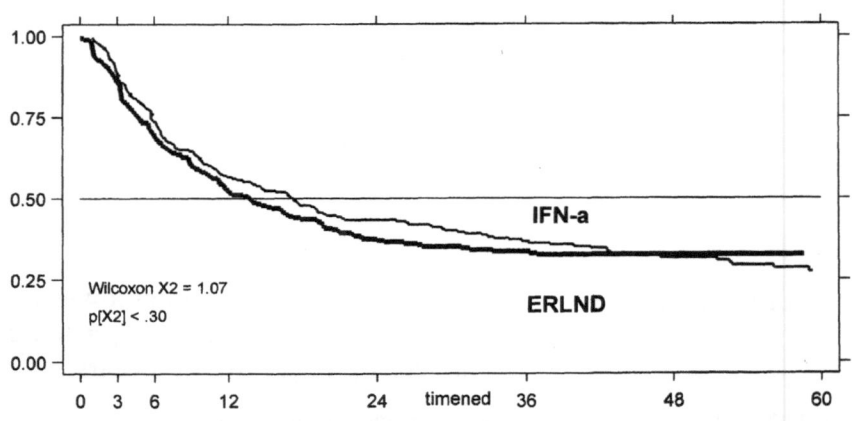

Fig. 3. Disease-free survival of 443 evaluable patients according to treatment in WHO Melanoma Programme Clinical Trial 16 (IFN 225 pts - ERLND 218 pts)

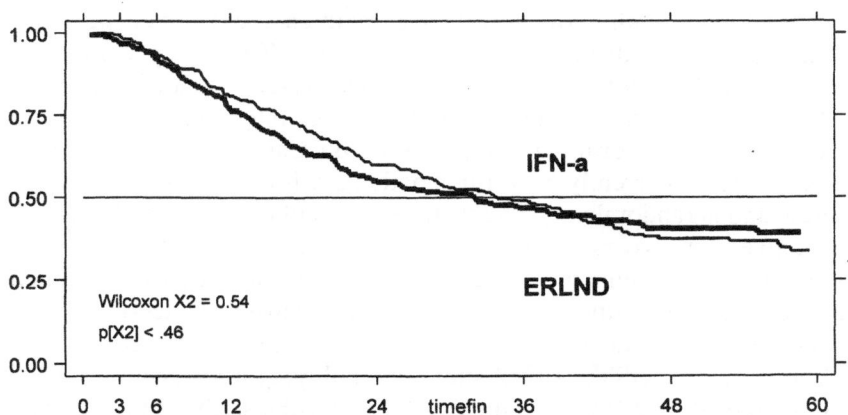

Fig. 4. Overall survival of 443 evaluable patients according to treatment in WHO Melanoma Programme Clinical Trial 16 (IFN 225 pts - ERLND 218 pts)

that commonly many of these effects tended to reduce or disappear after 2 or 3 weeks of therapy and that at sixth month even minor toxicity was practically absent. After the first month of therapy most patients stopped any type of medication eventually taken for controlling fever or other toxic signs.

The excellent tolerance to the treatment was confirmed by a parallel study on the quality of life of these patients carried out in our Institute by a separate staff of neurologists and psychologists. This evaluation demonstrated that the adopted schedule of therapy was well tolerated by the large majority of patients and that it did not produce any negative impact or influence the quality of life or the daily activities of treated patients even after many months of treatment [22].

Ongoing studies

Having established the potential efficacy of high-dose IFN-α in stage III disease, a number of phase III studies are currently investigating whether less aggressive regimens may be equally active (Table 2). This is important in view of the toxicity associated with high-dose IFN-α therapy, and may lead to the establishment of better tolerated regimens for patients with stage III disease.

The ECOG EST 1690 study was planned as a follow-up to the ECOG EST 1684 study and is comparing the high-dose regimen employed in the

EST 1684 study with a low-dose IFN-α regimen, 3 MU given s.c. t.i.w. for 2 years and with no maintenance therapy. This study completed accrual of 642 patients in 1995 and will be analysed at maturity in 1998.

Two further studies are investigating low- or intermediate-dose regimens. The UK Coordinating Committee on Cancer Research (UKC-CCR) study is currently recruiting patients with stage II or stage III disease and is randomizing patients to receive either IFN-α2a, 3 MU s.c. t.i.w., given for 2 years or until relapse; or no treatment. The study aims to recruit 1000 patients over 5 years, in order to detect a 10% difference between the two groups. To date, 190 patients have been accrued. This study also includes an analysis of quality of life and cost-benefit.

The ongoing EORTC 18952 study is employing a lower-dose induction regimen than that used in the ECOG EST 1684 study and is comparing two maintenance regimens [23]. This study, which plans to recruit 1000 patients, includes a control group of 200 patients who are randomized to observation. In this three-arm trial, patients are randomized between induction treatment with IFNα at 10 MU/day subcutaneously 5 days/week for 4 weeks followed by 10 MU three times a week for 1 year, the same induction regimen followed by IFNα 5 MU/day three times a week for 2 years, and observation. The total planned dose of IFNα for the entire treatment period in both treatment arms is thus 1760 MU [23].

Lastly, the currently ongoing ECOG no. 1694 trials is comparing the no. 1684 high dose IFNα schedule with treatment with a ganglioside vaccine in the same group of patients.

Conclusions

An important point in the adjuvant treatment of melanoma has been achieved by the encouraging results of high dose IFNα in the ECOG no.1684 trial. However, in consideration of the significant toxicity of the treatment it should be questioned whether the results of a single study should change clinical practice in melanoma patients. The results of the confirmatory ECOG no. 1690 study, as well as the EORTC no. 18952 study will probably provide important additional information.

Despite all these puzzling and in some ways controversial clinical data, the crucial point necessary for a correct interpretation of the results deriving from these studies remains unsolved: the biologic mechanism of activity of αIFN against cancer cells. In this field some information is now emerging but the exact modality of interaction between αIFN and the tumor target is presently not clear.

Therefore in our opinion, until all these clinical and biological results become available, no definite recommendations can be made for adjuvant treatment with IFNα in high-risk melanoma patients in routine practice.

References

1. Gresser I (1985) How does interferon inhibit tumor growth? In: Gresser I (ed) Interferons.Academic Press, New York, 6:93-126
2. Creagan ET, Ahamann DL, Green SJ et al (1984) Phase II study of recombinant leukocyte A interferon (rIFN-alpha A) in disseminated malignant melanoma. Cancer 54: 2844-2849
3. Cunningham TT, Schoenfeld D, Nathanson L et al (1979) A controlled ECOG study of adjuvant therapy in patients with stage I and II malignant melanoma. In: Programme and Abstracts of the Second International Conference on the Adjuvant Therapy of Cancer, Tucson
4. Kirkwood JM, Ernstoff M (1985) Melanoma therapeutic options with recombinant interferons. Sem Oncol 12(4S5):7-12
5. Kirkwood JM, Ernstoff M (1986) Potential applications of the interferons in oncology: lessons drawn from studies of human melanoma. Sem Oncol 8(3, Suppl 2): 48-56
6.. Grob JJ, Dreno B, Delaunay M, Chastang C, Cupissol D, Guillot B, Souteyrand P, Sassolas B et al (1997) Long term results of an adjuvant therapy with low doses IFN-α2A in resected primary melanoma thicker than 1.5 mm without clinically detectable node metastases. Oral abstracts of the 4th World Conference on Melanoma. Melanoma Research 7 (suppl 1)
7. Grob JJ, Dreno B, De la SalmoniÈre P, Delaunay M, Cupissol D, Guillot B, Souteyrand P et al (1998) Randomised trial of interferon α-2a as adjuvant therapy in resected primary melanoma thicker than 1.5 mm without clinically detectable node metastases. Lancet 351:1905-1910
8. Grob JJ, Dreno B, Delaunay M et al (1996) Results of the French multicenter trial on adjuvant therapy with interferon alfa-2a in resected primary melanoma (> 1.5 mm). Proc Am Soc Clin Oncol 15: 437 (Abstract)
9. Pehamberger H, Soyer P, Steiner A, Kofler R, Binder M, Mischer P, Pachinger W, Aub^ck J, Fritsch P, Kerl H, Wolff K (1997) Adjuvant interferon alpha-2a treatment in resected primary cutaneous melanoma. Oral abstracts of the 4th World Conference on Melanoma. Melanoma Research 7 (suppl 1)
10. Pehamberger H, Soyer HP, Steiner A, Kofler R, Binder M, Mischer P, Pachinger W et al (1998) Adjuvant interferon alpha-2a treatment in resected primary stage II cutaneous melanoma. J Clin Oncol (in press)
11. Balch C et al (1981) A multifactorial analysis of melanoma. Ann Surg 193(3):377-388
12. Banzet P et al (1978) Adjuvant chemotherapy in the management of primary malignant melanoma. Cancer 41:1240
13. Cunningham TJ et al (1979) A controlled ECOG study of adjuvant therapy in patients with stage I and II malignant melanoma. In: Salamon SS, Jones SE (eds) Adjuvant Therapy of Cancer II. Grune & Stratton, New York p 507

14. Fisher RI et al (1981) Adjuvant immunotherapy or chemotherapy for malignant melanoma. Surg Clin North Am 61:1267
15. Kaiser LR et al (1981) Adjuvant therapy for malignant melanoma. Surg Clin North Am 61:1249
16. Veronesi U et al (1982) A randomized trial of adjuvant chemotherapy and immunotherapy in cutaneous melanoma. New Engl J Med 307(15):913-916
17. Kirkwood JM, Strawderman MH, Ernstoff MS, Smith TJ, Borden EC, Blum RH (1996) Interferon alfa-2b adjuvant therapy of high risk resected cutaneous melanoma: the Eastern Cooperative Oncology Group Trial EST 1684. J Clin Oncol 14(1):7-17
18. Cole BF, Gelber RD, Kirkwood JM, Goldhirsch A, Barylak E, Borden E (1996) Quality-of-life-adjusted survival analysis of interferon alfa-2b adjuvant treatment of high-risk resected cutaneous melanoma: an Eastern Cooperative Oncology Group Study. J Clin Oncol 14:2666-2673
19. Hillner BE, Kirkwood JM, Atkins MB, Johnson ER, Smith TJ (1997) Economic analysis of adjuvant interferon alfa-2b in high-risk melanoma based on projections from Eastern Cooperative Oncology Group 1684. J Clin Oncol 15:2351-2358
20. Creagan ET, Dalton RJ, Ahmann DL et al (1995) Randomized, surgical adjuvant clinical trial of recombinant interferon alfa-2a in selected patients with malignant melanoma. J Clin Oncol 13:2776-2783
21. Belli F, Cascinelli N (1998) Low dose interferon α 2A as adjuvant tretament after radical node dissection for cutaneous melanoma. Update of WHO Melanoma Programme Trial 16. Proceeding SSO 51st Annual Meeting, S. Diego (5):8
22. Caraceni A, Gangeri L, Martini C, Belli F, Brunelli C, Baldini M, Mascheroni L, Lenisa L, Cascinelli N (1998) Neurotoxicity of Interferon-α in Melanoma Therapy. Results from a randomized clinical trial. Cancer 83:482-489

Part VI
Infectious Agents and Cancers

Molecular Mechanisms of Hepatitis B and C Viruses Related Liver Carcinogenesis

C. Brechot

Introduction

Primary liver cancer is the eighth most frequent tumor world-wide but the incidence of this tumor significantly varies in different geographical areas, the highest incidence being shown in Sub-Saharian Africa and South east Asia. It is important to emphasize the heterogeneity of the histological background on which the tumor develops. Most HCCs will complicate the evolution of an active or inactive cirrhosis. However some tumors will occur on livers with minimal histological changes. A large number of epidemiological and molecular studies have indeed clearly indicated the major importance of environmental factors in the developpment of primary liver cancers in humans. Chronic infections by Hepatitis B (HBV) and C (HCV) are major risk factors (Figure 1). Although this review will mostly analyse the impact of HBV chronic infection it is important to emphasize that some chemical carcinogens are also involved, as well as, yet poorly defined, hormonal factors which would account for higher incidence of the tumor in man. Finally the role of genetic factors has been raised but is difficult to properly adress, due to several confounding variables such as intra familial transmission of HBV.

Liver cell proliferation and liver carcinogenesis (Figure 2)

Most hepatocytes in a normal liver are in a quiescent state. Constitutive induction of liver cell progression into the cell cycle can be however triggered by several factors: growth factors and cytokines stimulation, oncogenes overexpression, "suppressor" genes inactivation (such as the Retinoblastoma (Rb) protein and P53 encoding genes). As summarised in the Figure 2, this ongoing progression from a G0/G1, differentiated status, to S phase induced by chronic hepatitis B and C can overcome DNA repair mechanisms in the presence of mutational events. This may induce fixed DNA mutations and chromosomal rearrangements which

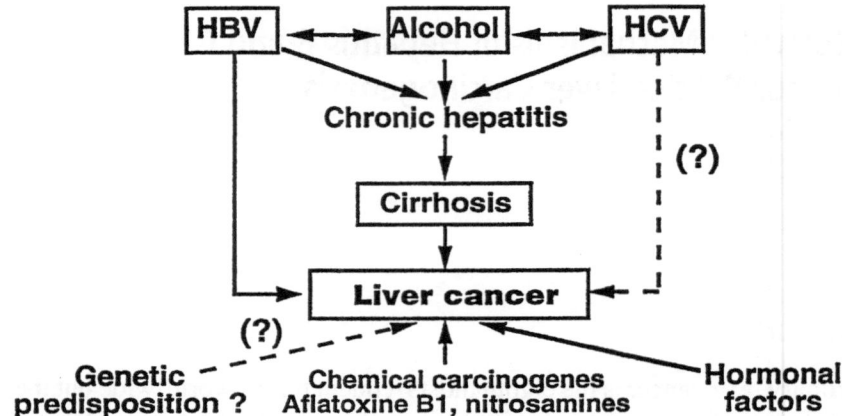

Fig. 1. Etiological factors of HCC

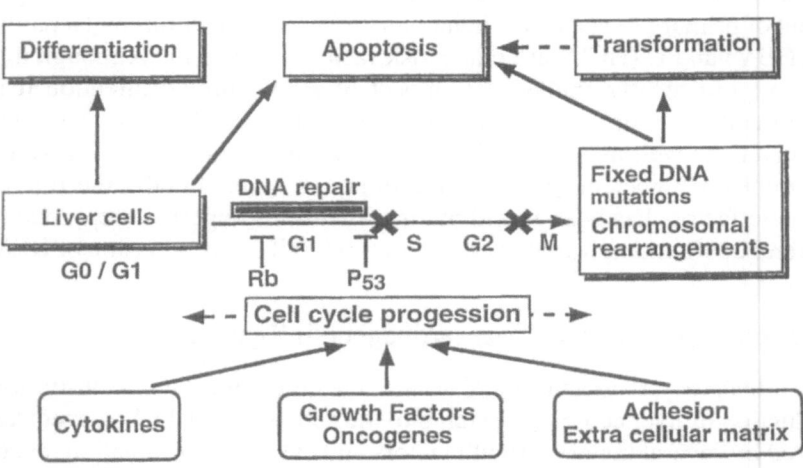

Fig. 2. Liver cell proliferation and HCC. The figure illustrates the critical role in liver carcinogenesis induced by various agents in generating DNA mutations, leading to liver cell transformation

are major determinants of cell transformation; under these conditions, if those cells escape elimination from programmed cell death [36, 48] and/ or immune response, they will become fully transformed. Progression of the tumor will then implicate a number of further genetic events, including angiogenesis which is a strict requirement for tumor growth and dissemination of metastatic tumor cells, both locoregionally and at distance. Thus any pathological condition associated to chronic stimulation of entry of quiescent liver cells into cell cycle should be viewed as a risk factor for liver cancer.

The role of hbv and hcv in liver cell carcinogenesis (Figures 3 and 4)

It is clear that both HBV and HCV induced CAH and cirrhosis are major factor in liver carcinogenesis. There is however also evidence for direct effects of HBV in this process and they should be viewed as having synergistic effects with chronic inflammation. In contrast there are presently only very preliminary informations regarding HCV.

HBV DNA integration into the cellular DNA allows persistence of the viral genome in the cell; inspection of the viral DNA sequences present in tumor cells has shown that, in a large proportion of the tumors, the

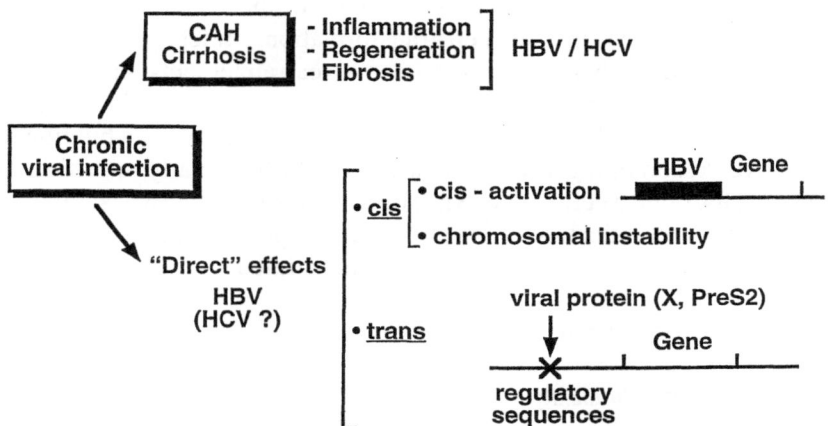

Fig. 3. Role of HBV in liver carcinogenesis. The figure summarises the different indirect and direct effects of HBV accounting for the impact of HBV in HCC

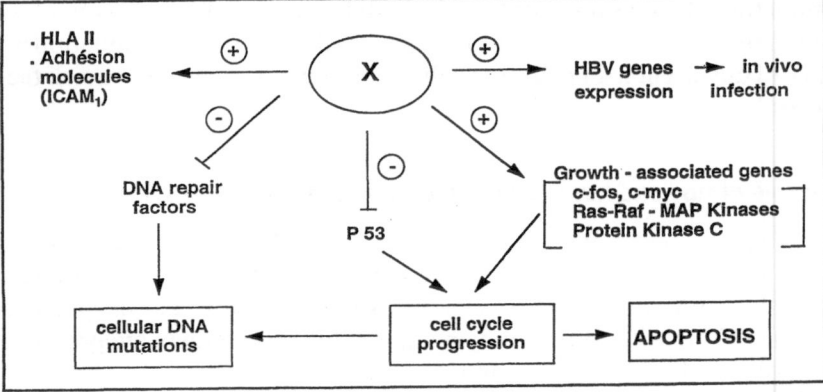

Fig. 4. Hypothetical biological effects of HBV X. The figure summarises the current hypotheses concerning the effect of X on cell signalling, cell cycle progression, apoptosis, as well as its potential role on viral cycle and antigen presentation

sequences encoding for the X and/or truncated enveloppe PreS2/S viral proteins are retained. In addition several reports are consistent with the involvement of these proteins, independently of the site of viral integration ("trans" effect), in liver cell transformation. Integration of HBV DNA can also directly induce chromosomal rearrangements; in fact it has been suggested that the viral DNA sequences encompassing the encapsidation signal might show intrinsic recombinogenic activity via binding to a putative "recombinogenic" cellular protein [40]. Finally, insertion of the viral DNA into a cellular gene has been shown in a few HCCs; in some of these cases modification of the target gene expression upon HBV integration (i.e: "cis" activation) could be demonstrated.

Consequences of HBV DNA integration

1) Chromosomal DNA instability

Several studies have investigated the pattern of chromosomal rearrangements in Hepatocellular carcinoma, independently of the presence or absence of HBV markers. There is no unique profile; still some of these chromosomal abnormalities cluster in some regions which are listed in the figure (For review see: [29, 32, 33, 49]). These findings suggest that activation or inactivation of cellular genes located in the vicinity of the breakpoints might be involved in some steps of liver cell transformation. In this regard "candidate" genes have been identified such as P53, Rb, and more recently the gene encoding for the Insulin-like growth factor II receptor (R-IGF II); in other cases the finding of rearrengement of the same locus in several tumors leads to speculate on the existence of presently unknown suppressor genes in this chromosomal domain. In this context, it is interesting to note that HBV DNA insertion has been identified at some of these loci. As an example, the viral DNA was shown in one tumor to integrate in 17 p13, a cytogenetic band where the P53 tumor suppressor gene is located.

2) Synthesis of the X and truncated PreS2/S proteins

HBV X

Despite the frequent rearrangements of integrated HBV DNA sequences, an intact X protein or a truncated form retaining its biological efects can be synthetised from a large number of integrants [35]. X is an essential gene for establishment of in vivo WHV infection in the woodchuck [50]. X is expressed at a low level throughout all stages of the viral infection, as evidenced by the detection of anti-X antibodies [20] and it is generally believed that the titers of anti-X will parallell level of viral multiplication.

There are several evidences which point to an important role for X in liver carcinogenesis [21]. Expression of X RNA has been shown to be maintained in tumorous hepatocytes, even though S and C viral transcripts were no more detectable. Some reports have also demonstrated presence of the protein in the tumorous hepatocytes but these studies have been hampered by the low performance of most available anti-X antibodies. There are in vivo studies in transgenic mice which showed developpment of HCCs in animals expressing the X protein at a high level under the control of the X promoter [24]. It is now clear, however, that such HCCs will only develop in mice with an intrinsic genetic susceptibility to tumors developpment [26]. Other studies of X transgenic mice, suggest a cooperative effect between HBV X and chemical carcinogens in HCC occurence. Finally the findings from a recent analysis of transgenic mice expressing both X and WHV/c-myc supports an in vivo transactivating activity of X and shows acceleration of myc induced liver carcinogenesis by X [41]. In vitro studies are also consistent with a role for X in some steps of cellular transformation. Expression of X can indeed induce foci in some experimental conditions in NIH 3T3 cells and transform immortalised FMH 202 cells [28]. The most convincing evidence however comes from studies in different cell types which demonstrated progression of the cell through G1/S and G2/M transitions upon X expression [23, 24]; these reports have also emphasized the importance of the ras-raf- MAP kinases transduction pathway in this phenotypic effect [2, 3, 23, 24]. There are however several other mechanisms which have been proposed to account for the induction by X of cell cycle progrssion and, in cooperation with other factors, transformation. Their respective impact is still debated since many results have been obtained in in vitro models which actual relevance is controversial; it is also important to emphasize that a major problem for such studies is the difficulty to obtain an efficient expression of the X protein. Yet, the available data can be summarised as follows: 1. There is evidence for transcriptional activation of several cellular genes upon X expression such as growth related c-fos and c-myc oncogenes but also genes encoding for adhesion (ICAM-1) and HLAII molecules [34]. This transcriptionnal activation is mediated by different transcription factors such as NF-KB [10], AP-1, CREB, but does not involve direct binding of X to DNA sequences; instead X might activate transcription by two distinct pathways: direct binding to elements of the transcriptional machinery such as TATA binding protein and RNA Polymerase II subunits and activation of transduction signals such as the ras-raf-MAP kinase and Protein Kinase C [22] cascades. In this view an important point to clarify is the precise subcellular localisation of X; while some recent studies have suggested a dual localisation: nuclear and cytoplasmic, with distinct biological effects [14], this is still debated and most evidences point to a major cytoplasmic signal.

There are however other interesting biochemical properties of X to consider: X has been shown to inhibit activity of some serine proteases inhibitors [39] and components of the proteasome complex [17]. One can therefore hypothesize that X might modulate the degradation and thus turn over of some cellular proteins involved in transcription and/or cell cycle progression regulation. Our group has recently presented data based on the use of the Green fluorescent protein as a Tag and confocal microscopy which demonstrates colocalisation of X with the proteasome in the cytoplasm and thus support the hypothesis of an interaction between X and proteasome subunits [1, 18, 37] X might also directly impair regulation of the G1/S transition by interacting with P53 [16, 42,

44]; Finally there are some recent evidences which would directly implicate X in apoptosis regulation although either sensitisation to apoptosis [27, 37] or, in contrast, inhibition of apoptosis [47] have been observed. Thus, altogether, there are now several directions to be thoroughly investigated and a major issue will be to demonstrate that these various molecular effects are relevant in vivo.

Insertional mutagenesis (cis-activation)

Table 1. Insertion of HBV DNA in cellular genes in the human and Woodchuck models

HBV and HCC
"Cis" activation of cellular genes

- **Human HCCs** = rare
  - (1) **Retinoic acid receptor** β
  - (2) **Cyclin A**
  - (3) **Epidemal growth factor**
  - (4) **Mevalonate kinase (PLC/PFR/5)**
  - (5) **Carboxypeptidase N related gene**
  - (6) **28s rRNA**
- **Woodchuck HCCs** = frequent
  - **C-myc**
  - **N-myc 2**

1. De Thé. Nature 1987;330:667
2. Wang. Nature 1990;343:555
3. Zhang. BBRC 1992;188:344
4. Graef. Oncogene 1995;208:696
5. Marchio Viral Hepatitis and liver disease 1994;730
6. Tsuei. J Virol Methods 1994;49:269

Two different situations must be distinguished: in HCCs developed in woodchucks infected by WHV, insertion of the WHV DNA into the *c-myc* or, predominantly, *N-my 2c* oncogenes is frequent (identified in at least half of the tumors so far analysed) [7, 8, 15, 19] (Table 2). There are convincing evidences, in vitro in cell culture and in vivo in transgenic mice, for the direct transforming property of constructs containing these integrants; these observations have also underlined that in these woodchuck tumors, the sites of integration of WHV DNA into c-myc are identical to those utilised by some oncogenic retroviruses in experimentally induced animal tumors.

Table 2. The table summarises the potential effects of HCV in liver carcinogenesis

HCV   AND   HCC

* Rare HCV related HCCs develop on livers with "minimal" CH[1]

* "Direct" effects of HCV (?)

- Cis = 0 (no integration of HCV genome)
- Transcriptional regulation of cellular and viral genes :

      . C-myc, c-fos   role of core proteins ?[2-4]
      . Rb   (deleted forms ?)[5]
      . IFNβ

- Transforming property of NS3 serine-protease ?[6]
- Lipid metabolism ?[7]
- Apoptosis (Fas ?) ?
         (TNF-R ?)

* Impact of HCV Genotype (1b) ?

[1]. De Mitri, Lancet., 1995 ; 345 = 413
[2]. Kim, Jpn.J.Med.Sci.Biol., 1994 ; 47 = 211
[3]. Ray, Virus Research, 1995 ; 37 = 209
[4]. Shih, J.Virol., 1995 ; 69 = 1160
[5]. Lo, Virology. 1995 ; 213 : 455
[6]. Sakamuro, J.Virol., 1995 ; 69 = 3893
[7]. Barba et al = submitted

In contrast, in human tumors, insertion of the HBV DNA into a cellular gene has only been shown in a few cases (listed in table 1); furthermore insertion in the same gene in different tumors has never been so far reported. Finally a direct cis-acting promoter insertion mechanism has only been definitely shown in two cases, and both tumors developed on a histologically non-cirrhotic liver with evidence of clonal proliferation of cells containing a single HBV integration site. In the first case, HBV DNA integration occurred in an exon of the retinoic acid receptor B gene (RAR B); 29 aminoacids of the viral PreS1 gene were fused to the DNA-binding and hormone-binding domains of the RAR, which is a member of the steroid-thyroid receptor gene family [11, 12].

In the second case, the human cyclin A-encoding gene was identified by our group in an early liver cancer developing on a histologically normal liver [45]. Integration of HBV DNA occured in the second intron of Cyclin A gene and (Figure 5) has modified the cyclin A expression pattern.

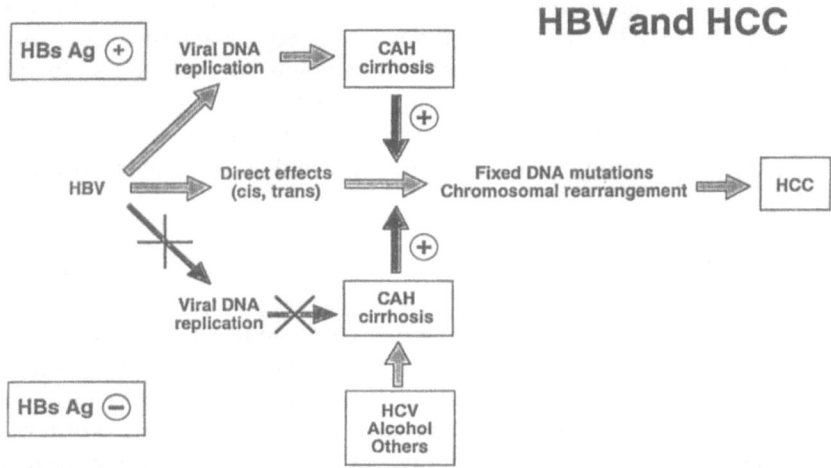

Fig. 5. HBV and HCV related liver carcinogenesis. The figure illustrates the proposed hypothesises and tentatively compares HBsAG positive and HBsAG negative patients

Cyclin A plays a major role in both G2/M and G1/S check-points of the cell cycle [13]. We have now obtained in vitro results which demonstrate the transforming property of the HBV-Cyclin A protein (Patil et al, in preparation).

Hepatocellular carcinoma in hepatitis b surface antigen-negative patients

There are striking geographical variations in the association between HCC and chronic infection by HBV. In Western countries (i.e Northern Europe, USA), and in Japan only 15 to 20% of tumors occur in HBsAg-positive patients, and other environmental factors such as alcohol and infection by hepatitis C virus (HCV) are clearly major risk factors. A number of epidemiological studies have shown a high prevalence of anti-HBs and anti-HBc antibodies in HBsAg-negative subjects (around 40 to 50% in France), indicating exposure to the virus [4]. These antibodies generally reflect resolved HBV infection; in HBsAg-negative subjects with HCC, however, HBV DNA sequences can be detected in the tumors, demonstrating the persistence of the viral infection and suggesting its implication in liver carcinogenesis [5]. It is important to realise that the improvement in the sensitivity of tests for HBsAg, together with the introduction of sensitive tests for HBV DNA, has modified the criteria for the diagnosis of HBV infection; there is indeed a spectum of chronic HBV infections with a low replication rate which, might be a risk factor for liver cancer [5]. These observations should be correlated with several studies showing persistence of HBV DNA long after recovery from acute viral hepatitis [31] and in patients with acute and chronic hepatitis [5, 9, 30, 43].

Conclusions

The data we have presented illustrate that viral agents (namely HBV and HCV) are major environmental etiological factors for human primary liver cancer. The available evidences demonstrate that HBV can trigger molecular mechanisms implicated in the control of liver cells proliferation and differentiation It will be therefore important to combine studies analysing the genetic of these tumors independently of HBV and HVC to those directly focussed on HBV and HCV related carcinogenesis.

References

1. Amsterdam, A., Pitzer, F., Santarius, U., Dantes, A. and Baumeister, W. Possible role of the multi catalytic proteinase (proteasome) in regulating of the cell cycle. 203-209 1994).
2. Benn, J. and Schneider, R.J. (1994). Hepatitis B virus HBx protein activates Ras-GTP complex formation ans establishes a Ras, MAP kinase signaling cascade. Proceedings of the National Academy of Sciences the U.S.A. 91, 10350-10354.
3. Benn, J. and Schneider, R.J. (1995). Hepatitis B virus HBx protein deregulates cell cycle checkpoint controls. Biochemistry. 92, 11215-11219.
4. Bréchot, C. (1987). Hepatitis B virus (HBV) and hepatocellular carcinoma. HBV DNA status and its implications. J. Hepatol. 4, 269-279.
5. Bréchot, C., Degos, F., Lugassy, C., et al. (1985). Hepatitis B virus DNA in patients with chronic liver disease and negative test for hepatitis B surface antigen. N Engl J Med. 312, 270-276.
6. Bréchot, C., Lugassy, C., Dejean, A., Pontisso, P., Thiers, V., Berthelot, P. and Tiollais, P. (1984). Hepatitis B virus DNA in infected human tissues viral hepatitis: in Viral hepatitis and liver diseases. 395-409.
7. Buendia, M.A. (1992). Hepatitis B viruses and hepatocellular carcinoma. Adv. Cancer Res. 59, 167-226.
8. Buendia, M.A., Paterlini, P., Tiollais, P. and Bréchot, C. Liver cancer: in Viral hepatitis: scientific basis and clinical management. (eds. Zuckerman, A.J. and Thomas, H.C.) 137-164 (Churchill livingstone, London, 1993).
9. Chazouillères, O., Mamish, D. and Kim, M.e.a. (1994). "Occult" hepatitis B virus as source of infection in liver transplant recipients. The Lancet. 343, 142-146.

10. Chirillo, P., Falco, M., Puri, P.L., Artini, M., Balsano, C., Levrero, M. and Natoli, G. (1996). Hepatitis B virus pX activates NF-kB dependent transcription through a Raf-independent pathway. Journal of Virology. 70, 641-646.

11. Dejean, A., Bougueleret, L., Grzeschik, K.H. and Tiollais, P. (1986). Hepatitis B virus DNA integration in a sequence homologous to v-erbA and steroid receptor genes in a hepatocellular carcinoma. Nature. 322, 70-72.

12. Dejean, A. and De Thé, H. (1990). Hepatitis B virus as an insertional mutagen in a human hepatocellular carcinoma. Mol. Biol. Med. 7, 213-222.

13. Desdouets, C., Sobczak-Thepot, J., Murphy, M. and Bréchot, C. (1995). Cyclin A: function and expression during cell proliferation. Progress in cell. (sous presse),

14. Doria, M., Klein, N., Lucito, R. and Schneider, R.J. (1995). The hepatitis B virus HBx protein is a dual specificity cytoplasmic activator of Ras and nuclear activator of transcription factors. EMBO J. 15, 4747-4757.

15. Etiemble, J., Degott, C., Renard, C.A., et al. (1994). Liver-specific expression and high oncogenic efficiency of a c-myc transgene activated by woodchuck hepatitis virus insertion. Oncogene. 9, 727-737.

16. Feitelson, M.A., Zhu, M., Duan, L.-X. and London, W.T. (1993). Hepatitis B x antigen and p53 are associated in vitro and in liver tissues from patients with primary hepatocellular carcinoma. Oncogene. 8, 1109-1117.

17. Fischer, M., Runkel, L. and Schaller, H. (1994). HBx Protein of Hepatitis B Virus Interacts with the C-Terminal Portion of a Novel Human Proteasome Alpha-Subunit. Virus Genes. 10, 99-102.

18. Fischer, M., Runkel, L. and Schaller, H. (1995). HBx protein of hepatitis B virus interacts with the C-terminal portion of a novel human proteasome alpha-subunit. 1995. 99-102,

19. Fourel, G., Tiollais, P. and Buendia, M.A. (1990). Nucleotide sequence of the woodchuck N-myc gene (WN-myc1). Nucl. Acids Res. 18, 4918.

20. Haruna, Y., Hayashi, N., Katayama, K., Yuki, N., Kasahara, A., Sasaki, Y., Fusamoto, H. and Kamada, T. (1991). Expression of X protein and hepatitis B virus replication in chronic hepatitis. Hepatology. 13, 417-421.

21. Kekulé, A. Hepatitis B virus transactivator proteins: the "trans" hypothesis of liver carcinogenesis: in Primary liver cancer: etiological and progression factors. (eds. Bréchot, C.) 191-210 (CRC Press, 1994).

22. Kekulé, A.S., Lauer, U., Weiss, L., Lüber, B. and Hofshneider, P.H. (1993). Hepatitis B virus transactivator HBx uses a tumor promoter signalling pathway. Nature. 361, 742-745.

23. Koike, K. (1995). Hepatitis B Virus HBx Gene and Hepatocarcinogenesis. Intervirology. 38, 134-142.

24. Koike, K., Moriya, H., Yotsuyanagi, H., Iino, S. and Kurokawa, K. (1994). Induction of cell cycle progression by hepatitis B virus HBx gene expression in quiescent mouse fribroblasts. Journal of Clinical Investigation. 94, 44-49.

25. Koike, K., Moriya, K., Iino, S., Yotsuyanagi, H., Endo, Y., Miyamura, T. and Kurokawa, K. (1994). High-level expression of hepatitis B virus HBx gene and hepatocarcinogenesis in transgenic mice. Hepatology. 19, 810-819.

26. Lee, T.-H., Finegold, M.J., Shen, R.-F., DeMayo, J.L., Woo, S.L.C. and Butel, J.S. (1990). Hepatitis B virus transactivator X protein is not tumorigenic in transgenic mice. Journal of Virology. 64, 5939-5947.

27. Levrero, M., Chirillo, P., Artini, M., Natoli, G., Costanzo, A. and Balsano, A. (1996). Induction of cell proliferation and apoptosis by HBV transactivation and HCC development: Rome, Italy.).

28. Luber, B., Arnold, N., Stürzl, M., Höhne, M., Schirmacher, P., Lauer, U., Wienberg, J., Hofschneider, P.H. and Kekulé, A.S. (1996). Hepatoma-derived integrated HBV DNA causes multi-stage transformation in vitro. Oncogene. 12, 1597-1608.

29. Marchio, A., Meddeb, M., Pineau, P., Danglot, G., Tiollais, P., Bernheim, A. and Dejean, A. (1997) Recurrent chromosomal abnormalities in hepatocellular carcinoma detected by comparative genomic hybridization. Gene, Chromosomes and Cancer. 8, 59-65.

30. Mason, A., Yoffe, B., Noonan, C., Mearns, M., Campbell, C., Kelley, A. and Perrillo, R.P. (1992). Hepatitis B virus DNA in peripheral-blood mononuclear cells in chronic hepatitis B after HBsAg clearance. Hepatology. 16, 36-41.

31. Michalak, T.I., Pasquinelli, C., Guilhot, S. and Chisari, F.V. (1994). Hepatitis B virus persistence after recovery from acute Hepatitis. Journal of clinical investigation. 93, 230-239.

32. Nagui, M., Pineau, P., Tiollais, P., Buendia, A. and Dejean, A. (1997). Comprehensive alleotyping of human hepatocellular carcinoma. Oncogene.14, 2927-2933.

33. Pineau, P., Marchio, A., Terris, B., Mattei, M.G., Tu, Z.U., Tiollais, P. and Dejean, A. (1996). A t (3;8) Chromosomal translocation associated with Hepatitis B virus integration involves the carboxypeptidase N locus. Journal of Virology. 70: (10) 7280-7284

34. Rossner, M.T. (1992). Hepatitis B virus X-gene product: a promiscuous transcriptional activator (review). Journal of Medical Virology. 36, 101-117.

35. Schluter, V., Meyer, M., Hofschneider, P.H., Koshy, R. and Caselman, W.H. (1994). Integrated hepatitis B virus X and 3' truncated preS/S sequences derived from human hepatomas encode functionally active transactivators. Oncogene. 9(11), 3335-3344.

36. Schulte-Hermann, R., Bursch, W. and Grasl-Kraupp, B. Active cell death (apoptosis) in liver Biology and disease: in Progress in Liver Disease. (eds. Boyer, J.L. and Ockner, R.K.) 1-35 Philadelphia, 1995).

37. Sirma, H., Rosmorduc, O., Kremsdorf, D. and Bréchot, C. (1996). Subcellular localisation of HBV X protein during the cell cycle in fixed and living mammalian cells: Rome, Italy.).

38. Takada, S., Gotoh, Y., Hayashi, S., Yoshida, M. and Koike, K. (1990). Structural rearrangement of integrated hepatitis B virus DNA as well as cellular flanking DNA is present in chronically infected hepatic tissues. Journal of Virology. 64, 822-828.

39. Takada, S., Kido, H., Fukutomi, A., Mori, T. and Koike, K. (1994). Interaction of hepatitis B virus X protein with a serine prorease, tryptase TL, as an inhibitor. Oncogene. 9, 341-348.

40. Tatzelt, J., Fechteler, K., Langenbach, P. and Doerfler, W. (1993). Fractionated nuclear extracts from hamster cells catalyse cell-free recombination at selective sequences between adenovirus DNA and a hamster preinsertion site. Genetics. 90, 7356-7360.

41. Terradillos, O., Renard, C., Billet, O., Molina, T., Briand, P., Tiollais, P. and Buendia, M.A. The HBV X gene accelerates liver carcinogenesis in WHV/C-myc transgenic mice: Rome, Italy.).

42. Truant, R., Antunovic, J., Greenblatt, J., Prives, C. and Cromlish, J.A. (1995). Direct Interaction of the Hepatitis B Virus HBx Protein with p53 Leads to Inhibition by HBx of p53 Response Element-Directed Transactivation. Journal of Virology. 69, 1851-1859.

43. Uchida, T., Aye, T.T., Becker, S.O., et al. (1993). Detection of precore/core-mutant hepatitis B virus genome in patients with acute or fulminant hepatitis without serological markers for recent HBV infection. Journal of Hepatology. 18, 369-372.

44. Ueda, H., Ullrich, S.J., Gangemi, J.D., Kappel, C.A., Ngo, L., Feitelson, M.A. and Jay, G. (1995). Functionnal inactivation but not structural mutation of p53 causes liver cancer. Nature Genetics. 9, 41-47.

45. Wang, J., Chenivesse, X., Henglein, B. and Bréchot, C. (1990). Hepatitis B virus integration in a cyclin A gene in a hepatocellular carcinoma. Nature. 343, 555-557.

46. Wang, J., Zindy, F., Chenivesse, X., Lamas, E., Henglein, B. and Bréchot, C. (1992). Modification of cyclin A expression by hepatitis b virus DNA integration in a hepatocellular carcinoma. Oncogene. 7, 1653-1656.

47. Wang, W., London, T. and Feitelson, M.A. (1991). Hepatitis B x antigen in hepatitis B virus carrier patients with liver cancer. Cancer Research. 51, 4971-4977.

48. White, E. (1996). Life, death, and the pursuit of apoptosis. Genes and Development. 10, 1-15.

49. Yamada, T., De Souza, A.T., Finkelstein, S. and Jirtles, R.L. (1997). Loss of the gene encoding mannose 6-phosphate/insulin-like growth factor II receptor is an early event in liver carcinogensis. Proc Natl Acad Sci USA. 94, 10351-10355.

50. Zoulim, F., Saputelli, J. and Seeger, C. (1994). Woodchuck hepatitis virus X protein is required for viral infection in vivo. Journal of Virology. 68, 2026-2030.

Epstein-Barr Virus and Malignant Diseases

B. E. Griffin

Preface and Acknowledgment

Epstein-Barr virus (EBV), a causal agent for infectious mononucleosis, is recognised as a carcinogenic agent for man, providing a major risk factor for a number of malignancies, including B-cell (Burkitt's, immunosuppression-related and Hodgkin's disease) and T-cell (sinonasal angiocentric) lymphomas, and poorly differentiated nasopharyngeal carcinoma. Over the past decade, although the data are less consistent, an association with a large number of other tumors has been identified, including many lymphoepithelial carcinomas. The expression pattern of EBV genes differs among the tumors, implying strong host cell control over viral gene expression; non-overlapping regions on the viral genome, specific for immortalization of either B-lymphocytes or epithelial cells in culture have been identified. Reports on tumor cells that initially possess, then lose EBV genetic information, point to a possible "hit and run" mechanism following on from viral infection, without significant loss of cell phenotype. As such an event may mimic tumor progression, identification of the initial pattern of viral gene expression, followed by alterations that result in genetic loss, should be a focus of research for the future, alongside new protocols for viral and/or tumor containment.

The author wishes to thank The Leverhulme Trust for support of her work.

Introduction

The International Agency for Research on Cancer (IARC; Lyon) has been evaluating carcinogenesis risks to humans since 1969, initially assessing chemical carcinogens, then extending the program to include life-style factors and biological agents, such as viruses. Their findings are published in monograph form. In 1997, one of the topics chosen for assessment was Epstein-Barr virus (EBV), together with the more recently discovered human herpesvirus, Kaposi's sarcoma virus (KSH, or HHV-

8). The conclusions from the evaluation of EBV were: "there is *sufficient evidence* for carcinogenicity of EBV in the causation of Burkitt's lymphoma, sinonasal angiocentric T-cell lymphoma, immunosuppression-related lymphoma, Hodgkin's disease and nasopharyngeal carcinoma. EBV is *carcinogenic to humans*" [1]. Such a strong conclusion - which is less strong where KSH is concerned - seems pertinent in the light of critical comments frequently made regarding any role for viruses in malignancy, particularly from individuals who find it difficult to accommodate the concept of "latency" where infectious agents, such as herpesviruses, are concerned. For EBV, such doubts are often expressed even with regard to poorly differentiated nasopharyngeal carcinoma and African (endemic) Burkitt's lymphoma, the two tumours where an EB viral association has now been studied extensively for more than 30 years, and correlative associations of 100% and > 95%, respectively, found. In the evidence accumulated and assessed by the IARC, some of these doubts may be silenced, at least for the present.

Background

EBV was first isolated and identified as a herpesvirus in the middle 1960s [2] from a B-cell line, EB (designated after its originators, Epstein and Barr), generated *in vitro* by co-culture of cells with a biopsy from an African Burkitt's lymphoma. Initially called EB virus (later Epstein-Barr virus), it was recognized as a contributor to infectious mononucleosis (IM), Burkitt's lymphoma (BL) and nasopharyngeal carcinoma (NPC) [3, 4]. Later studies with an animal model proved a causal relationship between EBV and IM [5].

Studies over the years have confirmed the continued strong association between EBV, (endemic) African BL, and NPC (as found in high prevalence among Chinese peoples in southern China and other parts of Asia). They have also identified about 90% of the world's population as being infected by this virus upon reaching adulthood, infection occurring at earlier ages in more crowded communities with poor, inadequate levels of hygiene, but often delayed into late adolescence in more sparsely populated areas of the world with higher standards of living. The latter areas serve as reservoirs for IM. One of the key outstanding problems where EBV and associated malignancies are concerned is, with such a high frequency of infection, why tumors develop in some individuals in a community and not in others of similar backgrounds with regard to age and sex, genetics, environmental exposure and habits; that is, within a particular high risk population, why do some individuals prove susceptible to tumor development and others do not? Many epidemiological studies have been carried out to resolve questions relating to cofactors in disease, but on the whole, these agents have proved elusive, although, as discussed below and elaborated elsewhere [1], for individual tumors some risk factors have been identified. Questions relating to virus strain variations have also been raised, and although alterations among viral sequences have been identified, and strains exhibiting different properties in *in vitro* experiments characterized, to date there is no compelling evidence in support of the existence of tumorigenic and non-tumorigenic wild type strains of virus. However, such studies are obviously much more difficult to carry out with large viruses, such as EBV (about 172-200 kilobase pairs), as compared with small viruses such as papilloma (8 kilobase pairs), where strain differences are known to be important to the pathology. With EBV, for the moment, strain variation as a significant component of disease, as well as the interesting problem of "viral load", remain open questions.

Herpesviruses contain double-stranded DNAs with varying amounts of genetic information and different sequence organizations [6]. In its structure, EBV DNA, more than the genomes of other herpesviruses, resembles its host chromosome in being composed of a linear arrangement of unique and repetitive sequences. However, unlike human chromosomal DNA where repetitive sequences are usually not translated into proteins, leading them even to be designed as "junk" DNA, the constraints in size and complexity on viruses - EBV being no exception - can result in repetitive regions being used as components of functionally relevant genetic information. With EBV, although the function of several of the proteins incorporating repetitive sequences have been defined, the best-characterized being EBNA1 (EBV nuclear antigen 1), responsible for maintaining the viral DNA as an extrachromosomal entity in most infected cells [7], the functions of proteins containing other repeats are essentially unknown. Some of them are not found expressed in latently infected cells, and presumably encode functions needed for other aspects of the virus life cycle.

The assignment of viral functions onto the DNA was considerably simplified when the complete sequence of EBV was determined in 1984 [8], using recombinant clones from restriction enzyme digests derived from B95-8 marmoset cells, themselves generated with virus from a mononucleosis patient. The B95-8 viral strain is competent to immortalize human B-lymphocytes in culture, and its genome has been adopted as representing a "prototype" strain against which other wild type and variant strains of virus are compared. Figure 1, taken from [9], contains a schematic diagram of a "composite" EBV genome showing the conventional restriction enzyme (BamHI)-derived physical map, the localization of major internal repetitive (IR) regions, some of the key viral functions associated with latency and the minimal immortalizing region (MIR) required for producing continuously proliferating cells *in vitro*, either from B cells (B) or epithelial cells (E). Notably, there is no overlap between MIR-B and MIR-E.

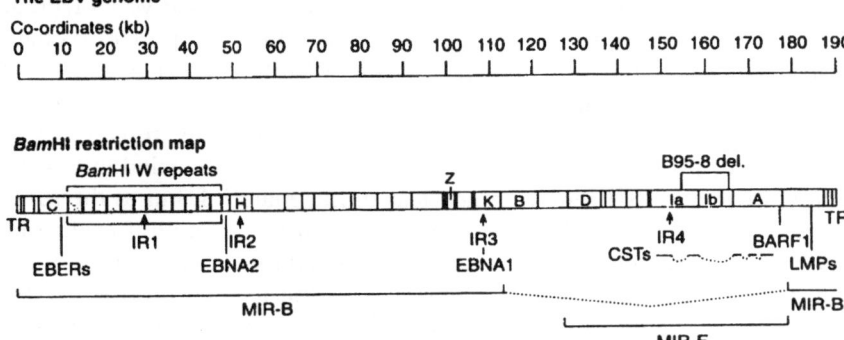

Fig. 1. The Epstein-Barr virus (EBV) genome.
Upper panel. Coordinates of a linearized version of a composite EBV genome which includes a region deleted in the 172 kilobase pair prototype viral strain (B95-8) whose complete DNA sequence has been determined [8]. Most EBV strains do not have this deletion and, depending upon the numbers of copies of internal and terminal repetitive sequences (IR1-IR4, and TR, respectively, see bottom figure), vary in size from about 172-200 kilobase pairs. In the virion, EBV exists in the linear form indicated, but in infected cells, the genome is circularized through the terminal repeats (TR).
Lower panel. Some landmarks on the viral genome, as discussed in the text. A physical map, based on fragments obtained by cleaving viral DNA with the restriction enzyme, *Bam*HI, ordering these as the sequences occur, but naming them according to size (*Bam*HI A being the largest, etc.) is given and location of some key viral functions indicated. EBNA, EBV nuclear antigen; LMP, latent membrane protein; EBERs, high level expression EBV-encoded RNAs; BARF1, rightward open reading frame 1, the conventional designation for EBV genes [8]; MIR-B [49, 50] and MIR-E [41, 42], minimum immortalizing regions for B-cells and epithelial cells, respectively. The complementary strand transcripts (CSTs) are a family of highly spliced viral transcripts encoded from *Bam*HI Ia up to the open reading frame for the BARF1 gene [28-31], as indicated. Their function(s) have yet to be determined. The viral latent origin of replication is located in *Bam*HI C, and two lytic replication origins are found in *Bam*HI H and Ia, the latter deleted in B95-8 cells. (Adapted from [9]).

EBV Associated Malignancies - New Discoveries

Until ten years or so ago, the range of tumors associated with EBV was thought to be restricted, confined mainly to endemic BL and poorly differentiated NPC. Although there were a few reports in the literature on EBV association with other malignancies, notably an early publication on EBV in lymphoepithelial carcinomas in Greenland eskimoes [10] and in a central nervous system lymphoma [11], and much general conjecture with regard to Hodgkin's lymphoma, the burst of information regarding other tumors has come more recently. One explanation for the many, newly discovered tumors carrying and expressing the EB viral genome comes from the newly developed, quicker and more sensitive molecular methods of analysis, notably procedures based on the polymerase chain reaction (PCR) and *in situ* hybridization (ISH). Whether these are equally (or more) accurate than the older methods of solution hybridization, or solid phase Southern and Northern blot protocols, remains to be determined; few if any comparative studies have been carried out. Certainly, PCR and ISH require much less tumor material, but at the same time are more at risk of errors due to sampling and fixation protocols. With PCR, an added complication is introduced by enzyme inhibitors in the tissues themselves which might, in addition to the notorious "false positives" introduced by contaminants, result in "false negative" results [12]. Thus, it may be understandable that the literature now contains apparently contradictory findings. Nonetheless, as assessed by the IARC committee, the consensus opinion is that a significant and pathologically relevant association exists between EBV and several other tumors, including immunosuppression-related lymphomas, and subgroups of T-cell lymphoma and the B-cell lymphoma, Hodgkin's disease (HD). With the latter, as suggested by earlier studies, a previous history of IM appears to be a risk factor for the development of disease in later life [13]. With sinonasal non-Hodgkin's lymphomas, studies come from a broad range of countries, involving for the most part small numbers of cases [1], where the majority of T- (but not B-) cells in the tumor population contain detectable EBV DNA and, when assessed, express viral genes. Notably, however, expression, where evaluated, has been limited to analyzing a few viral genes only. However, this seems less important where, as with this tumor, numerically high levels of positivity are generally obtained.

The present of EBV in HD was first reported in 1987 [14], and since then, where the virus is concerned, this pathology has been a major focus of attention with statistics reported for virus presence (and often expression) in up to 50% of HD among Western cases, and occasionally 100% in other settings [15]. Localization to the diagnostic Reed-Sternberg cells is found with high frequency. Seroepidemiological studies have shown elevated antibody titres to EBV antigens *prior to* and at the *onset* of tumor development [16], as observed earlier for BL and NPC. The variation in numbers of EBV positive tumors observed among different geographical areas leads again to the question of viral loads and whether they play a role in tumor genesis, or otherwise influence detection, particularly in cases where viral copy numbers and/or levels of transcription are low. Clearly, however, the recent data strongly support the conclusion that EBV is a risk factor for HD, as reviewed [17], as it is for lymphomas in general among transplant and immunosuppressed or immunocompromised individuals [1]. EBV-positive lymphomas in HIV-infected individuals, often assigned to different classifications, are nearly all of B-cell origin; whereas the retrovirus itself may act as a cofactor in this disease, it has not been detected alongside EBV in the tumors.

An interesting class of malignancies where EBV has been detected with varying frequency, but less consistency, are the lymphoepitheliomas. Studies of this class of carcinomas - infiltrated with large numbers of lymphocytes - was undoubtedly stimulated by the high frequency of association found between the tumor of poorly differentiated epithelial cells, NPC, itself originally designated as lymphoepithelioma, and EBV. In a recent analysis comparing poorly differentiated and other histological NPC types (squamous cell carcinoma and nonkeratinizing carcinoma), all were found to contain the EBV genome, although the levels and types of gene expression varied among them [18]. These and other [19] data emphasize the risk of EBV for tumors at this site, regardless of the state of differentiation of the epithelial cell. An article that reviews the literature up to 1995 with regard to an association of the virus with lymphoepithelioma-like carcinomas (LECs) that occur outside the nasopharynx, concludes that EBV is associated consistently, but not in 100% of cases, with only four anatomical sites, that is, stomach, thymus, salivary gland and lung, the latter two being restricted to Asian patients [20]. In the opinion of the authors, the data suggesting association (or lack thereof) with skin, uterine cervix, oral cavity, urinary bladder, or medullary carcinoma of the breast, were inconclusive. The data published on LECs since this review [1] appear to support the conclusions reached by its authors. It will be relevant in the future to see whether their overall assessment - that the presence or absence of EBV in LEC is not of prognostic importance since tumors associated with EBV are morphologically identical to those without the virus - withstands the test of time. LECs in association with EBV have only been studied over a short period and the case numbers are still small. The data should be reviewed when these tumors have received the same degree of detailed attention given, for example, to HD.

Whereas lymphoepithelial carcinomas of the stomach are a relatively rare type of tumor, EBV association was identified in 16% (22/38 cases) in a study in the USA, using PCR and ISH [21]. In certain parts of the world, especially in Japan, high incidences of gastric carcinomas occur. In larger scale studies by several investigators, involving over 2000 cases in Japan, EBV was detected in about 7% of them [1], whereas a single Korean study reported EBV positivity in 12/89 cases [22]. Although the frequency of association with gastric carcinoma is low, the consistency with which the virus is identified suggests that EBV may make some contribution to this tumor. Less consistent are the data on a major tumor in Western countries, breast cancer. With medullary carcinomas, EBV was not detected in 10 cases [23], nor in 60 invasive breast cancers [24] or, by hybridization, in 107 archival formalin-fixed samples in the USA [25], whereas in a larger scale study in the UK, using fresh samples and PCR and ISH protocols, 19/91 (21%) of the tumors scored positive for EBV, with the viral signal being localized to the epithelial cells by ISH [26]. A positive association has been reported by an international group who investigated 574 breast biopsies using tumors from North Africa, and Europe. Their overall findings were that 182 cases (32%) were positive for EBV, with the percentage of association paralleling viral load and being greater in high risk areas (Northern Africa: 46%) than in intermediate or low risk areas (33-28%) in Europe [27]. With the exception of poorly differentiated NPC, it is evident at this stage that associations between EBV and other carcinomas require not just further study, but a reevaluation of the methodologies used, a topic that is discussed below. At the moment, they are generally evaluated as if they differ little in terms of their viral components from the lymphomas, a concept that may or may not be valid.

EBV Gene Expression

Overall, six nuclear antigens [EBNAs 1, 2, 3A-C, and 5 (or leader protein, LP)], three membrane antigens (LMP 1, 2A and 2B) and two classes of RNAs, the EBERs and a family of complementary strand polyadenylated transcripts, (CSTs, or alternatively *Bam*HI A transcripts; see Fig. 1) have been associated with viral latency. The viral gene expression seen in the various EBV-associated malignancies vary, and for purposes of discussion, have been previously divided into three latency categories, designated I - III [1] - see also Table 1 - with only EBNA-1 and the CSTs [28, 29] and EBERs consistently observed in all three categories [28]. CSTs are by far the major polyadenylated transcripts seen in NPCs, but are generally only seen in B-cells when PCR methods are used in the search. They have the capacity to express a number of small polypeptides, only one of which has tentatively been identified to date [30, 31]. A more interesting role for them, in maintenance of latency is suggested by their location (see Fig. 1); they are found to be transcribed in an antisense orientation to a number of genes, such as the viral DNA polymerase, associated with the EBV lytic cycle [30].

As data evolve from further and more extensive studies into EB viral gene expression in tumors, the patterns will doubtlessly be found to alter. Already, as taken from limited information on gene expression in a smooth-muscle tumor [32], a separate category I-like expression pattern has been identified, which includes expression of the viral transcriptional transactivator function, EBNA-2, rarely found in other malignancies. Moreover, some gastric carcinomas, originally designated category I [1], have been shown to express the membrane associated function, LMP2A [33]. One viral function, BARF1, has been consistently ignored in categorizing EBV gene expression in the past. Although it has only been examined with regard to NPC [28, 34, T. Ooka, personal communication] where it is expressed at high frequency, this gene, which encodes a related pair of small proteins (31-33 kDaltons), has the capacity to stimulate the growth of established cells in culture, even to tumorigenecity if expressed at high level, and to immortalize epithelial cells in culture [35].

To raise a further problem, to date, studies on gene expression, drawn from the B-cell model, have mainly been focused on latent genes, since it might reasonably be assumed that any gene associated with later stages of the viral life cycle would be absent in tumors. This is not strictly the case, and some genes associated with loss of latency (such as the viral BZLF1 gene, whose protein product is designated 'ZEBRA') have been observed in tumor cells, for example, from BL and NPC [9, 36]. These have not been identified as coming from the tumor cells themselves, and they may reflect a reservoir of virus found in association with tumors. In a recent study of salivary gland tumors, intense DNA signals, identified as resulting from expression of lytic genes (even including those for the neutralizing viral gp350/220 proteins) were found in nonmalignant epi-

Table 1. Patterns of EBV latent gene expression[+]

Type of latency	Gene product	Co-stimulatory molecules	Examples
IA	EBERs, EBNA-1 CSTs		Burkitt's lymphoma
IB	EBERs, EBNA-1 CSTs, LMP2A		Gastric carcinoma
II	EBERs, EBNA-1, LMP-1, -2A, -2B, CSTs, BARF1*	CD30 CD23 CD40 B7.1 LFA-1, -3 1CAM-1	Hodgkin's disease Nasopharyngeal carcinoma T-cell lymphoma
III	EBERs, EBNA-1, -2, 3A -C, -LP, LMP-1, 2A, 2B	CD30 CD23 CD40 CD44 B7.1 LFA-1, -3 1CAM-1	Post-transplant lympho-proliferative disorder Infectious mononucleosis
Other	EBERs, EBNA-1, -2		Smooth-muscle tumors

[+]Adapted from [1, 48]. EBER, EBV-encoded RNA; EBNA, EBV nuclear antigen; LMP, latent membrane protein; LP, leader protein (also called EBNA5). *Only studied in NPC.

thelial cells in association with the T-cells of the tumor [37]. Magrath and colleagues identified replicative viral DNA in BL [38]. In our own studies on African BL biopsies, we have consistently found transcripts corresponding to intermediate early genes, which override latency, in high frequency (approaching 70%) in a minority of cells in the tumor, and in many cells in a smaller number of tumors [9, Labrecque et al., ms in press]. How lytic infection - if it occurs even in a minority of cells - and tumor cells coexist, and whether the former may even act as stimulants of the latter, is a topic that does not appear to have been addressed. Also, how cells carrying lytic genes survive in an immunocompetent host is not known, although one possible explanation could involve sequestering by a host protein; for example, ZEBRA both *in vitro* and *in vivo* has been shown to bind the cellular p53 function [39]. It is perhaps not surprising that when primary biological materials, instead of *in vitro*-generated cell lines, are characterized, viral gene expression is being consistently identified that falls outside the neat categories identified in cultured materials.

The paucity of materials usually available for study often restrict the degree to which tumors are scrutinized for gene expression, and over and over again, even when carcinomas are being examined for EBV presence and expression, the same genes - usually those known to be associated with B-cell latency or providing rapid, easy answers - are evaluated. These assays may not always be reliable, as recorded in recent literature in a model study where, although EBV DNA had clearly been identified, the authors could not find the generally assumed ubiquitous (except perhaps in virus-producing cells) EBERs in most tissues examined [40]. Might we be overlooking something? It would seem reasonable to suggest that before assuming the absence of EBV, at least two viral markers should be explored, and their choice should depend upon the cell type itself being explored. To emphasize the latter point, it is notable that the minimum immortalizing viral regions identified for B-lymphocytes and epithelial cells, by *in vitro* experiments, are different and non-overlapping (as shown, MIR-B and MIR-E, Fig. 1, and discussed, [9]). It is probably true that for carcinomas, it is not yet entirely clear which are the best probes to use in assessing viral expression, relevant to cell growth and malignancy, but this topic could be highly relevant for determining frequency of association with a particular tumor. In the one study where expression over the entire viral genome was evaluated, using an NPC xenograft [28], transcriptionally active regions were identified whose products have not yet even been characterized; whether they are crucial to tumorigenesis in epithelial cells is unknown. An obvious anomaly is why expression of BARF1 is not chosen for evaluation in carcinomas, when it appears to be an important function in NPCs. This would appear to be an important oversight in this field.

Hit and Run: an Alternative Scenario for EBV in Cells?

Not only is it possible that EB viral gene expression, under the control of its host cell, might differ among cell types in tumors, the possibility must be addressed that EBV, after providing an important "insult" to a cell, need no longer remain in the cell. That is, EBV might be critical for *initiating* events along the pathway to tumorigenesis, but not necessary for

maintenance of the altered phenotype. Were this so, the chances of finding viral information in a faster growing tumor, such as a lymphoma,
might be greater than in the slower proliferating carcinoma, where additional cofactors have a greater chance to contribute to malignancy, an
hypothesis consistent with the viral association frequencies observed
between lymphomas (high) and carcinomas (highly variable), as elaborated above.

There are now sufficient numbers of reports of apparent "hit and run"
in the literature to suggest that this scenario might at least be considered
for EBV, although it would be difficult to prove. For example, the process
that leads to cellular immortalization of epithelial cells *in vitro* results in
a continuously proliferating cell line, although once established, it was
difficult to find even traces of viral DNA (or RNA) in the culture [41, 42].
Similar findings have been reported on cell lines established from Chinese NPCs [43]. With BL, in a cell line isolated from a sporadic case of
a clonal Caucasian tumor, both EBV positive and negative cells were
identified [44], as similarly reported for a BL-derived cell line of Japanese origin after passage in culture [45]. Although separation into EBV
positive and negative cell lines revealed different growth properties in the
latter case, with EBV proving a positive asset for proliferation, nonetheless, both lines were viable. With a cell line of African origin, the complete loss of EBV episomal DNA was observed during long-term culture
[46]. Again, in a study of so-called EBV-negative sporadic cases of BL,
a more careful examination of several tumors showed the presence of
EBV components, although not the entire viral genome [47]. These findings may reflect tissue culture artifacts, with serum factors subsequently
replacing viral functions needed originally in the cells. Alternatively,
they may be mimicking events that occur in tumor progression, where
genetic instability of the host chromosome may result in alteration of
expression of cellular genes and concomitant loss of the viral chromosome, "with or without prior integration into the host chromosome" with
little change in the cellular phenotype. In the epithelial cell studies cited
[41, 42], gene amplification of a part of the input viral DNA was found
to precede viral genetic loss; in the study on sporadic BLs, integration
appears to have occurred, without as yet complete viral DNA loss,
although sufficient changes had taken place to allow these tumors to be
originally designed as EBV-negative [47]. The point of emphasizing
these data is that although they represent as yet only a few separate studies, they might provide explanations for apparently conflicting results
reported on the frequency of EBV association among specific tumors. If

valid with regard to what might, or does, occur *in vivo*, EBV may be of greater significance in tumorigenicity than yet appreciated.

Conclusions

As emphasized by the literature cited here, and more extensively elsewhere [1], the strong case for an association between EBV and a variety of malignancies has been made. Whether continued assessment of tumors, such as that seen over the last decade, will identify more cancers with this viral association, or whether we have reached the limit of tumor association, remains to be seen. The fact that EBV can stimulate the growth of cells, *in vivo* and *in vitro*, seems indisputable, as does the fact that suppression of the immune system is a risk factor for tumorigenesis in EBV-positive individuals. It also seems clear that certain populations are more susceptible to particular tumors than other populations, but whether this is a reflection of exposure to different environmental factors, to genetic susceptibility, or to the age of the individual at the time of initial infection and the viral loads encountered, are problems that must continue to be addressed. For now, they remain largely unsolved. There is no compelling evidence that EBV on its own is fully oncogenic, rather the reverse. One might argue that EBV encodes sufficient "oncogenes" - both nuclear and membrane associated - to impose a full tumorigenic phenotype onto a cell, but it seems clear that these are not all usually expressed in the tumor setting. Whether they were initially expressed during an initiation period, then repressed, for example by epigenetic events (promoter methylation and subsequent down-regulation, for example) is an interesting possibility. This would explain the apparent host cell control over viral gene expression that appears to occur with this virus. Then there are clear cases, such as with breast cancer, when equally compelling data exist for and against a viral association with disease. This may reflect the populations of cells and individuals being examined in specific cases, or be related to the methodologies used in assessing association. This is an important problem that also needs resolution and explanation.

The last ten years has seen an explosion in the literature of reports on EBV association with malignancy, but it now appears to be time to substitute in depth evaluations for what often seem to be mere data collecting exercises. The future would seem to lie either in developing a good vaccine against this virus which, like the hepatitis B vaccine, could be given early in the life of an individual, or to an EBV negative individual exposed to the virus during a susceptible period (for example, organ transplant or gene or immunotherapy). Turning off EBV genes may be useful for therapy. It may also prove that for immunocompetent individuals, turning on viral genes could also be advantageous. The next years may show us how useful adoptive immunotherapy with EBV-specific cytotoxic T lymphocytes [48], or other protocols that stimulate the immune system, will prove, but it is clear that for many continents where some of the major tumors seen are EBV-related, this will prove too laborious and costly a procedure to be practical. Cheaper therapies, antiviral or vaccine, are needed. If EBV can initiate carcinogenic events that progress toward tumorigenesis without a continuous need for the virus (or viral gene expression), then prevention of infection would be the preferred treatment route. After 40 or more years of struggling with this virus, it would seem that the scientific and medical communities are waking up to a need for controlling EBV as a partial containment against development of a variety of malignancies.

References

1. IARF Monographs on the evaluation of carcinogenic risks to humans (1997) Epstein-Barr virus and Kaposi's Sarcoma herpesvirus/Human Herpesvirus 8. Vol. 70, IARC Press, Lyon, pp 347-373
2. Epstein MA, Barr YM, Achong BG (1965) The behaviour and morphology of a second tissue culture strain (EB2) of lymphoblasts from Burkitt's lymphoma. Br J Cancer 12:108-114
3. Henle W, Henle G (1969) The relationship between the Epstein-Barr virus and infectious mononucleosis, Burkitt's lymphoma and cancer of the postnasal space. Proc Natl Acad Sci USA 59:94-101
4. Griffin BE (1998) Relation of Burkitt's tumor-associated herpes-type to infectious mononucleosis. Rev Med Virol 8:61-66
5. Wedderburn N, Edwards JMB, Desgranges C et al (1984) Infectious mononucleosis-like response in common marmosets infected with Epstein-Barr virus. J Infect Dis 150:878-882
6. Whitley RJ (1996) Herpes simplex viruses. In: Fields BN, Knipe DM, Howley PM (eds) "Virology". 3rd ed, Raven Press, New York, pp 2297-2342
7. Yates JL, Warren N, Sugden B (1985) Stable replication of plasmids derived from EBV in various mammalian cells. Nature 313:812-815
8. Baer R, Bankier AT, Biggin MD et al (1984) DNA sequence and expression of the B95-8 Epstein-Barr virus genome. Nature 310:207-211
9. Griffin BE, Xue S (1998) Epstein-Barr virus infections and their association with human malignancies: some key questions. Ann Med 30:249-259
10. Saemundsen AK, Albeck H, Hansen JPH et al (1982) Epstein-Barr virus in nasopharyngeal and salivary gland carcinomas of Greenland Eskimoes. Br J Cancer 46:721-728

11. Hochberg FH, Miller G, Schooley RT, Hirsch MS, Feorino P, Henle W (1983) Central-nervous-system lymphoma related to Epstein-Barr virus. New Engl J Med 309:745-748
12. Cox C, Chang S, Karran L, GriffinB, Wedderburn N (1996) Persistent Epstein-Barr virus infection in the common marmoset (Callithrix jacchus). J Gen Virol 77:1173-1180
13. Serraino D, Franceschi S, Talamini R et al (1991) Socioeconomic indicators, infectious diseases and Hodgkin's disease. Int J Cancer 47:352-357
14. Weiss LM, Strickler JG, Warnker RA, Purtilo DT, Sklar J (1987) Epstein-Barr viral DNA in tissues of Hodgkin's disease. Am J Pathol 129: 86-91
15. Weinreb M, Day PJ, Niggli F et al (1996) The consistent association between Epstein-Barr virus and Hodgkin's disease in children in Kenya. Blood 87:3828-3836
16. Mueller NE (1996) Hodgkin's disease. In: Schottenfeld D, Fraumeni JF (eds) Cancer Epidemiology and Prevention. 2nd ed, Oxford Univ Press, N Y, pp 893-919
17. Glaser SL, Lin RJ, Stewart SL et al (1997) Epstein-Barr virus-associated Hodgkin's disease: epidemiologic characteristics in international data. Int J Cancer 70:375-382
18. Pathmanathan R, Prasad U, Chandrika G, Sadler R, Flynn K, Raab-Traub N (1995) Undifferentiated, nonkeratinizing, and squamous cell carcinoma of the nasopharynx. Variants of Epstein-Barr virus-infected neoplasia. Am J Pathol 146:1355-1367
19. Zhang JX, Chen HL, Zong S et al (1998) Epstein-Barr virus expression within keratinizing nasopharyngeal carcinoma. J Med Virol 55:227-233
20. Iezzoni JC, Gaffey MJ, Weiss LM (1994) The role of Epstein-Barr virus in lymphoepithelioma-like carcinomas. Anatomic Pathol 103:308-315
21. Shibata D, Weiss LM (1993) Epstein-Barr virus-associated gastric adenocarcinoma. Am J Pathol 140:769-774
22. Shin WS, Kang MW, Kang JH et al (1996) Epstein-Barr virus-associated gastric adenocarcinomas among Koreans. Am J Clin Pathol 105:174-181
23. Lespagnard L, Cochaux P, Larsimont D, Degeyter M, Velu T, Heimann R(1995) Absence of Epstein-Barr virus in medullary carcinoma of the breast as demonstrated by immunophenotyping, in situ hybridization and polymerase chain reaction. Am J Clin Pathol 103:449-452
24. Chu JS, Chen CC, Chang KJ (1998) In situ detection of Epstein-Barr virus in breast cancer. Cancer Lett 124:53-57
25. Glaser SL, Ambinder RF, DiGuiseppe JA, Horn-Ross LPL, Hsu JL (1998) Absence of Epstein-Barr virus EBER-1 transcripts in an epidemiologically diverse group of breast cancers. Int J Cancer 75:555-558
26. Labrecque LG, Barnes DM, Fentiman IS, Griffin BE (1995) Epstein-Barr virus in epithelial cell tumors: a breast cancer study. Cancer Res 55:39-45
27. Fina F, Buisson M, Ouafik L, Morand P, Martin PM, Seigneurin JM (1996) Epstein-Barr virus and breast cancer: a PCR study of 574 cases from different geographical areas. In: 3rd Hong Kong International Cancer Congress and 7th International EBV Symposium, Hong Kong, p 157; in press
28. Hitt MM, Allday MJ, Hara T et al (1989) EBV gene expression in an NPC-related tumour. EMBO J 8: 2639-2651
29. Chen HL, Lung MML, Sham JST, Choy DTK, Griffin BE, Ng MH (1992) Transcription of BamHI-A region of the EBV genome in NPC tissues and B cells. Virol 191:193-201.
30. Smith PR, Gao Y, Karran L, Jones MD, Snudden D, Griffin BE (1993) Complex nature of the major viral polyadenylated transcripts in Epstein-Barr virus-associated tumors. J Virol 67:3217-3225

31. Fries KL, Sculley TB, Webster-Cyriaque J, Rajadurai P, Sadler RH, Raab-Traub N (1997) Identification of a novel protein encoded by the BamHI-A region of the Epstein-Barr virus. J Virol 71:2765-2771

32. Lee ES, Locker J, Nalesnik M et al (1995) The association of Epstein-Barr virus with smooth-muscle tumors occurring after organ transplantation. New Eng J Med 332:19-25

33. Sugiura M, Imai S, Tokunaga M et al (1996) Transcriptional analysis of Epstein-Barr virus gene expression in EBV-positive gastric carcinoma: unique viral latency in the tumour cells. Br J Cancer 74:625-631

34. Teng ZP, Ooka T, Huang DP, Zeng Y. Detection of Epstein-Barr virus DNA in well and poorly differentiated nasopharyngeal carcinoma cell lines. Virus Genes 13:53-60

35. Wei MX, deTurenne-Tessier M, Decaussin G, Benet G, Ooka T (1997) Establishment of a monkey kidney epithelial cell line with the BARF1 open reading frame from Epstein-Barr virus. Oncogene 14:3073-3081

36. Cochet C, Martel-Renoir D, Grunewald V et al (1993) Expression of the Epstein-Barr virus immediate early gene, BZLF1, in nasopharyngeal carcinoma tumor cells. Virol 197:358-365

37. Wen S, Mizugaki Y, Shinozaki F, Takada K (1997) Epstein-Barr virus (EBV) infection in salivary gland tumors: lytic EBV infection in nonmalignant epithelial cells surrounded by EBV-positive T-lymphocytes. Virol 227:484-487

38. Gutierrez MI, Bhatia K, Magrath I (1993) Replicative viral DNA in Epstein-Barr virus associated Burkitt's lymphoma biopsies. Leukemia Res 17:285-289

39. Zhang Q, Gutsch D, Kenney S (1994) Functional and physical interaction between p53 and BZLF1: implications for Epstein-Barr virus latency. Mol Cell Biol 14:1929-1938

40. Farrell PJ, Hollyoake M, Niedobitek G, Agathanggelou A, Morgan A, Wedderburn N (1997) Direct demonstration of persistent Epstein-Barr virus gene expression in peripheral blood of infected common marmosets and analysis of virus-infected tissues in vivo. J Gen Virol 78:1417-1424

41. Griffin BE, Karran L (1984) Immortalization of monkey epithelial cells by specific fragments of Epstein-Barr virus DNA. Nature 309:78-82 (1984)

42. Karran L, Teo CG, King D et al (1990) Establishment of immortalized primate epithelial cells with sub-genomic EBV DNA. Int J Cancer 45:763-772

43. Lin CT, Chan WY, Chen W et al (1993) Characterization of seven newly established nasopharyngeal carcinoma cell lines. Lab Invest 68:716-727

44. Trivedi P, Zhang Q-J, Chen F et al (1995) Parallel existence of Epstein-Barr virus (EBV) positive and negative cells in a sporadic case of Burkitt lymphoma. Oncogene 11:505-510.

45. Takada K, Ji Z, Fujiwara S, Shimizu N, Tanabe-Tochikura A (1992) Partial elimination of Epstein-Bar virus plasmids from Burkitt's lymphoma cells by transfecting the BZLF1 gene. J Virol 66:5590-5593

46. Srinivas SK, Sample JT, Sixbey JW (1998) Spontaneous loss of viral episomes accompanying Epstein-Barr virus reactivation in a Burkitt's lymphoma cell line. J Inf Dis 177:1705-1709

47. Razzouk BI, Srinivas SK, Sample CE, Singh V, Sixbey JW (1996) Epstein-Barr virus DNA recombination and loss in sporadic Burkitt's lymphoma. J Inf Dis 173:529-535

48. Rooney CM, Smith CA, Heslop HE (1997) Control of virus-induced lymphoproliferation: Epstein-Barr virus-induced lymphoproliferation and host immunity. Mol Med Today 24-30

49. Kempkes B, Pich D, Zeidler R, Sugden B, Hammerschmidt W (1995) Immortalization of human B lymphocytes by a plasmid containing 71 kilobase pairs of Epstein-Barr virus DNA. J Virol 69:231-238
50. Robertson E, Kieff E (1995) Reducing the complexity of the transforming Epstein-Barr virus genome to 64 kilobase pairs. J Virol 69:983-993

Helicobacter pylori and Malignant Diseases

J.- Q. Huang, R. H. Hunt

Introduction

It has been 16 years since *Helicobacter pylori* was first successfully isolated from the stomachs of patients with gastritis [1]. Our understanding of the importance of the infection in the pathogenesis of many upper gastrointestinal diseases evolves rapidly. It is now well accepted that *H. pylori* infection is the cause of type B chronic active gastritis and the majority of peptic ulcer disease [2]. The infection is also correlated closely with the development of gastric adenocarcinoma [3, 4] and gastric B cell mucosa-associated lymphoid tissue lymphoma (maltoma) [5]. Eradication of *H. pylori* infection prevents recurrence of the intestinal type gastric adenocarcinoma in patients following endoscopic resection of early gastric cancer [6]. Furthermore, cure of the infection results in a complete histological regression of maltoma in 80% of the patients and prevents recurrence in virtually all cases [5]. The aims of this chapter are to review the current literature on *H. pylori* infection and its relationship with gastrointestinal malignancies, and to discuss several factors that influence the results of current epidemiology studies of the relationship between the infection and gastric cancer, gastric maltoma, and other gastrointestinal malignant diseases.

H. pylori Infection and Gastric Cancer

In 1994, the International Agency for Research on Cancer (IARC) of the World Health Organization concluded that *H. pylori* infection was a group I human carcinogen although experimental evidence from animal studies was lacking [3]. This conclusion was based on the results from 4 cohort and 9 retrospective case-control studies conducted in several countries with markedly different incidence of gastric cancer. Although the evidence supports a close association between the infection and gastric cancer, inconsistent or even conflicting results seen in the literature have made many clinicians and researchers skeptical of the relation of

H. pylori infection to gastric cancer. In the last three years, many epidemiology studies have been published to address the role of *H. pylori* infection as a risk factor for the development of gastric cancer. However, the results vary dramatically [4, 7]. More recently, a comprehensive meta-analysis has identified that the variations seen with different studies were due to several confounding factors including patient age, characteristics of gastric cancer and inappropriate selection of control groups [4]. By combining raw data from 19 studies statistically, we have estimated that the overall relative risk for gastric cancer is 2.29 (95% confidence interval 2.04-2.58, with Mantel-Haenszel method) for patients with *H. pylori* infection [4]. The relative risk is higher in patients with early gastric cancer than in those with advanced disease (Table 1). The infection is highly correlated with non-cardiac gastric cancer but not with cancer at the cardia (Table 1). Although study design was not considered as a source of the heterogeneity in the meta-analysis, the result of a combined analysis of three rigorously designed cohort studies and some unpublished data has suggested that there was a significant trend towards an increasing risk for gastric cancer with advancing duration of the infection [8].

Table 1. Summary of the key results of meta-analysis of *H. pylori* seropositivity in patients with gastric cancer

Subgroups	N	DerSimonian and Laird		Mantel-Haenszel		Z^2* (d.f.=1)	p value*
		OR	95% CIs	OR	95%CIs		
All studies	19	1.92	1.32-2.78	2.29	2.04 - 2.58		
Cohort	5	2.24	1.15-4.40	1.93	1.44 - 2.59	1.40	0.2
Case-control	14	1.81	1.16-2.84	2.37	2.08 - 2.69		
Intestinal GC	10	2.49	1.41-4.43	2.23	1.74 - 2.87	1.29	0.3
Diffuse GC	10	2.58	1.47-4.53	2.85	2.14 - 3.79		
Early GC	3	6.35	1.88-21.5	6.40	3.76 - 10.9	6.01	0.01
Advanced GC	3	2.13	0.42-10.7	2.20	1.51 - 3.21		
Cardiac GC	7	1.23	0.56-2.71	1.41	1.00 - 1.98	8.69	0.003
Cardiac GC[a]	6	0.92	0.61-1.38	0.93	0.62 - 1.38	20.4	< 0.001
Non-cardiac GC	10	3.08	1.78-5.31	2.77	2.20 - 3.50		
Population-based	13	2.11	1.30-3.43	2.89	2.51 - 3.43	29.9	< 0.001
Hospital-based	6	1.49	1.06-2.10	1.37	1.11 - 1.70		

GC, gastric cancer; N, number of studies; OR, odds ratio; 95% CIs, 95% confidence intervals; [a], one study excluded with unclear definition of the site of cancer; *comparison between two subgroups. Data were extracted from [4] with permission

Cohort Studies

Methodologically results from cohort studies provide the strongest evidence for a causal relationship between *H. pylori* infection and gastric cancer because it shows that the infection preceded by many years the development of gastric cancer. There were a total of eight prospective case-control studies published in full in the English literature by April 1998 with odds ratio ranging from 0.93 to 6.0 ([9-16], Fig. 1). Six of them showed consistently that the infection was significantly correlated with gastric cancer [8-10, 9-11, 13-15, 14-16]. Five of the 6 studies had a follow-up period of longer than 5 years from the time of blood sampling, suggesting the importance of the duration of infection for the development of gastric cancer. Indeed, the two negative studies had a follow-up period of only 2.4 and 3.1 years [12, 13], which is too short for the development of gastric cancer because gastric carcinogenesis is a long and complex process requiring 20-40 years for completion from atrophy, intestinal metaplasia, dysplasia, to cancer [17].

Three early studies conducted in the UK [9] and USA [10, 11] showed consistently that *H. pylori* infection increased the risk for gastric cancer

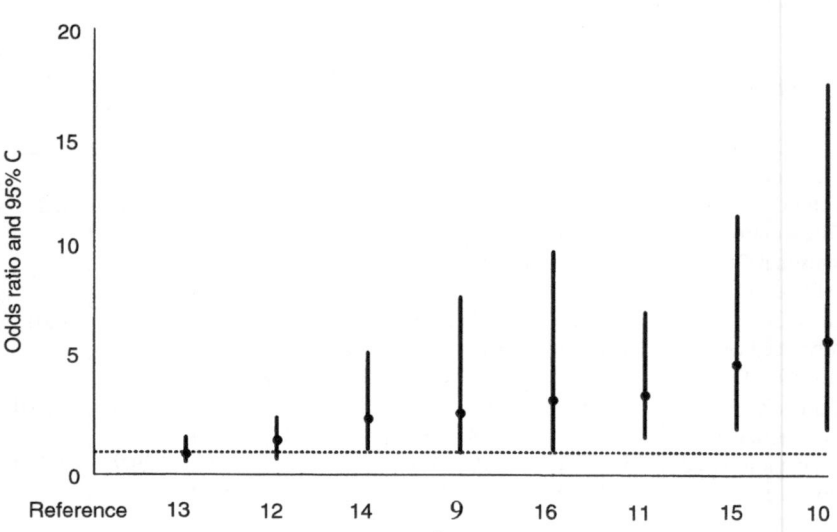

Fig. 1. Graphic display of individual odds ratio and 95% confidence interval of 8 cohort studies. The dotted line indicates OR = 1. OR = odds ratio, 95% CI = 95% confidence interval

with odds ratio ranging from 2.77 to 6.0. Since these studies have been discussed extensively elsewhere [3,18], only studies published in the last three years are discussed in this chapter.

In a study reported by Aromaa et al. from Finland, eighty-four gastric cancer patients were identified from 39,268 persons participating in a health check-up program during a mean follow-up of 9.5 years [14]. These patients were matched with 146 controls by age, sex and residence. *H. pylori* anti-IgA antibodies was positive in 89.3% of the cases and 76% of the controls, giving an odds ratio of 2.52 (95% confidence interval 1.14-5.57), suggesting a strong correlation between the infection and development of gastric cancer in this population [14]. There was also a significant difference in the concentration of pepsinogen I between gastric cancer patients and controls, indicating the existence of a severe gastric atrophy in the patients. This may explain the relatively low titers of IgG antibodies seen in gastric cancer patients due to loss of colonization by the bacteria over time [14]. Furthermore, the unusually high prevalence of *H. pylori* infection (82.9%) in the control group may have further underestimated the real risk [14].

Another study from Sweden included a cohort of 32,906 persons [15]. During an average of 5.7 years of follow-up, 56 incident cases were found. They were matched by age, date of birth and time of blood donation with 224 controls from the same cohort. *H. pylori* infection was diagnosed in 82.1% of the patients and 49.1% of the controls, yielding an odds ratio of 5.0 (95% confidence interval 2.2-11.5) [15]. A strong correlation was found between *H. pylori* infection and patients with non-cardiac gastric cancer but not with cancer at the cardia [15]. A significant correlation was also found in patients with and without previous history of gastric surgery [15].

A Japanese study reported by Watanabe et al. also found a significant correlation between *H. pylori* infection and gastric cancer in a mean of 3.2 years prospective case-control study with an odds ratio of 3.38 (95% confidence interval 1.15-9.9) [16]. However, after adjustment for atrophic gastritis, the infection was no longer correlated with gastric cancer (OR 1.84, 95% CI 0.59-5.72). Whereas, atrophic gastritis was strongly associated with gastric cancer (OR 3.38, 95% CI 1.54-7.42) [16]. The authors concluded that *H. pylori* infection was not directly associated with gastric carcinogenesis. There were several methodological flaws in this study. First, 78% of the patients were older than 60 years and 75.6% of the cases had atrophic gastritis. This might have caused a high false seronegativity of *H. pylori* infection in the patients. Second, the sample size was relatively small which might lack a statistical power to detect a possible difference between the cases and controls although *H. pylori* infection rate was 15.5% higher in the cases than in controls. Third, the way the data were analyzed is debatable since *H. pylori* infection is a well recognized cause for chronic atrophic gastritis, adjustment for atrophic gastritis would underestimate the real risk of *H. pylori* infection for gastric cancer. Fouth, the 3.2 years of follow-up may not be long enough to see the impact of *H. pylori* infection on gastric carcinogenesis.

Two other negative studies performed in China suffered from some methodological flaws including small sample size [12], diagnosis of gastric cancer based only on medical record [12,13], unclear characteristics of gastric cancer [12,13], no validation of the ELISA kit used to detect *H. pylori* antibody [13], and a short term of follow-up [12,13]. Thus, one must be cautious in interpreting the results of these studies, because the site and stage of gastric cancer have an important impact on the relative risk of *H. pylori* infection for gastric cancer measured as odds ratio as shown in our meta-analysis [4].

Retrospective Case-Control Studies

Unlike prospective cohort studies, retrospective case-control studies have many inherent methodological limitations. Since the diagnosis of *H. pylori* infection and gastric cancer was made at the same time, it is impossible to determine which one preceded the other. The presence of gastric atrophy and also intestinal metaplasia may reduce the density of the bacteria colonization causing false seronegativity. Furthermore, selection bias and other confounding factors are more difficult to control than in a prospective case-control study. Nevertheless, it is legitimate to assume that *H. pylori* infection anteceded the development of gastric cancer, because the infection was acquired in early childhood in almost all cases and persists for life if untreated. Therefore, a well-conducted positive case-control study performed in populations with a low risk for gastric cancer strongly suggests causation since the background prevalence of *H. pylori* infection is generally lower in these populations than in those with a high risk for gastric cancer.

In the last three years, there were three case-control studies published in full in the English language examining the relationship between *H. pylori* infection and gastric adenocarcinoma. All were from populations with high risk for gastric cancer [19-21]. The study reported by Kato et al. [18] showed that *H. pylori* infection was not associated with the development of gastric cancer with an odds ratio of 1.25 (95% CI 0.84-1.85). However, this study had a serious methodological problem because the authors included patients with peptic ulcer and gastritis in the control group, which are well known to be closely associated with the infection. Therefore, the negative association might result from the inappropriate control group used in this study. The other two studies from Mexico and Spain, in which a well-matched population-based control group was used, all showed a positive correlation between the infection and gastric cancer with odds ratio of 3 and 3.01, respectively [20,21].

It is clear that hospital-based control groups have a significantly higher background prevalence of *H. pylori* infection than population-based controls [4]. Case-control studies with hospital-based control group tend to give a small odds ratio and a negative correlation between *H. pylori* infection and gastric cancer [4,7], indicating the importance of the selection of controls.

H. pylori Infection and Gastric Maltoma

Gastric maltoma has been considered as a consequence of *H. pylori* infection. More than 90% of cases result from the infection with *H. pylori* in the stomach of patients [21] although very few systematic epidemiology studies have been conducted to determine the incidence and prevalence of maltoma in the general populations [22]. The results from a well conducted prospective case-control study reported by Parsonnet et al. [23] showed a strong correlation between *H. pylori* infection and non-Hodgkin's lymphoma with an odds ratio of 6.3 (95% CI 2.0-19.9). Our meta-analysis which combined two case-control studies with 49 cases and 195 controls showed that *H. pylori* seropositivity was 87.8% in the cases and 55.9% in the controls, giving a pooled odds ratio of 5.65 (95% CI 2.18-15.54) [5]. Therefore, the current information published in the literature supports a strong correlation between the infection and maltoma. The results from animal studies of a transplanted gastric lymphoma model also support this conclusion where the development of gastric lymphoma was seen only in animals infected with *H. pylori* but not in those without the infection [23].

The most supportive evidence for *H. pylori* infection as a possible risk factor for maltoma comes from clinical trials in which eradication of the infection regresses completely the lymphoma in 80% of the patient [5]. This will be discussed in detail later in this chapter.

The Importance of Cytotoxic Strains of *H. pylori*

Recent studies have suggested that *H. pylori* strains secreting the cagA and/or vacA proteins may be more important in the pathogenesis of gastric cancer. Four studies have examined the relationship between toxic strains of *H. pylori* and gastric cancer published in full [24-27]. Three showed an increased risk for gastric cancer in patients infected with cagA positive strains compared with those infected with cagA negative strains [24-26]. Blaser et al. [24] reported an OR of 1.9 (95% CI 0.9-4.0) in a nested case-control study conducted in a Japanese population in Hawaii including 103 *H. pylori*-infected gastric cancer cases and 103 matched *H. pylori*-infected controls. However, when subgroup analysis by histological type of cancer was performed, a significantly increased risk was found only in patients with the intestinal type gastric cancer (OR 2.3, 95% CI 1.0-5.2), but not in those with the diffuse type (OR 1.0, 95% CI 0.1-7.1). Another nested case-control study reported by Parsonnet et al. [25] consisted of 103 cases and 139 controls selected among 128,992 subjects in California. Those infected with cagA positive *H. pylori* strains were 5.8-fold more likely than uninfected subjects to develop gastric cancer (95% CI 2.6-13.0). This was true for both the intestinal and diffuse types of gastric cancer. When compared with *H. pylori*-infected controls, infection with cagA positive strains increased the risk by 3.3-fold for gastric cancer in general, 3.8-fold for the intestinal type and 2.1-fold for the diffuse type. However, statistical analysis did not show any significant difference for the diffuse type due to the small number of subjects [25].

The role of cytotoxic strains of *H. pylori* in the development of gastric cancer was confirmed further by a German study which included 90 cases and 90 matched controls [26]. Although the overall seroprevalence of *H. pylori* IgG antibodies was not significantly different between cases and controls, a two-fold increased risk was found in patients with antibodies against *H. pylori* cagA or vacA proteins (OR 2.00, 95% CI 1.18-3.39), suggesting the importance of testing cytotoxic strains of *H. pylori* in gastric cancer epidemiology studies. Similar results were also seen in another study from Estonia in which there was a significant difference in the seropositivity of anti-*H. pylori* cagA- antibodies between gastric cancer patients and controls (p = 0.004) although the overall seroprevalence of *H. pylori* IgG antibodies was similar between the cases and controls [27].

More recently, an inverse relation between cagA+ strains of *H. pylori* infection and cancer of the distal esophagus and gastric cardia was reported by Chow et al. [28]. In this study, cagA+ *H. pylori* infection was found in 31.6% of patients and 53.5% of controls, yielding an OR of 0.4 (95% CI 0.2-0.8). Infection with cagA+ strains of *H. pylori* also was not shown to increase the risk for non-cardiac gastric cancer (OR 1.4, 95% CI 0.7-2.8). Since this study had a selection bias for not including 30% of eligible cases and also the sample size was small (n = 33 cases), underestimation of the risk was possible.

The relation of cytotoxic strains of *H. pylori* to maltoma is more poorly studied than to gastric cancer. However, the results of a recent study showed that, in 67 *H. pylori* positive patients with low and high grade maltoma, 64 (95.5%) patients were infected with cagA+ strains of *H. pylori*, whereas cagA+ seropositivity was detected in only 67% (33 of 49) of the *H. pylori*-positive control group with chronic active gastritis (p = 0.000037), suggesting a crucial role of *H. pylori*, especially strains expressing cagA genes in the pathogenesis of gastric malt-type lymphoma [29], although some studies did not support this conclusion [30,31].

Eradication of *H. pylori* Infection and Gastric Malignancies

It is legitimate to assume that eradication of *H. pylori* infection would prevent or ultimately cure most cases of gastric cancer and maltoma since the infection plays a key role for the development of these two malignancies. The result of the first clinical trial examining the effect of eradication of *H. pylori* infection on the prevention of subsequent development of gastric cancer in patients following endoscopic resection of early gastric cancer was very promising [6]. In a study of 132 patients with early gastric cancer after endoscopic resection, sixty-five patients (group A) received *H. pylori* eradication therapy and 67 patients (group B) did not. After three years of endoscopic follow-up, none of the patients in group A developed a new cancer, whereas 6 (9%) of the 67 patients in group B had a new early intestinal-type gastric cancer diagnosed by endoscopy [6], suggesting the importance of *H. pylori* eradication therapy for gastric cancer. Furthermore, a significant improvement in gastritis and intestinal metaplasia was seen in patients receiving eradication therapy. This might have contributed to the prevention of subsequent development of any new cancer [6]. Although this study was not a randomized and controlled clinical trial, it provides us with important information on the role of *H. pylori* infection in the development of gastric cancer and warrants strongly further randomized controlled adequately-powered clinical trials.

Currently, there are several on-going long-term prospective random-ized intervention studies to examine the effect of *H. pylori* eradication in populations with high risk for gastric cancer with different endpoints such as progression or regression of pre-cancerous lesions or development of gastric cancer [32]. These studies can provide us with very useful infor-mation to clarify the role of *H. pylori* in the development of gastric cancer when they are finished. However, as with other cancer epidemiology studies, a long-term follow-up is crucial to determine the role of *H. pylori* infection in the process of gastric carcinogenesis, since there was no sig-nificant change in the gastric pre-cancerous lesions one year after eradi-cation of *H. pylori* infection in a randomized population-based endoscopic study in China [33].

Several studies have shown excellent results in the treatment of patients with maltoma following eradication of *H. pylori* infection. In a pooled analysis, Stolte et al. [34] reported a complete histological regres-sion of maltoma in 74.3% of 171 patients. In a meta-analysis of 12 treat-ment arms with 300 patients, we have found that histological regression of maltoma was successfully achieved in 84% of the patients, with com-plete regression in 90% and partial regression in 10% of the patients [5]. Recurrence of maltoma is generally very low if eradication of *H. pylori* infection is truly obtained. In 146 patients after a follow-up of 9 to 24 months, only 2 (1.4%) patients had recurrent lymphoma. *H. pylori* rein-fection was documented in one patients [5].

It is important to point out that histological regression of maltoma does not necessarily mean a cure of the disease since most patients who had complete remission after cure of *H. pylori* infection displayed evidence of monoclonal B cells during a median follow-up of 24 months [35]. B cell clone may be related with the development of gastric maltoma in patients with *H. pylori*-associated chronic gastritis [36]. Therefore, his-tological regression of maltoma is not equal to "molecular remission". Long-term follow-up of patients with histological remission after cure of the infection is needed.

H. pylori Infection and Other Malignant Diseases

H. pylori Infection and Esophageal Cancer

The prevalence of *H. pylori* infection in patients with reflux esophagitis or Barrett's esophagus is about 30% [37]. Most reports show that the infection correlates inversely with reflux esophagitis or Barrett's esophagus [37, 38]. There were few published well-conducted epidemiology studies in the literature to address the relationship between *H. pylori* infection and esophageal cancer. Chow reported a case-control study of 129 patients with esophageal and cardia cancer, which were compared with age, sex and race-matched population-based controls [28]. An inverse relationship was seen between infection with *H. pylori* or strains expressing cagA proteins and patients with esophageal and cardia cancer (OR 0.7 and 0.4, respectively) [28]. This is also true with several case-series studies in which *H. pylori* infection was found to be negatively correlated with increasing esophageal mucosa dysplasia [38], or to be even absent in the mucosa of Barrett's esophagus in patients with esophageal adenocarcinoma [39]. Therefore, the current information do not support a causal association between *H. pylori* infection and esophageal cancer. However, the infection may be associated with Barrett's MALT as shown in a study where the prevalence of *H. pylori* infection was significantly higher in patients with Barrett's MALT than in those with Barrett's but without MALT (57.1% vs. 23.3%, p < 0.007) [40].

H. pylori Infection and Colon Cancer

The prevalence of *H. pylori* infection in patients with colon cancer has been poorly studied. Three case-control studies all did not find any significant difference in the prevalence of *H. pylori* infection between patients with colon or colorectal cancer and controls [41-43]. The study by Moss et al. [41] found that *H. pylori* seropositivity was 56% (23/41 patients) in patients with colorectal carcinoma and 63% (26/41) in the controls, which were matched by age, sex, race and social class to the cases. Another case-control study showed no significant difference in *H. pylori* seropositivity between patients with colon cancer and the controls (55.3% vs. 49%, p = 0.32) although the overall prevalence of *H. pylori* infection including patients with colorectal polyps was significantly higher than that of controls (64% vs. 49%, p < 0.02) [43]. Thus, currently there is no evidence to suggest that *H. pylori* infection plays a role in the development of colon cancer.

H. pylori Infection and Pancreatic or Hepatic Cancer

One recent study claims that *H. pylori* infection is significantly associated with pancreatic cancer [44]. Ninety-two patients with histologically confirmed diagnosis of pancreatic adenocarcinoma were compared to 62 mixed controls (35 patients with colorectal cancer and 27 healthy volunteers). *H. pylori* seropositivity was present in 65% of the patients and 45% of the mixed controls, giving an OR of 2.1 (95% CI 1.1-4.1). However, microscopic examination of pancreactic specimens did not reveal any evidence of the bacteria [44]. There are several methodological problems in this study, which might have biased the results. First, the study was not well matched by frequency; second, a mixed control group was used, which lacks of representativity to the base population; third, it is not known if the patients with pancreatic cancer had any previous history of peptic ulcer or gastritis. It is possible that the high prevalence of *H. pylori* infection seen in the patient group might result from concurrent gastric diseases. Therefore, one needs to be cautious in interpreting the results generated from poorly-designed studies, especially *H. pylori* epidemiology cancer studies [4,7].

References

1. Warren JR, Marshall B (1983) Unidentified curved bacilli on gastric epithelium in active chronic gastritis. Lancet 1:1273-1275
2. Huang JQ, Hunt RH (1997) Eradication of Helicobacter pylori: problems and recommendations. J Gastroenterol Hepatol 12:590-598
3. International Agency for Research on Cancer (1994) Schistosomes, liver flukes and Helicobacter pylori IARC Monographs on the Evaluation of Carcinogenic Risks to Humans. Vol 61, IARC Lyon
4. Huang JQ, Sridhar S, Chen Y, Hunt RH (1998) Meta-analysis of the relationship between Helicobacter pylori seropositivity and gastric cancer. Gastroenterology 114(6):1169-1179
5. Huang JQ, Sheldon A, Hunt RH (1997) Is there a causal relationship between H. pylori infection and gastric maltoma ? A meta-analysis of evidence from epidemiological studies and clinical trials. Gut 41(Suppl 1):A49(04/179)
6. Uemura N, Mukai T, Okamoto S, Yamaguchi S, Mashiba H, Taniyama K, Sasaki N, Haruma K, Sumii K, Kajiyama G (1997) Effect of Helicobacter pylori eradication on subsequent development of cancer after endoscopic resection of early gastric cancer. Cancer Epidemiol Biomarkers Prev 6(8):639-642
7. Huang JQ, Hunt RH (1998) An overview of Helicobacter pylori epidemiology studies. In: Hunt RH, Tytgat GNJ (eds) Helicobacter pylori: Basic Mechanisms to Clinical Cure. Kluwer Academic Publishers, Lancaster, (in press)
8. Forman D, Webb PM (1994) H. pylori and gastric cancer: the significance of the problem. In: Hunt RH, Tytgat GNJ (eds) Helicobacter pylori: Basic mechanisms to clinical cure. Kluwer Academic Publishers, Lancaster, 461-468
9. Forman D, Newell DG, Fullerton F, Yarnell JWG, Stacey AR, Wald N, Sitas F (1991) Association between infection with Helicobacter pylori and risk of gastric cancer: Evidence from a prospective investigation. Br Med J 302:1302-1305
10. Nomura A, Stemmermann GN, Chyou PH, Kato I, Perez-Perez GI, Blaser MJ (1991) Helicobacter pylori infection and gastric carcinoma among Japanese Americans in Hawaii. N Engl J Med 325:1132-1136

11. Parsonnet J, Friedman GD, Vandersteen DP, Chang Y, Vogelman JH, Orentreich N, Sibley RK (1991) Helicobacter pylori infection and the risk of gastric carcinoma. N Engl J Med 325:1127-1131

12. Lin JT, Wang LY, Wang JT, Wang TH, Yang CS, Chen CJ (1995) A nested case-control study on the association between Helicobacter pylori infection and gastric cancer risk in a cohort of 9775 men in Taiwan. Anticancer Res 15:603-606

13. Webb PM, Yu MC, Forman D, Henderson BE, Newell DG, Yuan JM, Gao YT, Ross RK (1996) An apparent lack of association between Helicobacter pylori infection and risk of gastric cancer in China. Int J Cancer 67:603-607

14. Aromaa A, Kosunen TU, Knekt P, Maatela J, Teppo L, Heinonen OP, H‰rk‰nen M, Hakama MK (1996) Circulating anti-Helicobacter pylori immunoglobulin A antibodies and low serum pepsinogen I level are associated with increased risk of gastric cancer. Am J Epidemiol 144(2):142-149

15. Siman JH, Forsgren A, Berglund G, Florèn CH (1997) Association between Helicobacter pylori and gastric carcinoma in the city of Malmˆ, Sweden. A prospective study. Scand J Gastroenterol 32:1215-1221

16. Watanabe Y, Kurata JH, Mizuno S et al (1997) Helicobacter pylori infection and gastric cancer: A nested case-control study in a rural area of Japan. Dig Dis Sci 42(7):1383-1387

17. Asaka M, Takeda H, Sugiyama T, Kato M (1998) What role does Helicobacter pylori play in gastric cancer? Gastroenteorlogy 113(6):S56-S60

18. Kato S, Onda M, Matsukura N, Tokunaga A, Matsuda N, Yamashita K, Shields PG (1996) Genetic polymorphisms of the cancer related gene and Helicobacter pylori infection in Japanese gastric cancer patients. An age and gender matched casecontrol study. Cancer 77(Suppl 8):16541-661

19. Barreto Zuniga R, Maruyama M, Kato Y, Aizu K, Ohta H, Takekoshi T, Bernal SF (1997) Significance of Helicobacter pylori infection as a risk factor in gastric cancer: serological and histological studies. J Gastroenterol 32(3):289-294

20. Martinde Argila C, Boixeda D, Redondo C, Alvarez I, Gisbert JP, Garcia Plaza A, Canton R (1997) Relation between histologic subtypes and location of gastric cancer and Helicobacter pylori. Scand J Gastroenterol 32(4):303-307

21. Thiede C, Morgner A, Alpen B et al (1997) What role does Helicobacter pylori eradication play in gastric MALT and gastric MALT lymphoma? Gastroenterology 113:S61-S64

22. Parsonnet J, Hansen S, Rodriquez L et al (1994) Helicobacter pylori infection and gastric lymphoma. N Engl J Med 330:1267-1271

23. Enno A, O'Rourke J, Howlett CR, Lee A (1996) Mouse to mouse resuscitation of low-grade MALT lymphoma induced by prolonged Helicobacter infection. A preliminary study of transplanted tumors. Gastroenterology 110:A536

24. Blaser MJ, Perez-Perez GI, Kleanthous H, Cover TL, Peek RM, Chyou PH, Stemmermann GN, Nomura A (1995) Infection with Helicobacter pylori strains possessing cagA is associated with an increased risk of developing adenocarcinoma of the stomach. Cancer Res 55:2111-2115

25. Parsonnet J, Friedman GD, Orentreich N, Vogelman H (1997) Risk for gastric cancer in people with cagA positive or cagA negative Helicobacter pylori infection. Gut 40:297-301

26. Rudi J, Kolb C, Maiwald M, Zuna I, Herrbay AV, Galle PR, Stremmel W (1997) Serum antibodies against the Helicobacter pylori proteins cagA and vacA are associated with increased risk for gastric adenocarcinoma. Dig Dis Sci 42(8):1652-1659

27. Vorobjova T, Nilsson I, Kull K et al (1998) CagA protein seropositivity in a random sample of adult population and gastric cancer patients in Estonia. Eur J Gastroenterol Hepatol 10:41-46

28. Chow WH, Blaser MJ, Blot WJ, Gammon MD, Vaughan TL, Risch HA, Perez Perez GI, Schoenberg JB, Stanford JL, Rotterdam H, West AB, Fraumeni JF Jr (1998) An inverse relation between cagA+ strains of Helicobacter pylori infection and risk of esophageal and gastric cardia adenocarcinoma. Cancer Res 58(4):588-590

29. Eck M, Schmau(er B, Haas R, Greiner A, Czub S, M(ller-Hermelink HK (1997) Malt-type lymphoma of the stomach is associated with Helicobacter pylori strains expressing the CagA protein. Gastroenterology 112:1482-1486

30. De Jong D, van der Hulst RWM, Pals G et al (1996) Gastric non-Hodgkin lymphomas of mucosa-associated lymphoid tissue are not associated with more aggressive Helicobacter pylori strains as identified by cagA. Am J Clin Pathol 106:670-675

31. De Jong D, van Dijk WC, van der Hulst RWM (1997) CagA+ H. pylori strains and gastric lymphoma. Gastroenterology 113(6):2022-2023 (letter)

32. Forman D (1998) Lessons from on-going intervention studies. In: Hunt RH, Gytgat GNJ (eds) Helicobacter pylori: Basic Mechanisms to Clinical Cure. Kluwer Academic Publishers, Lancaster (in press).

33. Sung JY, Lin SR, Ching JYL, Zhou LY, To KF, Wang RT, Leung WK, Wang LX, Ng EKW, Lee YT, Lau JYW, Chao W (1998) Effects of curing Helicobacter pylori infection on pre-cancerous gastric lesions: one-year follow-up of a prospective randomized study in China. Gastroenterology 114(4, Part 2):A296(G1215)

34. Stolte M, Morgner A, Meining A, Thiede C, Neubauer A, Seifert E, Bayerd(rffer E. Clinical presentation, diagnosis and treatment of Helicobacter pylori-related gastric lymphoma. In: Hunt RH, Gytgat GNJ (eds) Helicobacter pylori: Basic Mechanisms to Clinical Cure. Kluwer Academic Publishers, Lancaster, 222-231

35. Neubauer A, Thiede C, Morgner A et al (1997) Cure of Helicobacter pylori infection and duration of remission of low-grade gastric mucosa-associated lymphoid tissue lymphoma. J Natl Cancer Inst 89:1350-1355

36. Zucca E, Bertoni F, Roggero E et al (1998) Molecular analysis of the progression from Helicobacter pylori-associated chronic gastritis to mucosa-associated lymphoid-tissue lymphoma of the stomach. N Engl J Med 338(12):804-810

37. Xia HH-X, Talley NJ Helicobacter pylori infection, reflux esophagitis, and atrophic gastritis: an unexplored triangle. Am J Gastroenterol 93(3):394-400

38. Wright TA, Myskow M, Kingsnorth AN (1997) Helicobacter pylori colonization of Barrettís esophagus and its progression to cancer. Dis Esophagus 10(3):196-200

39. Quddus MR, Henley JD, Sulaiman RA, Palumbo TC, Gnepp DR (1997) Helicobacter pylori infection and adenocarcinoma arising in Barrett's esophagus. Hum Pathol 28:1007-1009

40. Weston AP, Cherian R, Horvat RT, Lawrinenko V, Dixon A, McGregor D (1997) Mucosa-associated lymphoid tissue (MALT) in Barrett's esophagus: prospective evaluation and association with gastric MALT, MALT lymphoma, and Helicobacter pylori. Am J Gastroenterol 92(5):800-804

41. Moss SF, Neugut AI, Garbowski GC, Wang S, Treat MR, Forde KA (1995) Helicobacter pylori and colorectal neoplasia: evidence against an association. Gastroenterology 108(4):A511

42. Thorburn CM, Friedman GD, Orentreich N, Vogelman JH, Parsonnet J (1995) High gastrin levels increase risk for colorectal carcinoma. Gastroenterology 108(4):A

43. Meucci G, Tatarella M, Vecchi M, Ranzi ML, Biguzzi E, Beccari G, Clerici E, de Franchis R (1997) High prevalence of Helicobacter pylori infection in patients with colonic adenomas and carcinomas. J Clin Gastroenterol 25(4):605-607
44. Raderer M, Wrba F, Kornek G, Maca T, Koller DY, Weinlaender G, Hejna M, Scheithauer W (1998) Association between Helicobacter pylori infection and pancreatic cancer. Oncology 55(1):16-19

Part VII
Advances in solid tumors

High Risk Soft Tissue Sarcoma: an Overview

R. E. Pollock

Introduction

Soft tissue sarcoma is a cluster of extremely rare solid tumor malignancies. In the United States approximately 6,000 new diagnoses of this disease are rendered annually, and it constitutes less than 1% of adult solid tumors. In the pediatric age group, the overall incidence of soft tissue sarcoma is approximately 7%, where the predominate histology is rhabdomyosarcoma. The aggregate overall incidence is approximately equivalent to that of multiple myeloma or carcinoma of the salivary gland. About 10% of soft tissue sarcomas are in the head and neck area, 30% in the trunk and retroperitoneum, 15% in the upper extremity, and 45% in the lower extremity. Ten percent of the patients will present synchronous distant disease, and the pattern of relapse is primarily pulmonary. About 50-60% of patients relapse as an isolated pulmonary lesion, 30% relapse as an isolated local recurrence, and 10% relapse at other or multiple sites. In the extremity, about 75% of the failures are pulmonary, whereas in the trunk and retroperitoneum 50% of the failures are local. This points to the relative difficulty of obtaining biologically secure negative margin resections in the central body axis as compared to the extremity where amputation may be an ultimate salvage procedure. Approximately 80% of the local and distant recurrences in this disease occur within two years of initial diagnosis. In this chapter we will consider three different components of the high risk soft tissue sarcoma problem. These include:
1. defining high risk soft tissue sarcoma;
2. treating high risk soft tissue sarcoma;
3. outcomes for high risk soft tissue sarcoma patients.

Defining High Risk Soft Tissue Sarcoma

This past year the AJCC/UICC unified revision of soft tissue sarcoma staging was published [1]. This revision incorporates several noteworthy alterations compared to previous staging algorithms. Most important is that while the staging system is still a T (primary tumor), N (regional lymph nodes), M (distant metastasis), G (histopathologic grade), the concept of an A/B discriminator has been introduced. A status is accorded to superficial tumors, whereas B status signified a tumor deep to the investing muscle fascia. Accordingly, staging classification can be clustered such that stage I tumors are low grade lesions without nodal or distant metastases, superficial in location and of any size. Stage I lesions are generally treatable by wide local excision alone. The stage II soft tissue sarcomas are low grade, large and deep; high grade, small, superficial or deep; or high grade, large, superficial lesions. Stage II tumors are free of distant dissemination and are generally treated by combinations of surgery with radiation and the occasional use of chemotherapy. The stage III lesions are the high grade deep tumors greater than 5 cm without dissemination. The stage III lesions are usually treated by combinations of surgery, chemotherapy, and radiotherapy. This tumor stage will be the focus of this chapter. The stage IV lesions are tumors of any grade, size, or location in which dissemination to regional lymph nodes or distant sites has occurred. In these patients, treatment is primarily systemic therapy and surgery and radiation therapy are reserved for palliative purposes.

Several problems exist with the current staging system. The presence of nodal disease as a potential staging criteria is open to challenge in that only 3% of soft tissue sarcomas metastasize to lymph nodes. In this regard, the two most common histologic subtypes malignant histiocytoma (40%) and liposarcoma (25%) account for only 5% and 1% of the nodal metastases, respectively. Several relatively rare forms of adult soft tissue sarcoma (epithelioid, synovial, and rhabdomyosarcoma) account for the majority of the nodal metastases. However, their respective incidence is less than 1%, 8%, and 3%, respectively.

The staging system is further complicated by problems in assigning histopathologic grade. Discordancy studies have been conducted in which expert sarcoma pathologists have been asked to assign grade and histopathologic subtype to a standard sarcoma slide set. Inter-pathologist discordancy rates for grade and histology designations as high as 40% have been observed in these studies [2].

Prognostic factors are also useful in describing high risk soft tissue sarcoma. Tumors that are high grade, greater than 5 cm in size, deeply located, resected with positive margins, presenting as a recurrence, and/or located in the lower extremity tend to have poorer prognosis than lesions devoid of these adverse considerations [3]. The French Federation of Cancer Centers Sarcoma Group recently published the results of an exhaustive multivariant regression analysis that focused on the issue of prognostic factors. The prognosis and local disease-free survival was increased in patients in whom adequate surgery was performed, in tumors of low grade, or tumors in a superficial location. The use of adjuvant radiotherapy significantly improved strictly local recurrence rates. Distant metastasis was governed by some of the same factors including grade III, size ≥ 10 cm, and deep location. Grade I status was associated with a decreased incidence of distant metastasis as was the use of adjuvant chemotherapy [4].

Much of the difficulty inherent in assigning grade on the basis of light microscopic characteristics will be resolved by an enhanced understanding of the molecular determinants driving soft tissue sarcoma proliferation and metastasis. Towards that end, an elegant study conducted by Levine et al. [5] considered a large group of high grade extremity soft tissue sarcomas analyzed for the presence or absence of several molecular factors. Overall survival was significantly enhanced in those patients in whom the drug eflux pump protein Pgp was not expressed. Likewise, prognosis was improved in those patients whose tumors were diploid as compared to aneuploid, had low expression of MDR-1 (multidrug resistance gene), and low expression of Ki-67, a tumor cell proliferation marker. As information of this type is gathered for larger clusters of soft tissue sarcoma, it will almost certainly be possible to improve overall staging via more accurate grading systems that will include molecular determinants. An application of this process is depicted in Figure 1, which shows two patients whose tumors as well as peri-tumoral adjacent normal tissue have been aspirated using a fine needle. The fine needle aspirates have then been disaggregated, the DNA retrieved and PCR amplified, with subsequent probing for several molecular constructs. As can be seen, patient 69 has amplification of the p53 regulatory molecule MDM2 as compared to either autologous normal tissue or in comparison to patient 89 (Fig. 1).

Treating High Risk Sarcoma

For many decades it has been clear that maximally effective soft tissue sarcoma management requires a multimodality approach. A research report co-authored by Drs. Clark, Martin, and White, who were three of the former Chairs of the Department of Surgery at the University of Texas M. D. Anderson Cancer Center, appeared in 1959 [6]. This manuscript is

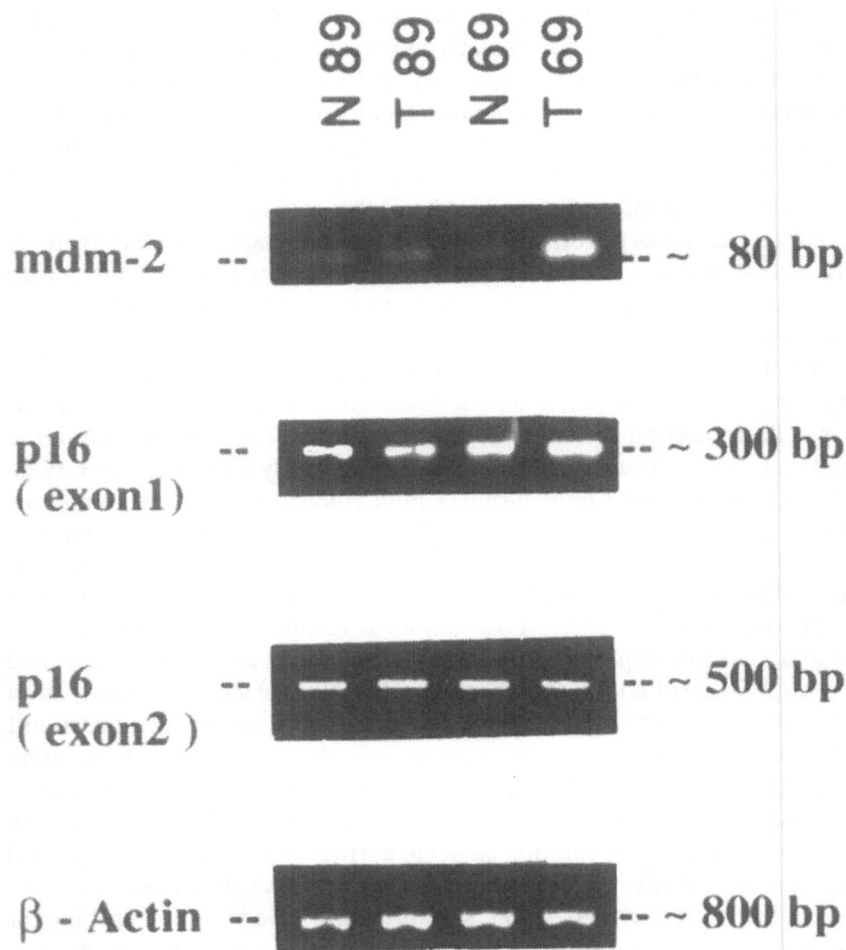

Fig. 1. Two tumors (T) and autologous normal tissues (N) were probed for the amplification of MDM2 oncogene or p16 (multiple tumor suppressor gene, which has two exons). DNA from all tissues was obtained by fine needle aspiration with subsequent PCR expansion prior to probing

noteworthy as the apparently first paper in the medical literature to demonstrate the efficacy of systemic chemotherapy in human soft tissue sarcoma treatment. It is pertinent to note that in this manuscript Dr. Clark wrote "since most soft tissue sarcomas are radioresistant, roentgen therapy as definitive treatment or in conjunction with surgical treatment is not used". Several years later, the use of external beam radiotherapy was introduced in soft tissue sarcoma at the University of Texas M. D. Anderson Cancer Center by Drs. Lindberg, Fletcher, and Martin [7].

There are several important radiotherapy controversies that have yet to be resolved in soft tissue sarcoma. These include appropriate fraction size, interval between fractions, the duration of each fraction, the timing of radiation vis-à-vis surgery (pre-, peri-, or postoperative), and the role of radiosensitizers (drugs, genes, etc.). Among the several standard radiotherapy approaches each have advantages and disadvantages. For example, preoperative treatment can be delivered via smaller radiotherapy fields, and results in possibly less mutilating surgery if tumor cytoreduction has occurred. There is no delay in the start of radiation therapy, and there is theoretically less likelihood of viable sarcoma cells implanting or embolizing at the time of surgical resection. Postoperative radiotherapy also has contrasting advantages and disadvantages. For example, there is no delay in surgical resection which poses a distinct psychological advantage in many patients, and there are no problems with radiotherapy-induced wound complications which can be quite problematic [9]. Moreover, the entire sarcoma specimen and adjacent normal tissue is available for pathologic and research analysis, leading to a very accurate assessment of size and extent of tumor. Typically, preoperative radiation therapy is delivered over the course of five weeks (5000 rads) as compared to postoperative radiation therapy which generally requires six to seven weeks and 6000-6500 rads due to the postsurgical hypoxic wound environment. Because the postoperative field must encompass the entire surgical site, the postoperative radiotherapy port generally is approximately 40% larger than would be necessary were the tumor radiated preoperatively [8].

It is intriguing that while external beam radiotherapy has been in use in this disease since the early 1960's, the two modalities have never been directly compared in a prospective randomized trial. The University of Toronto Princess Margaret Hospital Radiotherapy Group is currently conducting such a trial in which patients are being randomized to receive preoperative radiation followed by surgical resection with radiotherapy boost if residual disease remains, versus surgical resection followed by postoperative radiation with a radiotherapy boost dictated by the presence or absence of residual disease. Enrolled patients will also be followed prospectively for durable quality of extremity function, and patient accrual for this trial is nearing completion.

An additional context in which radiation therapy is particularly helpful occurs when a sarcoma involves critical neurovascular structures.

Figure 2 depicts a large posterior thigh sarcoma with sciatic nerve ingress and egress directly into and out of the tumor, as encompassed by vascular loops. The surgeon is confronted with the dilemma of either resecting the sarcoma en bloc in continuity with the sciatic nerve, thereby rendering the extremity insensate distal to the knee, versus bivalving the tumor, sparing the nerve, yet potentially leaving residual sarcoma on the neurovascular structure. Interstitial radiotherapy as an additional adjunct to surgical resection is extremely valuable in helping to resolve these problems. The interstitial radiotherapy experience at the Memorial Sloan-Kettering Cancer Center demonstrates that in this specific context there is an approximately 20% local recurrence rate which may be acceptable given the extreme consequences attendant to resecting a critical neurovascular structure [10]. Interstitial radiotherapy has additional advantages compared to pre- and postoperative external beam radiation. For example, the entire treatment can be delivered over the course of a ten day interval such that the entire surgical and radiotherapy intervention sequence requires approximately two weeks as compared to three months when external beam radiotherapy is utilized.

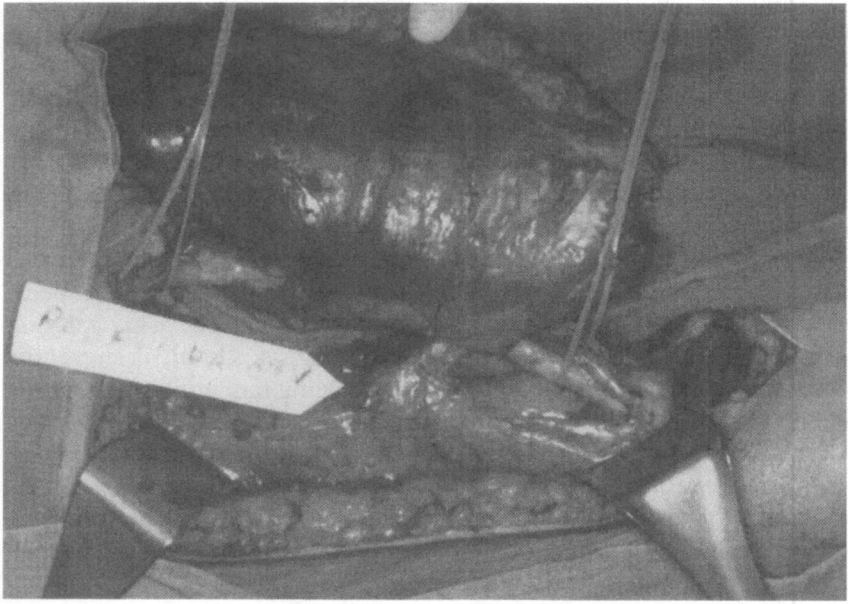

Fig. 2. Posterior thigh high grade sarcoma entrapping the sciatic nerve. The nerve is isolated proximally and distally with vessel loops

In addition, the cost of interstitial radiotherapy is significantly less than external beam radiotherapy [11]. The combination of surgery and radiotherapy as a limb salvage program must also be appreciated in the program of the lifetime financial and quality of life cost of an amputation. Grimer and colleagues have considered the cost effectiveness of limb salvage as compared to amputation for bone sarcomas [12]. While this experience may not be directly extrapolatable to soft tissue sarcoma, it is clear that a limb salvage procedure is significantly less expensive over the lifetime of a patient as compared to amputation and prothesis fitting in either the private or the public medical service sector.

It is also not clear that all patients with high grade extremity sarcomas require radiation therapy. Studies have demonstrated effective local control using surgery alone in selected high grade patients [13]. The investigation conducted by Rydholm and colleagues of the Scandinavian Sarcoma Group is particularly noteworthy. In this experience, 119 extremity soft tissue sarcomas were diagnosis using an initial fine needle aspiration, and no open biopsies were performed. Forty of the study tumors were subcutaneous, 30 were intramuscular, and 49 were in an extramuscular location. Wide margins of resection were obtained defined in subcutaneous tumors as a cuff of fat plus underlying muscle fascia and in intramuscular tumors defined as an unbroken muscular cuff. Seventy patients had subcutaneous and intramuscular lesions; 56 of 70 were resected with a wide negative margin as per the above criteria, and no radiation therapy was therefore offered. Of these latter 56 patients, 47 had high grade lesions. With a five year median follow-up (range 3.5 ñ 10 years) only 4 of the 56 (7%) had a local recurrence.

A similar question was recently addressed by Yang and colleagues [14] at the United States National Cancer Institute where a prospective randomized trial was conducted to assess the long term risk benefit profile of adjuvant radiation therapy in treatment of extremity soft tissue sarcoma. In these patients who were followed for at least 12 years, the addition of radiotherapy had a positive and statistically significant impact on local recurrence-free survival. However, radiotherapy had no impact on overall survival. The impact of radiation was also assessed using a quality of life measure which quantified several different criteria including muscle strength, joint motion, and edema. When these parameters were assessed at the early post-radiation therapy time points of 6 months there was significant impairment in joint motion with marked extremity edema. However, the edema subsequently resolved such that at 36 months after a radiation the only impairment in quality of life was decreased joint motion in those patients who had been randomized to receive radiation. The overall quality of life was measured using the Functional Living Index-Cancer (FLIC) score. The FLIC score was not significantly different comparing the radiated and the non radiated patients at any study time point.

While radiation therapy has certain definable long term toxicities, these are generally well tolerated by patients. However, not all high grade sarcoma patients may derive oncologic control benefits from adjuvant radiotherapy. As per the above experiences, in the future more selective applications of radiotherapy can be anticipated. The use of chemotherapy is also currently undergoing re-assessment. The approach at the University of Texas M. D. Anderson has been to use chemotherapy in the neoadjuvant setting, knowing that the toxicities of drugs active in this disease are remarkable [15,16]. The underlying hypothesis is that patients who respond to neoadjuvant chemotherapy may have an improved prognosis and could benefit from further chemotherapy in spite of the toxicities. In contrast, nonresponding patients who have a poorer prognosis could then be crossed over to second line drugs or placed in observation, thereby avoiding further toxicity. This approach has yielded sufficient cytoreduction in some responding patients such a limb salvage surgery could be performed in lieu of amputation.

Our current practice incorporates a high dose neoadjuvant doxorubicin/ifosfamide approach [17]. Doxorubicin is administered at 90 mg/m^2 over 72 hours by continuous infusion and ifosfamide is administered at 2.5 g/m^2 over 3 hours qd x 4 days. In an interim analysis of 79 treated patients, the overall response rate to date is 63%. For primary tumors at all sites, the overall response rate is 76% (23/37); in primary tumor of the extremity the overall response rate achieved to date is 80% (20/25). For metastatic tumor, 52% of patients (22/42) have responded. While these results are encouraging, at this time it is too early to know if these response rates will result in a more durable disease-free overall survival. A prospective randomized phase I trial has recently been initiated at the University of Texas M. D. Anderson Cancer Center to evaluate preoperative concurrent chemoradiation with doxorubicin for high risk primary and locally recurrent soft tissue sarcoma patients. Entry into this trial requires that patients have not received more than 450 mg total doxorubicin previously or any previous radiotherapy.

The use of chemotherapy may potentially impact on overall survival as well as local recurrence. For example, a recent report from the EORTC evaluated the use of adjuvant doxorubicin-based chemotherapy in adult high grade soft tissue sarcoma [18]. While there was no improvement in overall survival in the chemotherapy treated group, there was significantly decreased local recurrence. Comparable benefits may likewise be demonstrable in other trials such as the high dose M.D. Anderson experience when evaluated after appropriate follow-up intervals in the future.

The retroperitoneum remains a very difficult site in which to achieve durable local disease control. However, several studies have demonstrated enhanced retroperitoneal disease control using multimodality approaches. Sindelar et al. [19] utilized a combination of intraoperative radiation and postoperative external beam radiotherapy to achieve significantly improved local only control in patients who had complete resection of their retroperitoneal sarcomas. Toma et al. [20] reported a phase I/II trial experience which demonstrated the relative safety of doxorubicin administered with concurrent external beam radiation therapy. A 56% overall objective response rate was obtained in this retroperitoneal study. Towards a similar end, we have initiated a phase I trial evaluating the use of preoperative doxorubicin-based chemoradiation for localized resectable grade II and grade III retroperitoneal sarcomas. Patients who have experienced prior external beam radiotherapy or are radiographically unresectable are excluded from this trial. In the trial, patients receive doxorubicin at an escalating dose with concurrent external beam radiation therapy, followed by subsequent exploratory laparotomy with sarcoma resection and intraoperative radiation therapy. This trial is nearing completion of phase I accrual with minimal measurable toxicities at therapeutic radiation dose levels.

Most chemotherapy trials in high grade soft tissue sarcoma have considered drug administration in the postoperative adjuvant setting. The majority of the 14 major adjuvant chemotherapy trials for soft tissue sarcoma have failed to demonstrate an improvement in either overall survival or other survival parameters. Because of this problem, a meta-analysis was recently performed utilizing the aggregate patient entry data of the above 14 adjuvant chemotherapy trials [21]. The accrual periods for these trials ranged from initiation in 1973 to completion in 1990. All trials used doxorubicin as either a single or multidrug agent administered at varying total and per cycle doses. Disease sites tended to be the extremity but also included other anatomic sites in several trials. Trial accrual was variable and ranged from 29 to 468 patients.

In addition to the above potentially confounding variabilities, there are additional problems in several of the trials that render the meta-analysis approach problematic. For example, only 74% of the patients had primary sarcoma. Information on tumor status was not available for 13% of patients, and 11% of trial patients had recurrent disease. The disease site was likewise not homogenous in that only 58% of the patients had lesions limited to the extremity. Histologic diagnosis was not available for 18% of the tumors. Moreover, the grade was not available for 28% of the patients. Five percent of the patients included in the meta-analysis had low grade lesions, and the actual grading parameters varied in that four different grading schema were utilized in the 14 trials. The tumor size was also very heterogeneous: 18% of the tumors were less than 5 cm and the tumor was not available for 37% of the patients. The extent of resection was also a potentially confounding issue in that only 76% of patients had a margin negative resection. In 15% of the patients the margin of resection was involved with tumor, and for 9% of the patients margin information was not available. In a similar manner, radiotherapy was administered to 47% of the patients whereas 51% did not receive radiation.

With these caveats in mind, nonetheless it is pertinent that the local distant recurrence-free interval and the overall recurrence-free survival was significantly improved in the group that received adjuvant chemotherapy. The overall survival tended towards significantly improved status ($p = 0.12$); however, significance for this parameter was not demonstratable at the 95% confidence interval. As per the meta-analysis, the overall survival benefit for patients receiving adjuvant chemotherapy was a modest 4% at 10 years. It is relevant that there was no inter-trial heterogeneity for chemotherapy effects; i.e., none of the component trials nor the meta-analysis itself demonstrated that chemotherapy had a negative impact on any survival parameter. Subgroup analysis demonstrated no specific chemotherapy-related advantages for any of the standard clinical groupings considered. However, the extremity subgroup demonstrated a significant overall survival benefit in those patients receiving chemotherapy as did its use in patients whose tumors were between 5 and 10 cm in size. In addition, both malignant fibrous histiocytoma and liposarcoma as histologic subsets appeared to also benefit from adjuvant chemotherapy.

There are several problems that are inherent in a meta-analysis, and these have been extensively reviewed by LeLorier [22] and Pogue [23]. To add credence to the meta-analysis approach, Pogue has recommended that meta-analyses be performed prospectively. In this conception, trialists would prospectively discuss the criteria for a trial inclusion in the subsequent meta-analysis. Upon completion of accrual all trials that met these previously agreed upon criteria would then be included in the meta-analysis, which would remain open-ended to incorporate subsequent trials that also met inclusion criteria. In this way, the meta-analysis results could be continuously recalculated as part of an ever expanding prospective trial pool. As a consequence, iteratively over time beneficial therapeutic interventions can be more precisely defined for rare diseases such as soft tissue sarcoma using the meta-analysis approach. At this time it is prudent to conclude that chemotherapy is highly toxic, very expensive, and has minimal definable efficacy. For this reason, systemic chemotherapy in soft tissue sarcoma should not be administered outside of prospective randomized clinical trials, and it is clear that better systemic approaches need to be developed.

Outcomes for High Risk Soft Tissue Sarcoma

Soft tissue sarcoma patients who present with local recurrence only have a significantly improved overall survival relative to patients who present with either distant metastases or a combination of local recurrence and distant metastasis [24]. In those patients who are candidates for pulmonary metastasectomy, a 32% five year overall survival rate has been achieved at the University of Texas M. D. Anderson Cancer Center with a 26 month median overall survival [25].

Several experiences in treating local only recurrence have now been reported in the literature. Our own study analyzed 36 high grade soft tissue sarcoma patients who were treated for isolated local only recurrence at the M. D. Anderson [26]. A 12 year 75% overall survival was achieved in this selected group of patients, 44% of whom developed no further sarcoma recurrence. The majority of these patients were treated with a combination of aggressive surgery and chemotherapy, most having already received definitive radiotherapy at the time of initial treatment. An additional study was recently published by the University of Toronto Princess Margaret group, where a further attempt at limb salvage was made after failure of a prior combined modality limb salvage approach [27]. In this experience, freedom from systemic relapse was achieved in 70% of patients followed for a total of 340 months. Similar to the M. D. Anderson experience, the treatment for these individuals consisted of conservative surgery and interstitial reirradiation. This approach resulted in significantly improved long term disease-free and overall survival as compared to further surgery alone. In this study, brachytherapy catheters were placed in all patients. Patients were retreated with interstitial radiation if margins of less than one cm were achieved at the time of resection.   A total treatment dose of 45 Gy was utilized.   To avoid complications of possible wound breakdown, critical neurovascular structures were protected using autologous unirradiated normal tissue rotational or free tissue transfer flaps.   The cumulative radiotherapy dose to these critical neurovascular structures was limited to less than 95 Gy. The majority of patients (70%) had a demonstrably good to excellent post treatment functional results could as per the criteria of the Musculoskeletal Tumor Society extremity functional outcomes scale.

The biologic importance of positive surgical margins is an area of controversy that is being reconsidered at this time.   Our own experience with this problem was published several years ago when we examined the influence of positive surgical margins on local and distant failure in high grade sarcoma patients who received preoperative radiation [28].   This study considered 106 consecutive high grade sarcoma patients treated at the University of Texas M. D. Anderson Cancer Center between 1970 and 1987.   All of these individuals received preoperative radiation therapy with or without chemotherapy, and then underwent limb sparing surgery with or without postoperative adjuvant chemotherapy.   In 81 of the 106 patients a margin negative resection was obtained; however, 25 patients had a microscopically positive margin on final pathologic analysis.   It is intriguing that while the overall survival rate in both positive and negative margin patients was equivalent (68% vs. 65%), the rate of local recurrence was much different.   The negative margin patients had a 7% local recurrence rate.   The positive margin patients had a 32% local recurrence, meaning that 68% of the patients with positive margins never developed a local recurrence even after a minimum of 10 years of followup.   This perhaps surprising result suggests that not all margin positive patients have disease of equivalent biologic aggressiveness.   In the Memorial Sloan-Kettering interstitial radiotherapy prospective randomized trial, a positive margin was highly significant and constituted the dominant factor associated with local recurrence for large, deep, high grade soft tissue sarcoma patients who were part of this brachytherapy experience [29].   In this trial, positive margin patients who received brachytherapy enjoyed a 75% overall survival which was identical to the overall survival rate of the negative margin patients who did not receive brachytherapy.   In contrast, the positive margin group that did not receive brachytherapy had only a 40% survival, whereas the negative margin group that received brachytherapy enjoyed a 100% overall survival.

The issues of margin positivity, selective use of radiotherapy, and applications of chemotherapy to achieve local control may become clearer as our understanding of the molecular determinants driving sarcoma proliferation and metastasis develops. Our own research experience studying autologous pairs of high grade primary and metastatic soft tissue sarcoma has demonstrated remarkable clonal heterogeneity observable in both primary and metastatic tumor sites [30]. We have focused our attention on the p53 suppressor gene mutational status in high grade soft tissue sarcoma. It has been possible to demonstrate that primary sarcoma p53-mutated clones are markedly advantaged in successfully developing into and dominating metastatic soft tissue sarcoma deposits. This observation is particularly pertinent in soft tissue sarcoma given the emerging awareness that the hypoxic tumor environment typical of soft tissue sarcoma favors the induction of p53 mutations [31]. Our challenge for the future is to utilize this type of information in developing innovative molecularly-based sarcoma treatment systems either as stand alone therapy or in combination with other treatment modalities. If this ambitious goal can be realized, what could result are new multimodality treatment strategies for soft tissue sarcoma. Such treatment approaches might overcome problems of chemo- and radioresistance in this disease, while limiting patient treatment toxicities. Working together this goal can be achieved, thereby hopefully improving the outlook for patients burdened with high grade sarcoma.

References

1. American Joint Committee on Cancer (1997) AJCC cancer staging manual. Fifth Ed, Lippencott-Raven, Philadelphia
2. Alvegard TA, Berg NO (1989) Histopathology peer review of high-grade soft tissue sarcoma: the Scandinavian Sarcoma Group experience. J Clin Oncol 7(12):1845-1851
3. Singer S, Corson JM, Demetri GD, Healey EA, Marcus K, Eberlein TJ (1995) Prognostic factor predictive of survival for truncal and retroperitoneal soft-tissue sarcoma. Ann Surg 221(2):185-195
4. Coindre JM, Terrier P, Bui NB et al (1996) Prognostic factors in adult patients with locally controlled soft tissue sarcoma: a study of 546 patients from the French Federation of Cancer Centers Sarcoma Group. J Clin Oncol 14(3):869-877
5. Levine EA, Halzmayer T, Bacus S et al (1997) Evaluation of new prognostic markers for adult soft tissue sarcomas. J Clin Oncol 15(10):3249-3257
6. Clark RL, Martin RG, White EC (1959) A critical review of the management of soft-tissue sarcomas. Lancet 79(7):327-331
7. Lindberg RD, Fletcher GH, Martin RG (1975) The management of soft tissue sarcomas in adults: surgery and postoperative radiotherapy. J Radiol Electrol 56:761-767
8. Nielsen OS, Cummings B, O'Sullivan B, Catton C, Bell RS, Fornasier VL (1991) Preoperative and postoperative irradiation of soft tissue sarcomas: effect on radiation field size. Int J Radiation Oncol Biol 21:1595-1599

9. Skibber JM, Lotze MT, Seipp CA, Salcedo R, Rosenberg SA (1987) Limb-sparing surgery for soft tissue sarcomas: wound related morbidity in patients undergoing wide local excision. Surgery 102(3):447-452
10. Zelefsky MJ, Nori D, Shiu MH, Brennan MF (1990) Limb salvage in soft tissue sarcomas involving neurovascular structures using combined surgical resection and brachytherapy. Int J Radiation Oncol Biol 19:913-918
11. Janjan NA, Yasko AW, Reece GP et al (1994) Comparison of charges related to radiotherapy for soft-tissue sarcomas treated by preoperative external-beam irradiation versus interstitial implantation. Ann Surg Onc 1(5):415-422
12. Grimer RJ, Carter SR, Pynset PB (1997) The cost-effectiveness of limb salvage for bone tumors. J Bone Joint Surg 79:558-561
13. Rydholm A, Gustafson P, Rooser B et al (1991) Limb-sparing surgery without radiotherapy based on anatomic location of soft tissue sarcoma. J Clin Oncol 9(10):1757-1765
14. Yang JC, Chang AE, Baker AR et al (1998) Randomized prospective study of the benefit of adjuvant radiation therapy in the treatment of soft tissue sarcomas of the extremity. J Clin Oncol 16(1):197-203
15. Pezzi CM, Pollock RE, Evans HL et al (1990) Preoperative chemotherapy for soft-tissue sarcomas of the extremities. Ann Surg 21:476-481
16. Patel SR, Vadhan-Raj S, Papadopolous N et al (1997) High-dose Ifosfamide in bone and soft tissue sarcomas: results of phase II and pilot studies ñ dose-response and schedule dependence. J Clin Oncol 15(6):2378-2384
17. Patel SR, Vadhan-Raj S, Burgess MA, Papadopoulos NE, Plager C, Benjamin RS (1996) Dose-intensive chemotherapy in soft-tissue sarcomas (STS). Proc American Society of Clinical Oncology 15:552
18. Bramwell V, Rouesse J, Steward W et al (1994) Adjuvant CYVADIC chemotherapy for adult soft tissue sarcoma – reduced local recurrence but no improvement in survival: a study of the European Organization for Research and Treatment of Cancer Soft Tissue and Bone Sarcoma Group. J Clin Oncol 12(6):1137-1149
19. Sindelar WF, Kinsella TJ, Chen PW et al (1993) Intraoperative radiotherapy in retroperitoneal sarcomas: final results of a prospective, randomized, clinical trial. Arch Surg 128:402-410
20. Toma S, Palumbo R, Vincenti M et al (1995) Concomitant doxorubicin (DOXO) by continuous infusion (C.I.) and radiotherapy (RT) at low doses in locally advanced and/or metastatic soft tissue sarcomas (STS): long-term results of a phase II study. Proc of American Society of Clinical Oncology 14:520
21. Sarcoma Meta-analysis Collaboration (1997) Adjuvant chemotherapy for localised resectable soft-tissue sarcoma of adults: meta-analysis of individual data. Lancet 350:1647-1654
22. LeLorier J, Gregoire G, Benhaddad A, Lapierre J, Derderian F (1997) Discrepancies between meta-analyses and subsequent large randomized, controlled trials. N Eng J Med 337:536-542
23. Pogue J, Yusuf S (1998) Overcoming the limitations of current meta-analysis of randomised controlled trials. Lancet 351:47-52
24. Brennan MF (1997) Presidential Address ñ The enigma of local recurrence. Ann Surg Oncol 4(1):1-12
25. Casson AG, Putnam JB, Natarajan G et al (1992) Five-year survival after pulmonary metastasectomy for adult soft tissue sarcoma. Cancer 69(3):662-668
26. Midis GP, Pollock RE, Chen NP et al (1998) Locally recurrent soft tissue sarcoma of the extremities. Surgery (in press)

27. Catton C, Davis A, Bell R et al (1996) Soft tissue sarcoma of the extremity. Limb salvage after failure of combined conservative therapy. Radiotherapy and Oncology 41:209-214
28. Tanabe KK, Pollock RE, Ellis LM, Murphy A, Sherman NE, Romsdahl MM (1994) Influence of surgical margin on outcome on preoperatively irradiated extremity sarcomas. Cancer 73:1652-1659
29. Pisters PWT, Harrison LB, Leung DHY, Woodruff JM, Casper ES, Brennan MF (1996) Long-term results of a prospective randomized trial of adjuvant brachytherapy in soft tissue sarcoma. J Clin Oncol 14(3):859-868
30. Pollock RE, Lang A, Luo J, El-Naggar AK, Yu D (1996) Soft tissue sarcoma metastasis from clonal expansion of p53 mutated tumor cells. Oncogene 12:2035-2039
31. Graeber TG, Peterson JF, Tsai M, Monica K, Fornace AJ, Giaccia AJ (1994) Hypoxia induces accumulation of p53 protein, but activation of a G1-phase checkpoint by low-oxygen is independent of p53 status. Mol Cell Biol 14(9):6264-6277

Advances in the Management of Pancreatic Cancer

M. TEMPERO

Introduction

Adenocarcinoma of the exocrine pancreas remains a profound therapeutic challenge. Incremental improvements in overall survival have been small and the current 5 year survival of patients with pancreatic cancer is only 4% [1]. In the United States, this disease is a the fourth leading cause of cancer death in men and the fifth cause of cancer death in women.

In counterpoint to these discouraging statistics, it is important to note that progress has occurred in the palliative management of patients with pancreatic cancer and a remarkable decrease in the perioperative mortality of patients undergoing pancreatectomy has now been appreciated. In addition, noninvasive staging and diagnostic procedures have improved our ability to select patients most likely to benefit from surgical resection. This chapter will focus on selected strategies for nonoperative management of pancreatic cancer and includes a section on developing biologically based strategies for treatment.

Adjuvant Therapy

Surgical resection remains the only potentially curative form of therapy for pancreatic cancer. Less than 15% of patients who present with this disease have localized disease potentially resectable for cure [2]. Fortunately, for those who do undergo resection, the perioperative mortality rate is now 5% or less in experienced centers [3, 4].

Traditionally, adjuvant therapy for resected adenocarcinoma of the pancreas has been generally held to be the standard of care. In the US, this was based on a trial performed more than 15 years ago by the Gastrointestinal Tumor Study Group (GITSG) in which patients were randomized following resection to either observation or radiation therapy combined with 5-fluorouracil (5-FU) [5]. In this study, a total dose of 4000 cGy was given in a split course and 5-FU was given as a bolus infusion (500 mg/m^2/daily) for 3 days at the beginning of each 2 week radiation cycle. Following completion of radiation, 5-FU was administered weekly for 2 years. The treated group had a two year actuarial survival of 43% which was significantly higher than the 18% two year survival observed in the control group. These results were later upheld in a follow-up single arm trial in which patients were randomized to the treatment arm [6].

Surprisingly, there have been no confirmatory trials attempted until recently. The European Organization for Research and Treatment of Cancer (EORTC) has now completed a trial in patients with both ampullary carcinoma and adenocarcinoma of the pancreas. These patients were randomized to observation or a split course of radiation combined with 5-FU in a manner similar to that used by the GITSG, but were not given maintenance weekly 5-FU therapy. At the time of this writing, the final results of this trial have not yet been published in the peer-reviewed literature. Data presented at the European Cancer Conference meeting in the fall of 1997 suggested a trend for benefit in the subset of patients with adenocarcinoma of the pancreas [7].

Contemporary approaches for adjuvant therapy have focused primarily on preoperative treatment in the hope of increasing the resection rate and improving overall survival [8, 9]. While a number of studies have suggested that chemoradiation may be able to convert selected patients with unresectable disease to a resectable status or possibly even increase the overall resection rate, it is not yet clear whether this approach is superior to a standard post-operative regimen. Spitz et al. [10] analyzed results of 142 patients treated with either pre- or postoperative chemoradiation. This retrospective analysis showed no difference in survival between patient groups. However, the authors concluded that preoperative rapid fractionation chemoradiation could be delivered over a shorter period of time. In addition, up to one-fourth of eligible patients could not receive post operative adjuvant therapy because of prolonged recovery after resection. Thus, there may be practical advantages to preoperative adjuvant chemoradiation.

Therapy for Localized Unresectable Pancreatic Adenocarcinoma

Chemoradiation is often considered to be the standard of care for patients with locally unresectable adenocarcinoma of the pancreas. This approach was inaugurated by a GITSG trial in which patients with surgically confirmed locally unresectable adenocarcinoma of the pancreas were randomized to radiation alone (6000 cGy) or 5-FU combined with radiation doses of 4000 or 6000 cGy [11]. A two-fold improvement in median survival was observed in the chemoradiation arms and the regimen combining 5-FU and 4000 cGy produced the best survival with the least toxicity. In addition, the GITSG also demonstrated that chemotherapy with streptozotocin, mitomycin and 5-FU was inferior to the same drug combination plus radiation (one year survival 19% vs. 41%) [12]. Other contemporary approaches to improving these results have included alternate routes of administration of 5-FU as well as the evaluation of new radiation sensitizing drugs. For instance, Ishii et al. [13] have evaluated protracted infusion 5-FU and external beam radiation (54 cGy in 28 fractions over 5.5 weeks). However, the median survival of 10 months and the one year survival of 42% does not suggest improvement over regimens employing bolus 5-FU schedules. Other radiation sensitizing drugs in phase I evaluation include bromodeoxyuridine [14], paclitaxel [15], cisplatin [16], and gemcitabine [17]. Intraoperative radiotherapy (IORT) has also been studied as an adjunct to external beam radiation. A review of 159 Mayo clinic patients who received external beam radiation with or without an intraoperative electron boost. While there was no significant difference in survival, improved local control was seen in patients treated with IORT (82% vs. 48%) [18].

The role of chemotherapy alone in locally unresectable pancreatic adenocarcinoma has not yet been clarified. With the exception of the trial noted above, there have been no other randomized trials comparing single or combination chemotherapy regimens to chemoradiation. However, many patients with locally unresectable pancreatic adenocarcinoma are included in phase I and phase II chemotherapy studies which will be discussed below.

Systemic Chemotherapy

We have recently reviewed the efficacy data for single agent and combination chemotherapy [19]. In the past, chemotherapy regimens have been accepted or rejected based on their ability to produce an objective response. This approach may be somewhat hazardous as it is becoming increasingly accepted that it is difficult to measure objective response for both technical and biologic reasons in this disease [20]. Other endpoints of significant interest are overall survival and quality of life or symptom control.

Of the vast number of single agent chemotherapy drugs or other agents that have been tested in the therapy of pancreatic adenocarcinoma, only four agents have been shown in more than one trial to be associated with the median survival of greater than five months. These include 5-FU [21] and gemcitabine [22, 23] and two hormonal agents, tamoxifen [24, 25] and goserelin [26, 27], an LHRH agonist. 5-FU has been studied alone and with biochemical modulation using leucovorin [28], and/or alpha interferon [29, 30] with similar survival results. Gemcitabine, (difluoro-deoxycitidine) was noted in early phase II trials to improve symptoms out of proportion to the number of objective responses observed [22]. This lead to a randomized trial comparing 5-FU (600 mg/m^2 weekly) to gemcitabine (1000 mg/m^2 weekly) for up to 7 weeks followed by a week of rest, then weekly X3 every 4 weeks thereafter [23]. Endpoints of symptom improvement (termed "clinical benefit") and survival were analyzed. While the objective response rates were indistinguishable, gemcitabine improved symptoms in almost 24% of the patients compared to less than 5% with 5-FU, and a small but statistically significant improvement in median survival (5.7 vs. 4.4 months) was observed. Based on this trial, gemcitabine has commonly been accepted in the US as appropriate first-line therapy for patients with pancreatic adenocarcinoma particularly in symptomatic patients.

Several potentially promising combination chemotherapy regimens have now been studied in pancreatic adenocarcinoma. These include 5-FU, adriamycin, and mitomycin (FAM) [31], with or without streptozotocin [32], and a modification of this regimen of 5-FU, mitomycin-C, and streptozotocin (SMF) [33]. Another potentially promising regimen, cisplatin, cytosine arabinoside, and caffeine was eventually compared to SMF and shown not to be superior [34]. A review of all published combination chemotherapy regimens in pancreatic adenocarcinoma suggests that there are, at best, small differences in median survival and there does not appear to be a single superior combination regimen. An important study conducted by the North Central Cancer Treatment Study Group (NCCTG) compared combination therapy with FAM or 5-FU and adriamycin to monotherapy with 5-FU [35]. The survival curves were completely overlapping suggesting that no benefit was conferred with combined agents.

Four studies have now been conducted comparing combination chemotherapy to best supportive care. All of the studies have the common feature of the use of 5-FU containing regimens. Three of these studies using FAM [36], 5-FU and leucovorin with or without etoposide [37], and a complicated five drug regimen using 5-FU, mitomycin-C, methotrexate, vincristine, and cyclophosphamide [38] all showed some survival benefit over no therapy at all.

Thus, in 1998, it is probably safe to conclude that pancreatic adenocarcinoma remains a relatively chemoresistant disease. While chemotherapy may offer an advantage to best supportive care, combination chemotherapy does not appear to be superior to monotherapy with 5-FU. While gemcitabine may be superior to 5-FU treatment, a confirmatory trial has not been done and any actual improvement in median survival with gemcitabine or any other treatment is small. Thus, continued effort is needed in the development of new strategies for this disease.

Novel Approaches

One important area of study involves optimization of treatment with gemcitabine. Gemcitabine is a prodrug which requires intracellular phosphorylation. The triphosphate metabolite is the most active moiety and, when incorporated into DNA, causes premature DNA chain termination. The formation of the phosphorylated metabolites is both dose and dose rate dependent. Plunkett et al. [39] have demonstrated that a fixed rate infusion of gemcitabine (10 mg/m^2/min) results in more optimal formation of the triphosphate form of the active drug. A phase I trial using the fixed rate infusion has been conducted demonstrating the maximum tolerated dose to be 1500 mg/m^2 weekly X3 every 4 weeks [40]. A randomized trial is currently in progress comparing this regimen to a higher bolus dose of gemcitabine (2200 mg/m^2) given over a 30 minute infusion. In addition, there are now preclinical mechanistic studies which favor synergy between gemcitabine and cisplatin [41]; this doublet combination is now under active clinical investigation.

A common molecular hallmark of pancreatic cancer involves a k-ras mutation of the 12th or 13th codon. Since ras proteins require farnesylation in order to localize on the plasma cell membrane, another approach has been to develop inhibitors to farnesyl transferase as antineoplastic agents. Many of these agents have shown encouraging preclinical results [42,43] and at least three agents are now in phase I clinical trials. Another approach to take advantage of k-ras mutation has been to use antisense oligonucleotide constructs. Preclinical studies using liposome encapsulated antisense constructs for *in vivo* gene transfer have been used to successfully treat human pancreatic cancer cells inoculated intraperitoneally in athymic mice [44].

Another common molecular alteration in pancreatic cancer involves the tumor suppressor gene p53. In addition to the possibility of using mutated p53 as a target for synthetic antisense oligonucleotides, a ribozyme strategy to suppress growth of cancer cells transformed by mutant p53 is also under study [45]. Another novel approach involves an oncolytic adenovirus which multiples preferentially in mutant p53 cells [46]. Clinical trials using this virus have already been initiated using an intratumural approach in pancreatic adenocarcinoma.

Mucin-associated antigens are particularly common in adenocarci- noma of the pancreas. These can be exploited for active immunotherapy or conceivably used as a target for antibody mediated delivery of cyto- toxic agents. The antigen sialyl-Tn is highly expressed in pancreatic ade- nocarcinoma and a synthetic form of the antigen is currently in clinical trials in patients with breast and colon cancer [47]. If successful, this vac- cine could theoretically be applied to pancreatic cancer. An alternate approach has been selected by Jaffee et al. [48] who have developed allo- geneic pancreatic cell lines transfected with GM-CSF. This vaccine approach is currently in study in a phase Ib trial at Johns Hopkins Uni- versity.

In GI malignancy, antigens targeted for antibody mediated therapy have included 17-1A, TAG-72 (which shares some similarity with sialyl- TN) and CEA. Passive immunotherapy using MAb 17-1A represented an initial approach in patients with various gastrointestinal cancers includ- ing pancreatic adenocarcinoma [49]. This antibody participates in anti- body dependent cellular cytotoxicity which was the rationale for study. While passive immunotherapy did not appear to be a successful strategy in patients with advanced disease, new data in the setting of minimum residual disease in colorectal cancer suggests therapeutic benefit [50] offering some hope that this approach could potentially be useful as in the setting of minimal residual disease in pancreatic adenocarcinoma.

Our studies have focused on targeting TAG-72 with MAbs conjugated to beta-emitting redionuclides. By targeting TAG-72 which is not expressed in normal glandular tissue with the exception of secretory endometrium, it may be possible to deliver high radiation doses without detrimental effect to normal tissues. Our studies to date have shown that systemic delivery to MAb CC49 (a high affinity antibody against TAG-72) can achieve absorbed radiation doses of up to 3300 cGy in metastatic sites with ^{131}Iodine [51]. Studies with ^{90}Yttrium (^{90}Y) conjugated anti- body can achieve similar absorbed radiation doses with less myelosup- pression [52]. The development of a human anti-MAb against these murine antibodies are prompting us to turn to a humanized form of MAb CC49 which is predicted to be nonimmunogeneic allowing for sequential administration and higher cumulation of radiation in tumor targets. Incidental myelosuppression which occurs with systemic radioimmunoconjugate therapy and potential liver toxicity, which has been predicted by our dosimetry studies of ^{90}Y conjugated MAb-CC49, may potentially be overcome in the future by pretargeting strategies. A unique pretargeting strategy using streptavidin and biotin is currently under study with NR-LU-10 [53], an antibody which recognizes an epithelial antigen similar to 17-1A. In this approach, streptavidin conjugated antibody is first administered and targeted to tumor. Circulating streptavidin is cleared by biotin bound albumin. Biotin bound ^{90}Y is then administered to localize to streptavidin conjugated antibody. Studies with this approach are now being carried out in colorectal cancer and may eventually be applied to pancreatic adenocarcinoma.

Finally, matrix metalloproteinases (MMP) are a family of proteolytic enzymes that have a role in tumor invasion, metastasis, and angiogenesis. A MMP inhibitor (BB25160, Marimastat) has been developed and phase I and II trials in pancreas cancer have been completed [54]. A phase III trial comparing 5-FU to 5-FU and Marimastat has completed accrual, and results of this trial are eagerly awaited.

Summary

Progress in therapeutic strategies to improve survival in pancreatic cancer has been slow. Cautious optimism is raised for the future role of chemotherapy drugs in this disease with the introduction of gemcitabine, a novel nucleoside analog which has been shown to be modestly effective in the palliative management of these patients. It is likely that new successful systemic therapeutic approaches will be based on an appropriate understanding of the molecular and biologic perturbations that occur in this disease.

References

1. Landis SH, Murray T, Bolden S, Bolden S, Wingo PA (1998) Cancer Statistics CA Can J Clinicians 48:6-29
2. Warshaw AL, Fernandez-del C (1992) Pancreatic carninoma. N Engl J Med 326:455-465
3. Crist DW, Cameron JL (1994) The current status of the Whipple operation for periampullary carcinoma. Adv Surg 25:21-49

4. Trede M, Schwall G, Saeger HD (1990) Survival after pancreatoduodenectomy. Ann Surg 211:447-58
5. Kalser MH, Ellenberg SS (1985) Pancreatic cancer: Adjuvant combined radiation and chemotherapy following curative resection. Arch Surg 120:899-903
6. Gastrointestinal Study Group (1987) Further evidence of effective adjuvant combined radiation and chemotherapy following curative resection of pancreatic cancer. Cancer 59:2006-2010
7. ECCO9 (1997) The European Cancer Conference (Hamburg, 14-18 September) Abstracts, Eur J Cancer 33(Suppl 8):1-380
8. Hoffman JP, Weese JL, Solin LJ, Engstrom P, Agarwal P, Barber LW, Buttmann MC, Litwin S, Salazar H, Eisenberg BL (1995) A pilot study of preoperative chemoradiation for patients with localized adenocarcinoma of the pancreas. Am J Surg 169:71-77
9. Evans EB, Rich TA, Byrd DR, Cleary KR, Connelly JH, Levin B, Charnsangavej C, Fenoglio CH, Amers FC (1992) Preoperative chemoradiation and pancreaticoduodenectomy for adenocarcinoma of the pancreas. Arch Surg 127:1335-1339
10. Spitz FR, Abbruzzese JL, Lee JE, Pisters PW, Lowy AM, Fenoglio CJ, Cleary KR, Janjan NA, Goxwitz MS, Rich TA, Evans DB (1997) Preoperative and postoperative chemoradiation strategies in patients with pancreaticoduodenectomy for adenocarcinoma of the pancreas. J Clin Oncol 15:928-937
11. Moertel CG, Frytak S, Hahn RG, O'Connell MJ, Reitemeier RJ, Rubin J, Schutt AJ, Weiland LH, Childs DS, Holbrook MA, Lavin PT, Livstone E, Spiro H, Knowlton A, Kalser M, Barkin J, Lessner H, Mann-Kaplan R, Ramming K, Douglas HO, Thomas P, Nave H, Bateman J, Lokich J, Brooks J, Chaffey J, Corson JM, Zamcheck N, Novak JW (1981) Therapy of locally unresectable pancreatic carcinoma: A randomized comparison of high dose (6000 rads) radiation alone, moderate dose radiation (4000 rads + 5-fluorouracil), and high dose radiation + 5-fluorouracil. Cancer 48:1705-1710
12. Gastrointestinal Tumor Study Group (1988) Treatment of locally unresectable carcinoma of the pancreas: Comparison of combined modality therapy (chemotherapy plus radiotherapy) to chemotherapy alone. J Natl Cancer Inst 80:751-755
13. Ishii H, Okada S, Tokuuye K, Nose H, Okusaka T, Yoshimori M, Nagahama H, Sumi M, Kagami Y, Ikeda H (1997) Protracted 5-Fluorouracil infusion with concurrent radiotherapy as a treatment for locally advanced pancreatic carcinoma. Cancer 79:1516-1520
14. Robertson JM, Ensminger WD, Walker S, Lawrence TS (1997) A phase I trial of intravenous bromodeoxyuridine and radiation therapy for pancreatic cancer. Int J Radiat Oncol Biol Phys 37:331-335
15. Safran H, King TP, Choy H, Hesketh PH, Wolfe B, Altenhein E, Sikov W, Rosmarin A, Akerly W, Radie-Keane K, Cicchetti G, Lopez F, Bland K, Wanebo HJ (1997) Paclitaxel and concurrent radiation for locally advanced pancreatic and gastric cancer: A phase I study. J Clin Oncol 153:901-907
16. Boz G, DePaoli A, Roncadin M, Franchin G, Galligioni E, Arcicasa M, Bortolus R, Gobitti C, Minatel E, Innocente R et al (1991) Radiation therapy combined with chemotherapy for inoperable pancreatic carcinoma. Tumori 77:61-64
17. Lawrence TS, Chang EY, Hahn TM, Hertel LW, Shewach DS (1996) Radiosensitization of pancreatic cancer cells by 2', 2'-difluoro-2'-deoxycytidine. Int J Radiat Oncol Biol Phys 34:867-872

18. Roldan GE, Gunderson LL, Nagorney DM, Martin JK, Ilstrup DM, Holbrook MA, Kvols LK, McIlrath DC (1988) External beam versus intraoperative and external beam irradiation for locally advanced pancreatic cancer. Cancer 61:1110-1116
19. Tempero M (1998) Chemotherapy of Pancreatic Cancer. *In: Reber H (ed) Pancreatic Cancer: Pathogenesis, Diagnosis, and Treatment* Humana Press, Totowa, NJ pp 265-280
20. Rothenberg ML, Abbruzzese JL, Moore M, Portenoy RK, Robertson JM, Wanebo JH (1996) A rationale for expanding the endpoints for clinical trials in advanced pancreatic carcinoma. Cancer 78:627-632
21. Ahlgren JD (1996) Chemotherapy for pancreatic carcinoma. Cancer 78:654-663
22. Casper ES, Green MR, Kelsen DP, Heelan RT, Brown TD, Flombaum CD, Trochanowski B, Tarassoff PG (1994) Phase II trial of gemcitabine (2,2'-difluorodeoxycytidine) in patients with adenocarcinoma of the pancreas. Invest New Crugs 12:29-34
23. Burris HA, Moore MJ, Andersen J, Green MR, Rothenberg ML, Modiano MR, Cripps MC, Portenoy RK, Storniolo AM, Tarassoff P, Nelson R, Dorr FA, Stephens CD, Von Hoff DD (1997) Improvements in survival and clinical benefit with gemcitabine as firstline therapy for patients with advanced pancreatic cancer: A randomized trial. J Clin Oncol 15:2403-2413
24. Wong A, Chan A, Arthur K (1987) Tamoxifen therapy in unresectable adenocarcinoma of the pancreas. Cancer Treat Rep 71:749-750
25. Keating JJ, Johnson PJ, Cochrane AMG, Gazzard BG, Krasner N, Smith PM, Trewby PN, Wheeler P, Wilkinson SP, Williams R (1989) A prospective randomised trial of tamoxifen and cyproterone acetate in pancreatic carcinoma. Br J Cancer 60:789-792
26. Allegretti A, Lionetto R, Saccomanno S, Paganuzzi M, Onetto M, Martinoli C, Rollandi G, Marugo M, Fazzuoli L, Pugliese V (1993) LH-RH analogue treatment in adenocarcinoma of the pancreas: A phase II study. Oncology 50:77-80
27. Philip PA, Carmichael J, Tonkin K, Buamah PK, Britton J, Dowsett M, Harris AL (1993) Hormonal treatment of pancreatic carcinoma: a phase II study of LHRH agonist goserelin plus hydrocortisone. Br J Cancer 67:379-382
28. DeCaprio JA, Mayer RJ, Gonin R, Arbuck SG (1991) Fluorouracil and high-dose leucoverin in previously untreated patients with advanced adenocarcinoma of the pancreas: Results of a phase II trial. J Clin Oncol 9:2128-2133
29. Scheithauer W, Pfeffel F, Kornek G, Marczell A, Wiltschke C, Funovics J (1992) A phase II trial of 5-fluorouracil, leucovorin, and recombinant alpha-2b-interferon in advanced adenocarcinoma of the pancreas. Cancer 70:1864-1866
30. Pazdur R, Ajani JJ, Abbruzzese JL, Belt RJ, Dakhil SR, Dubovsky D, Graham S, Pilat S, Winn R, Levin B (1992) Phase II evaluation of fluorouracil and recombinant α-2a-interferon in previously untreated patients with pancreatic adenocarcinoma. Cancer 70:2073-2076
31. Smith FP, Hoth DF, Levin B, Karlin DA, Macdonald JS, Woolley PV, Schien PS (1980) 5-fluorouracil, adriamycin and mitomycin-C(FAM) chemotherapy for advanced adenocarcinoma of the pancreas. Cancer 46:2014-2018
32. Bukowski RM, Schacter LP, Groppe CW, Hewlett JS, Weick JK, Livingston RB (1982) Phase II trial of 5-fluorouracil, adriamycin, mitomycin-C, and streptozotocin (FAM-S) in pancreatic carcinoma. Cancer 50:197-200
33. Gastrointenstinal Tumor Study Group (1986) Phase II studies of drug combinations in advanced pancreatic carcinoma: Fluorouracil plus doxorubicin plus mitomycin C and two regimens of streptozotocin plus mitomoycin C plus fluorouracil. J Clin Oncol 4:1794-1798

34. Kelsen D, Hudis C, Niedzwiecki D, Dougherty J, Casper E, Botet J, Vinciguerra V, Rosenbluth R (1991) A phase III comparison trial of streptozotocin, mitomycin, and 5-fluorouracil with cisplatin, cytosine and arabinoside, and caffeine in patients with advanced pancreatic carcinoma. Cancer 68:965-969

35. Cullinan SA, Moertel CG, Fleming TR, Rubin JR, Krook JE, Everson LK, Windschitl HE, Twito DI, Marschke RF, Foley JF, Pfeifle DM, Barlow JF (1985) A comparison of three chemotherapeutic regimens in the treatment of advanced pancreatic and gastric carcinoma. JAMA 253:2061-2067

36. Palmer KR, Kerr M, Knowles G, Cull A, Carter DC, Leonard CF (1994) Chemotherapy prolongs survival in inoperable pancreatic carcinoma. BR J Surg 81:882-885

37. Glimelius B, Hoffman K, Sjödén PO, Jacobsson G, Sellström H, Enander LK, Linné T, Svensson C (1996) Chemotherapy improves survival and quality of life in advanced pancreatic and biliary cancer. Ann Oncol 7:593-600

38. Mallinson CN, Rake MO, Cocking JD (1980) Chemotherapy in pancreatic cancer. Br Med J 281:1589-1591

39. Plunkett W, Huang P, Searcy CE et al (1996) Gemcitabine: preclinical pharmacology and mechanisms of action. Semin Oncol 10:3-15

40. Brand R, Capadano M, Tempero M (1997) A phase I trial of weekly gemcitabine administered as a prolonged infusion in patients with pancreatic cancer and other solid tumors. Invest New Drugs 15:331-341

41. Kawai Y, Yang LY, Plunkett W (1998) Inhibition of repair of cisplatin-induced DNA damage in human colon carcinoma cells by gemcitabine. AACR Proc 39:156, Abst #1068

42. Ura H, Obara T, Shudo R, Itoh A, Tanno S, Fujii T, Nishino N, Kohgo Y (1998) Selective cytotoxicity of farnesylamine to pancreatic carcinoma cells and Ki-ras-transformed fibroblasts. Mol Carcinog 21:93-99

43. Moasser MM, Sepp-Lorenziono L, Kohl NE, Oliff A, Balog A, Su DS, Danishefsky SJ, Rosen N (1998) Farnesyl transferase inhibitors cause enhanced mitotic sensitivity to taxol and epothilones. Proc Natl Acad Sci USA 95:1369-1374

44. Aoli K, Yoshida T, Sugimura T et al (1995) Liposome-mediated in vivo gene transfer of antisense K-ras construct inhibits pancreatic tumor dissemination in the murine peritoneal cavity. Cancer Res 55:3810-3816

45. Cai DW, Mukhopadhyay T, Roth JA (1995) Suppression of lung cancer cell growth by ribozyme-mediated modification of p53 pre-mRNA. Cancer Gene Ther 2:199-205

46. Bischoff JR, Kirn DH, Williams A, Heise C, Horn S, Muna M, Ng L, Nye JA, Sampson-Johannes A, Fattaey A, McCormick F (1996) An adenovirus mutant that replicates selectively in p53-deficient human tumor cells. Science 274:373-376

47. MacLean GD, Reddish MA, Koganty RR, Longenecker BM (1996) Antibodies against mucin-associated sialyl-Tn epitopes correlate with survival of metastatic adenocarcinoma patients undergoing active specific immunotherapy with synthetic Stn vaccine. J Immunother Emphasis Tumor Immunol 19:59-68

48. Jaffee EM, Pardoll DM (1997) Considerations for the clinical development of cytokine gene-transducted tumor cell vaccines. Methods 12:143-153

49. Tempero MA, Sivinski C, Steplewski Z, Harvey E, Klassen L, Kay HD (1990) Phase II trial of interferon gamma and monoclonal antibody 17-1A in pancreatic cancer: Biologic and clinical effects. J Clin Oncol 12:2019-2026

50. Reithmüller G, Schneider-Gädicke E, Schlimok G, Schmiegel W, Raab R, Höffken K, Gruber R, Pichlmaier H, Hirche H, Pichlmayr R, Buggisch P, Witte J, and the German Cancer Aid 17-1A Study Group (1994) Randomised trial of monoclonal anti-

body for adjuvant therapy of resected Dukes'C colorectal carcinoma. Lancet 343:1177-1183

51. Tempero MA, Leichner P, Dalrymple G, Harrison K, Augustine S, Schlom J, Wisecarver J, Colcher D (1997) High dose therapy with ^{131}I labeled monoclonal antibody CC49: A phase I trial. J Clin Oncol 15:1518-1528

52. Leichner PK, Akabani G, Colcher D, Harrison K, Hawkins W, Eckblade M, Baranowska-Kortylewicz J, Augustine SC, Wisecarver J, Tempero M (1997) Patient-specific dosimetry of indium-111-and yttrium-90-labeled monoclonal antibody CC49. J Nucl Med 38:512-516

53. Breitz HB, Weiden PL, Vanderheyden JL et al (1992) Clinical experience with Rhenium 186 labeled monoclonal antibodies for radioimmunotherapy: Results of Phase 1 trials. J Nucl Med 33:1099-1109

54. Bramhall S (1997) The matrix metalloproteinases and their inhibitors in pancreatic cancer. Int J Pancreatology 2:1-12

CET OUVRAGE A ÉTÉ ACHEVÉ
D'IMPRIMER EN JANVIER 1999
SUR LES PRESSES DE L'IMPRIMERIE DE L'INDÉPENDANT
53203 CHÂTEAU-GONTIER - FRANCE
DÉPÔT LÉGAL : 1er TRIMESTRE 1999